Pathophysiology of Hypertension
in Blacks

CLINICAL PHYSIOLOGY SERIES

Pathophysiology of Hypertension in Blacks

Edited by

JOHN C. S. FRAY

Department of Physiology
University of Massachusetts Medical School
Worcester, Massachusetts

JANICE G. DOUGLAS

Division of Endocrinology and Hypertension
Case Western Reserve University
Cleveland, Ohio

New York   Oxford
Published for the American Physiological Society
by Oxford University Press
1993

Oxford University Press

Oxford   New York   Toronto
Delhi   Bombay   Calcutta   Madras   Karachi
Kuala Lumpur   Singapore   Hong Kong   Tokyo
Nairobi   Dar es Salaam   Cape Town   Madrid
Melbourne   Auckland

and associated companies in
Berlin   Ibadan

Published for the American Physiological Society by
Oxford University Press, 200 Madison Avenue, New York, New York 10016

Oxford is a registered trademark of Oxford University Press

Library of Congress Cataloging-in-Publication Data
Pathophysiology of hypertension in Blacks /
   edited by John C.S. Fray, Janice G. Douglas.
      p.   cm.—(Clinical physiology series)
   ISBN 0-19-506720-7
   1. Hypertension—Pathophysiology.   2. Afro-Americans—Diseases.
   3. Blacks—Diseases.   I. Fray, John C. S.   II. Douglas, Janice G.   III. Series.
   [DNLM: 1. Blacks.   2. Hypertension—ethnology.   3. Hypertension—physiopathology.
   4. Hypertension—psychology.   WG 340 P2978]
   RC685.H8P34   1993   616.1'32'008996073—dc20   DNLM/DLC   for Library of Congress   92-18761

9 8 7 6 5 4 3 2 1

Printed in the United States of America
on acid-free paper

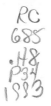

Dedicated to the healers who have devoted their best talents to relieving the suffering of so many people; to the black men and women who have so courageously suffered in silence; to our teachers, without whom this project would have been impossible; to the *students,* for it is you who must accept and execute the challenge.

Foreword

A. CLIFFORD BARGER

This authoritative and comprehensive volume, *Pathophysiology of Hypertension in Blacks,* written by leaders in the field and edited by Drs. Fray and Douglas, two eminent black scientists, is appearing at a most opportune time. In both the public and the private sector research emphasis is on the need to provide further information to solve the problem of hypertension, which afflicts 60 million Americans and has a disproportionately high incidence, severity, and mortality in the growing minority population. In their strategic planning for the next decades, Dr. Louis Sullivan, Secretary of Health and Human Services, Dr. Bernardine Healy, Director of the National Institutes of Health, and officers of the Robert Wood Johnson Foundation, the Rockefeller Foundation, and others, assign a high priority to the improvement of health care of minorities.

Fortunately, black students of the biological sciences are becoming more aware of the impact of hypertension on the health of their families and friends and of the future role of students in resolving the problem of high blood pressure. As a Visiting Professor of the Porter Development Program of the American Physiological Society at Spelman College, I was impressed by the quality of the questions the students raised about the physiological regulation of blood pressure, by their poignant vignettes of the pathological consequences of hypertension in their parents and grandparents, and by their probing queries about the role of genetics, emotional and psychological factors, evolutionary influences during slavery that may have led to increased salt sensitivity, and other nutritional and cultural factors in the pathogenesis of hypertension, all topics superbly covered by the authors of this book.

The history of hypertension and its possible relation to salt intake goes back a long way. In the *Yellow Emperor's Classic of Internal Medicine,* which appeared before 2500 B.C., an aphorism states that if too much salt is taken in food, the pulse hardens, a statement we would interpret today as evidence of elevated blood pressure. Derek Denton has written that there was no such surfeit of salt in West Africa. In fact, because of its scarcity, salt was an important element in the slave trade; it is said that children were sold into slavery in return for this precious commodity. Twice a year, caravans of 2,000 camels brought salt from the Taoudeni salt swamp in the Sahara Desert to Timbuktu for limited distribution to the wealthy in West Africa.

Grim and Wilson have hypothesized that during the slavery period of history, high mortality from salt depletion as a result of diarrhea and sweating during passage to the West may have selected individuals who had an enhanced ability to conserve salt and that their descendants in the United States today are at a risk for salt-sensitive hypertension. In contrast, early evidence compiled by Donnison in 1929 and by Kaminer in 1960 of blood pressure in African natives suggested that little or no hypertension existed in the rural areas and that blood pressure did not rise with aging. In this book, however, Mufunda and Sparks report an increasing prevalence of hypertension as rural Africans move to urban areas and adopt the living patterns of the Western world. They postulate that among the changes associated with Westernization that may be responsible in some degree for the elevated blood pressure are the increased intake of simple sugars (with resultant obesity), the higher consumption of salt and alcohol, and a new variety of psychosocial stresses. Mufunda and Sparks conclude that a better understanding of the cause of the rising morbidity of hypertension in urban Africa could provide valuable clues to the pathogenesis of hypertension of blacks in America.

In other chapters, Falkner, Dressler, Anderson and McNeilly, and Myers and McClure explore ways in which psychosocial, cultural, and economic stresses may induce physiological changes that lead to chronic elevation of blood pressure in blacks. The emphasis of these authors is primarily on the role of the sympathetic nervous system and its changing reactivity in increasing systemic vascular resistance and retention of salt by the kidneys. Their hypotheses are consonant with the earlier studies of Walter B. Cannon on emotional factors in disease, with a marked increase in sympathoadrenal activity in stressful situations. Moreover, the localization of the center for sham rage in the hypothalamus by Bard and Cannon now assumes even greater significance in view of the recent demonstration by Fernald that behavior may alter the histology of the hypothalamus in certain African fish, inducing striking physiological changes. These findings may help resolve the age-old arguments in the nature-nurture debate in hypertension. It may be a long time before these observations can be translated to humans, but the report of LeVay of differences in the architecture of the hypothalamus in male sexual behavior suggests a new avenue of research in normotensive and hypertensive patients.

Fray has already begun to explore the hypothalamic-hypophyseal influence on renin secretion and its role in the regulation of blood pressure. In addition, with the recent impressive advances in the molecular biology of the renin system, we may soon have a better understanding of the hormonal alterations in black hypertensives. In light of the rapid expansion of our knowledge of renin and its importance in the pathogenesis of hypertension, it is well to recall the skepticism with which Tigerstedt's pioneering publication of 1898, announcing the discovery of renin, was received. He had set out to determine whether substances released from the kidney may influence the circulatory system in view of the well-known relationship between renal and cardiac diseases. The experiments demonstrating a pressor agent in the kidney were extraordinarily successful, but they brought Tigerstedt nothing but criticism, even scorn. Most early investigators were unable to repeat his experiments. Within one year of the publication of Tigerstedt's paper, Lewandowsky of Berlin wrote a scathing and sarcastic rebuttal of the report, emphasizing that the adrenal medullary extract of Oliver and Schafer was far more powerful than the substance supposedly extracted from the kidney. And Janeway, the doyen of American clinical nephrologists, concluded in 1913 that Tigerstedt's report should be dismissed out of hand. According to his personal friends, Tigerstedt no longer mentioned the renin studies and may have wished that his 1898 paper would be forgotten, since it had brought him nothing but grief. In the 1924 obituary of Tigerstedt, in the *Skandinavische Archive Physiologie*, the journal he had edited for many years, no reference to renin was made by his long-time colleague, Santesson.

In contrast to the disbelief shown for the work of Tigerstedt, the scientific world greeted Goldblatt's production of experimental hypertension in the dog with accolades when his reports began to appear in 1934. Cannon, Houssay, Pickering, and others acclaimed his production of hypertension by reduction of renal blood flow as opening a significant new field of research. However, Goldblatt was probably unaware of Tigerstedt's earlier report, for renin had disappeared from the literature of the teens and twenties.

Goldblatt's research did serve to renew the quest for a renal pressor agent. By 1938, Landis and co-workers in the United States, and Pickering and Prinzmetal in England, had independently extracted and purified renin from the normal kidney, thus laying the groundwork for our understanding of the role of renin in the production of renovascular hypertension. Houssay and co-workers reported that the grafting of an ischemic kidney in the neck of a nephrectomized dog raised the blood pressure of the recipient animal; transplanting a normal kidney did not induce hypertension. They also demonstrated that the canine renal venous pressor agent produced vasoconstriction in the perfused hind limb of the toad, *particularly if the blood was removed from dogs whose hypertension was only of a few days' duration,* the first suggestion that the ischemic kidney released more pressor agent during the initiation of renovascular hypertension than during the chronic stage of the syndrome.

Following the development by Haber of radioimmunoassays for renin and aldosterone, Gutmann and Miller reported that systemic plasma renin activity (PRA) began to rise within minutes after renal artery compression in the conscious, uninephrectomized dog on a normal salt diet, with concomitant elevation of blood pressure. Systemic PRA continued to rise over the first two to three days, with a parallel retention of sodium and water and increase in plasma volume. Although the renal perfusion pressure was maintained at a constant level, PRA and aldosterone concentration returned to control values over several days, while blood pressure remained high. These data suggested that the elevated renin levels were responsible for the initial rise in blood pressure but that sustained hypertension was due to other factors, such as the salt and water retention and increased plasma volume, a view championed by Guyton.

As Fray has emphasized, in the chronic stage, the canine model resembled the low renin and salt-sensitive hypertensive black. To delineate further the interaction of renin and sodium balance in renovascular hypertension, Rocchini repeated the experiments in the uninephrectomized dog but kept the animals on a low-salt diet to preclude sodium retention. Under these circumstances, PRA remains high throughout the period of renal artery compression, as does the blood pressure. Thus in the salt-depleted dog, in which salt and water retention does not occur, renin appears to play a major role in both initiation and maintenance of renovascular hypertension.

It is unfortunate that Tigerstedt is not alive to see the further vindication of his views on renin provided by molecular biologists. For example, Mullins, Peters, and Ganten have reported that transgenic rats, bearing an extra gene for renin, develop hypertension even though PRA does not rise. Perhaps, as Dzau has suggested, local tissue renin plays a role as important as systemic PRA and may also help explain certain features of Fray's equilibrium model. In addition, several groups (Jacobs and co-workers, and Hilbert et al.), using linkage analysis, have mapped genes in the hereditary hypertensive rat that are linked to the elevated blood pressure and are closely linked to the gene encoding angiotensin-converting enzyme, an enzyme that plays a major role in blood pressure homeostasis. Thus, we have increasing evidence concerning genetic control of renin in hypertension and the interaction of renin with other hormonal, metabolic, ionic, and nutritional factors, as discussed by Sowers et al. and Cooper and Borke. How these may be manipulated by drug therapy provides a rational approach to the treatment of hypertensive blacks as reported in the chapter written by Wright and Douglas.

The most important problem that remains is the development of a rational preventive program for this polygenic disease in which the kidney plays such an important role. This important and timely text provides the physiological foundation for progressive research on the pathogenesis of hypertension in the black population. In 1916, as a surgical resident, Goldblatt watched a nephrectomized patient die when a single, anomalous, half-horseshoe kidney was inadvertently removed. Although uremia developed, blood pressure did not rise, and he concluded, "no kidneys, no hypertension."

Preface

Over 15 million adult black Americans have hypertension. The disease is associated with a decline in life expectancy among blacks. Hypertension often leads to stroke, heart disease, and kidney failure, and blacks have a higher incidence than whites of stroke (50%), heart disease (30%), and generalized kidney disease (50%). Hypertension is the primary cause of the over 18-fold higher incidence of end-stage renal disease among blacks compared to whites. Although effective treatment of hypertension and related disorders is increasing considerably in the general population, it is decreasing in the black population. The main reasons for this decline may be lack of appreciation of the profound effects of socioeconomic and psychosocial factors in the pathogenesis of the disease in blacks, lack of adequate physiological knowledge of the disease in blacks, and lack of adequate conceptual paradigms by which future research must be guided. This book seeks to fill these gaps by documenting available evidence of the pathogenesis, consistent diagnosis, and appropriate treatment of hypertension in blacks.

We gratefully acknowledge the many people who have contributed to this book. Several chapters were first presented at the Federation of American Societies of Experimental Biology Meeting in April 1991, at a symposium sponsored by The American Physiological Society (APS) and partially supported by Abbott Laboratories and American Cyanamid Co. The APS Clinical Physiology Subcommittee provided the opportunity to publish the symposium proceedings with the approval of the APS Publications Committee. We especially acknowledge the enthusiastic support of Dr. John S. Cook, Chair of the Publications Committee, and Dr. Julien Biebuyck, Chair of the Clinical Physiology Subcommittee. At various stages Edith Barry, Susan Hannan, and the production staff at Oxford University Press offered valuable suggestions and editorial assistance. Finally, the expert secretarial assistance of Cheryl Barry is gratefully acknowledged.

Worcester, Massachusetts   J.C.S.F.
Cleveland, Ohio   J.C.D.
January 1992

Contents

PART V   THEORY AND THERAPY . . . THE VOLUME-VASOCONSTRICTION SPECTRUM

Contributors

Norman B. Anderson, Ph.D.
Department of Psychiatry
Duke University Medical Center
Durham, North Carolina

A. Clifford Barger, M.D.
Department of Cellular and Molecular
*   Physiology*
Harvard Medical School
Boston, Massachusetts

James L. Borke, Ph.D.
Department of Physiology and
*   Pharmacology*
Loyola University School of Dentistry
Maywood, Illinois

Richard S. Cooper, M.D.
Department of Preventive Medicine and
*   Epidemiology*
Loyola University Stritch School of
*   Medicine*
Maywood, Illinois

Janice G. Douglas, M.D.
Division of Endocrinology and
*   Hypertension*
Case Western Reserve University
Cleveland, Ohio

William W. Dressler, Ph.D.
Department of Behavioral and
*   Community Medicine*
University of Alabama
Tuscaloosa, Alabama

Bonita Falkner, M.D.
Division of Pediatric Nephrology and
*   Hypertension*
Medical College of Pennsylvania
Philadelphia, Pennsylvania

J.C.S. Fray, Ph.D.
Department of Physiology
University of Massachusetts Medical
*   School*
Worcester, Massachusetts

Clarence E. Grim, M.D.
Department of Medicine
Charles R. Drew University of Medicine
*   and Science*
Los Angeles, California

Faith H. McClure, Ph.D.
Department of Psychology
California State University,
*   San Bernardino*
San Bernardino, California

Maya McNeilly, Ph.D.
Department of Psychiatry
Duke University Medical Center
Durham, North Carolina

Jacob Mufunda, M.D., Ph.D.
Department of Physiology
University of Zimbabwe
Harare, Zimbabwe

Hector F. Myers, Ph.D.
Department of Psychiatry
Charles R. Drew University of Medicine
*   and Science*
Los Angeles, California

James R. Sowers, M.D.
Division of Endocrinology, Metabolism,
*   and Hypertension*
Wayne State University School of
*   Medicine*
Detroit, Michigan

Harvey V. Sparks, Jr., M.D.
Department of Physiology
Michigan State University
East Lansing, Michigan

Thomas W. Wilson, Ph.D.
Department of Medicine
Charles R. Drew University of Medicine
  and Science
Los Angeles, California

Jackson T. Wright, Jr., M.D., Ph.D.
Division of Endocrinology and
  Hypertension
Case Western Reserve University
Cleveland, Ohio

Michael B. Zemel, Ph.D.
Division of Endocrinology, Metabolism,
  and Hypertension
Wayne State University School of
  Medicine
Detroit, Michigan

Paula C. Zemel, Ph.D.
Department of Nutrition
University of Tennessee
Knoxville, Tennessee

I
INTRODUCTION

1

Hypertension in Blacks: Physiological, Psychosocial, Theoretical, and Therapeutic Challenges

J.C.S. FRAY

Blacks constitute only 12% of the U.S. population, but a variety of factors expose this group to the greatest health risk. Members of this group, chiefly descendants of African slaves, are unfavorably represented in all the major demographic topologies: one-third live in poverty, a value threefold higher than whites; one-half live in urban communities typified by poverty, inadequate and overcrowded schools, overcrowded housing, unemployment, constant exposure to a pervasive drug subculture and periodic street violence, and in general a high level of stress. Life expectancy is rising for the general population, but falling for blacks. Although indistinguishable from whites in causes of death by chronic diseases, blacks are distinguished by increased severity and greater prevalence of such diseases. Of the estimated 60 million hypertensive cases reported, blacks represent 25% (almost twofold higher than representation in the general population). Not only are blacks more likely to develop hypertension, but the disorder develops earlier, is often more severe, and is more likely to be fatal at an earlier age. Stroke is 50% greater in blacks compared with whites; ventricular hypertrophy is 30% greater in blacks; death in middle-aged blacks is sixfold greater; and kidney failure or end-stage renal disease in blacks is threefold higher than whites. End-stage renal disease is also more pervasive in blacks with diabetes and hypertension and is generally less prevalent in diabetic whites than diabetic blacks. Socioeconomic and psychosocial factors, plus inadequate scientific knowledge, preclude black hypertensives from getting early and aggressive therapy; consequently the majority of black hypertensives go untreated or are treated unsuccessfully. These facts prompted the recent observation that while the treatment of hypertension is improving considerably in the general population and while the morbidity and mortality from hypertension-related diseases are rapidly declining in the general population, treatment proposals (and programs) and morbidity and mortality rates remain impoverished in black communities (31).

One reason for the lack of attention to the disease in blacks is the paucity of hard scientific data from which to develop rational and efficacious therapies. Although it is generally agreed that black hypertensives are more resistant to treatment than whites, we still have only a very limited understanding of the

3

disease. The margins of essential hypertension as it occurs in blacks need to be provided. The origin of the disorder in blacks, its genetic basis, and its evolution need to be described, at least in physiological terms. The important role of chronic psychosocial stressors needs to be brought into any conceptualization of pathogenesis, as does the important role of diet from slavery to today. The importance of abnormal ion metabolism as well as renal renin hyporesponsivity need examination in blacks. This book sets at least a partial description of the physiological basis of the disease in blacks and offers more than a few successful therapeutic strategies, based upon what is now known of the pathophysiological basis of the disease.

The book is divided into four parts. The first considers the proposals for the origin of hypertension in the black population, especially those out of Africa. Grim and Wilson (19) present arguments that support their view that blacks developed hypertension as a consequence of the slave trade, particularly the "middle passage." The hypothesis rests on the foundation that heightened "salt sensitivity" in blacks is a Darwinian drive to select adaptable strategies for survival during evolutionary pressures. In this hypothesis the derangement is localized to sodium-transporting systems. The first part also considers pathogenesis in black children. Falkner (10) argues that a genetic defect may be involved, but that it may reside in the insulin-stimulated glucose uptake systems. The resultant insulin resistance or hyperinsulinemia in black children may have profound effects on the sympathetic nervous system's ability to regulate blood pressure and salt and water balance.

The second part of the book considers models that bring sociocultural and psychosocial factors to bear on physiological processes. It is now generally agreed that the primary physiological manifestation of psychosocial stressors is the liberation of stress response molecules that alter blood pressure. Therefore, one end product of sociocultural and psychosocial stressors is to raise blood pressure by increasing cardiac output and (or) total peripheral resistance. Dressler (8) suggests underlying mechanisms for the social and cultural dimensions; Meyers and McClure (26) make the case for an "interactions" approach when considering the psychosocial stressors; Anderson and McNeilly (2) point toward a "contextual model" in which augmented autonomic reactivity may play a significant role. The contextual model is considered not only rigorously physiological but also high in predictive value.

Part III returns to the physiological consequences of salt sensitivity, improper diet, intracellular ionic changes, and the improper processing of renin. Mufunda and Sparks (28) take a closer look at the problem of salt sensitivity in Africans in the homeland and in the diaspora. Their observations answer some concerns about the salt-sensitivity theory, but also raise new questions, especially about diet and ions other than salt. Sowers et al. (34) address these issues, and Cooper and Borke (5) present a comprehensive review of the evidence implicating ionic changes at the (intra)cellular level. The final chapter in Part III examines the issue of plasma renin activity (PRA), calls attention to the complex series of steps involved in the renin-secretory process, and points to mechanisms of impairment in blacks.

The fourth part of the book outlines a theory of the initiation, development, and maintenance of hypertension, and rational therapeutic strategies for successful diagnosis and treatment. The theoretical approach is an extension of the original mosaic model advanced by Page (29), which coupled with Laragh's views of "volume-vasoconstriction" analysis (22,23) gives new meaning to the underlying biophysical processes at the level of the resistance vessels (14). Since the data are incomplete for black hypertensives, experimental renovascular hypertension is used as a model (12). Wright and Douglas (39) focus on effective therapeutic strategies to lower blood pressure in black hypertensives. They call attention to the effectiveness of diuretics, beta blockers, non–beta blocker sympatholytic drugs, angiotensin converting enzyme inhibitors, and calcium channel blockers. It is concluded that diuretics coupled with calcium channel blockers are the most effective therapeutic strategy for black hypertensives, particularly those diagnosed as "low-renin hypertensives." A more detailed summary of each of the four parts follows.

THE MIDDLE PASSAGE . . . THE EARLY YEARS
GENETIC SHIFTING GROUND

Historically, there is scarcely any evidence supporting the hypothesis that blacks were prone to hypertension in preslavery times. All of the earlier reliable studies, from Donnison's (7) work on, show hypotension in endogenous communities. Even today, as demonstrated by Mufunda and Sparks (28), rural Africans are less prone to develop hypertension than their more urban counterparts. Several approaches have been used to understand passage from the physiologic state of constant hypotension to the malignant stage of chronic hypertension.

Two directions have been pursued. In one direction, some workers have ascribed the evolution of an increased "salt sensitivity" to the slave trade. Grim and Wilson (19) have been the main proponents of this view. The general thesis is that evolutionary pressure, which forced captured Africans living in a salt-deprived environment to adapt to the many ramifications of slavery, subsequently manifested itself physiologically as an enhanced genetic expression of a salt-transporting system. In another direction, other workers give some priority to insulin. Falkner (10) suggests that the primary genetic defect is in the insulin-stimulated glucose uptake system, giving rise to hyperinsulinemia or insulin resistance. The excess insulin then interacts with the sympathetic nervous system and sodium-transporting processes in the kidney and vasculature. Insulin excess also triggers structural changes that, collectively, lead to an increased total peripheral resistance, a parameter higher in black children than in whites (10).

Grim and Wilson (21) advance the hypothesis that hypertension developed in Western Hemisphere blacks because the middle passage and other periods of entrenched slavery were characterized by excessive sodium depletion from sweating, diarrhea, and vomiting. Africans in their traditional societies were low salt consumers; therefore they evolved enhanced sodium-conservation mechanisms, chiefly the renin–angiotensin–aldosterone system (RAAS). The general view is that evolutionary pressure, the Darwinian drive, forced the development of a genetic machinery to conserve salt beyond normal levels during the slavery period and that this genetic machinery expresses itself in the descendants of slaves by decreasing the responsiveness of RAAS. Grim and Wilson (19) show the strong logical link between physiological adaptation to salt and Darwinian evolution. For many centuries salt was a major item of trade, commerce, and taxes. Being a savored "Western addiction," it was inaccessible to the indigenous peoples of Africa. The point may be made that the knowledge of the addictiveness of salt prompted slave traders to give captured Africans pickled, spoiled meats. The novel diets containing foreign foods and excess salt had deleterious effects. In fact, at first, as Grim and Wilson (19) point out, over 70% of the slaves died of maladies closely linked to their physiological rejection of rotten animal flesh (diarrhea and vomiting leading to hypernatremia).

The genetic predisposition model predicts certain children at risk. Falkner (10) concludes that black children are expected to have a greater rate of risk, based solely on family history. When these children are exposed to mental stress, they exhibit a rise in blood pressure within minutes, a response triggered by the sympathetic drive to increase total peripheral resistance. Falkner further observes that the major determinants of resting blood pressure in black children are body size and growth rates, i.e., bigger and fatter children have higher blood pressure, in general. The reason for the higher pressure may not be increased cardiac output but increased total peripheral resistance, which may be achieved by hypertrophy of the vasculature or increased reactivity. Although the issue of differences in peripheral vascular structure is attractive, it remains unconfirmed by concrete evidence. On the other hand, the available evidence is in line with the view that black children have greater vascular reactivity (10). Falkner (10) advances the hypothesis that insulin may play a major role in the development of hypertension among black children. There is, she postulates, a primary genetic defect in insulin-dependent stimulation of glucose uptake, which leads to hyperinsulinemia. Although the exact origin of the defect and its link to the slave trade have not been established, insulin excess, it is postulated, powers the sympathetic nervous system and retards sodium transport in kidney and vascular smooth muscle cells and forms the basis for the initial step of increased salt sensitivity (10). Insulin excess may also promote vascular growth directly through its own anabolic effect or through insulinlike growth factor I. Falkner (10) concludes that although these ("hypothetical") pathways are not unique to blacks, they may play an important role in the development of hypertension in black children.

The shifting ground of the genetic history of hypertension in blacks needs restudy. From what has been said thus far (and from what is to follow), it must be concluded that the history of the prevalence of hypertension among blacks began at the exact time (no more than 400 years ago) when the stress of ingesting salt entered the African diet. The salt-sensitivity hypothesis suggests how the evolutionary pressure may be Darwinian and supports the view of the genetic strength of blacks to adapt to severe environmental stress. What is interesting is that in young black children we see these genetic traits manifesting themselves in a variety of ways, including impairment of sugar metabolism. Taken together, the evidence suggests that in the beginning the genetic capability of blacks to defend against physiological cardiovascular stress was very much intact, particularly as it relates to sodium conservation and responsiveness of RAAS (see Chapter 7, this volume), but the compounded artificial (and addictive) additional stress with salt and pickled food caused adaptations that point to an unidentified genetic locus. That is, the genetic factor(s) responsible for the greater prevalence of hypertension in blacks remains to be identified.

THE CONTEXTUAL MODEL . . . SOCIOCULTURAL AND PSYCHOSOCIAL DIMENSIONS

Some practitioners argue that in addition to strong genetic influences, sociocultural and psychosocial factors play an important role in the pathogenesis of hypertension in blacks. Without a social and a cultural dimension to the afferent side of blood pressure–regulating mechanisms, any analysis of the pathophysiology of hypertension in blacks is incomplete. Dressler (8) advances a strong argument suggesting underlying mechanisms whereby a wide variety of social and cultural forces may interact with fundamental physiological responses to cause overall attenuated responsiveness. Meyers and McClure (26) propose a multidimensional analysis (or "interactional perspective") in an attempt to sort out and rank the psychosocial stressors involved. Similarly, in the framework of a contextual model, Anderson and McNeilly (2) summarize the evidence, suggesting a possible site of action of chronic psychosocial stressors in physiological terms. The contextual model shows promise because it attempts to look at the physiological mechanisms whereby sociocultural and psychosocial forces lead to a greater prevalence of hypertension in blacks.

An impressive amount of evidence implicates social and cultural dimensions as having a major role in black hypertensives. This role is over and above that of underlying genetic predisposition. Dressler (8) presents a working model whereby a wide variety of social and cultural influences may interact with fundamental physiological responses to cause an overall attenuated responsiveness. He makes the important point that unless future research includes social and cultural influences in analyses of black hypertensives, conclusions can only be tentative and, at best, partial. Dressler (8) postulates, and proceeds to show, that low occupational class blacks who maintain a "high status lifestyle" inevitably develop hypertension. In his studies of blacks in a Southern community he observed that the material benefits of a high status lifestyle were acquired by the most successful blacks, but the cultural status rewarded for the acquisition was denied (8), and this negative outcome sets in motion a pathophysiological sequence leading to hypertension. The physiological mechanism(s) responsible for the elevated pressure is increased total peripheral resistance triggered by physiological stress response molecules, a process independent of structural remodeling. Another pathway whereby psychosocial stressors influence blood pressure is to increase cardiovascular reactivity. Dressler (8) shows how risk of hypertension in blacks in the sociocultural context is caused by high status lifestyle, low class rank, and little perceived access to social support.

But the work of Dressler (8) makes an even more profound point. Genetic models of the disease should not focus on hereditary factors at the expense of ethnocentric bias. In any complete description of this particular disorder, the social dimension must be inclusive. That is why the issue of skin color has been such a problem. It is well known, as Dressler (8) points out, that pigmentation is a hereditary feature, and whereas most practitioners (and others interested in the debate) often make the association of dark pigmentation and hypertension as resulting from the genes dictating skin color, there is no evidence to suggest a causal relationship. The literature is replete with such assertions. But as Dressler points out, "skin color has been a contentious and divisive issue in Western culture for centuries; the color of skin has led to markedly different experiences for different segments of the population. It therefore seems just as 'natural' to look to the social implications of differences in skin color as the mediating influence on blood pressure." Dressler also makes a few suggestions as to how the sociocultural model of hypertension may be strengthened and enriched by influencing established physiological parameters. But this is far from the only approach to the social (or psychosocial) dimension.

Myers and McClure (26) make a case for an interactive approach to the psychosocial problems in black hypertensives. They begin with the premise of an underlying genetic predisposition and go on to show that hypertension develops in blacks as a consequence of interaction of a number of *psychosocial stressors:* socioeconomic status (SES), behavioral and lifestyle factors, psychological attributes, and family dynamics. At bottom is the search for a way of conceptualizing the problem so that we may approach the solution from one of its many angles. The evidence, reviewed by Myers and McClure (26), is compelling that blacks are at the bottom of the SES ladder and therefore are targeted to bear the bulk of the SES weight in terms of low SES background, less than desirable living conditions (a major stress in itself), and shattered families and communities. Understanding the underlying pathophysiological mechanisms in the pathogenesis of hypertension in the black population is the overall objective of all research strategies. But Myers and McClure (26) argue that without consideration of psychosocial stressors any analysis would be incomplete and that an interactive approach to psychosocial problems offers most promise. They point out the growing body of evidence that supports the theory that blacks "who cope with life demands by compensating for limited instrumental resources by increasing effort and determination ... also run additional cardiovascular risks" (26). The most successful blacks are those who use active coping skills *(John Henryism)* as a mechanism for defraying the abysmal life of broken dreams. The *price of the ticket* is to outdo steel. At the cellular level, the final manifestation of active coping is increased cytosolic calcium (see Chapter 11, this volume). Myers and McClure (26) review the notion suggesting that blacks, especially adult males, who respond to anger (and perhaps shame) with suppression or overreaction, are particularly at risk for hypertension. The evidence, though preliminary, suggests that anger (and, again, perhaps shame) provoked by "racially loaded experiences may be more cardiovascular dysregulating for blacks than anger provoked by more racially neutral encounters" (26). Without multidimensional consideration of the problem to incorporate psychosocial stressors, the solution will be necessarily incomplete. Myers and McClure (26) present a strong case for such consideration.

The contextual model developed by Anderson and McNeilly (2) takes these issues a few steps further to the site of ultimate determination of essential hypertensive blacks, the resistance vessels. This model offers promising lines of investigation that as they noted, should advance our knowledge by moving "beyond studies that simply *describe* racial group differences . . . toward experiments aimed at understanding the basis of the observed differences." The time may have come, Anderson and McNeilly (2) assert, when it may be more profitable to design studies that "ask what factors are responsible for the greater vascular reactivity observed among blacks relative to whites and more importantly, what variables are predictive of heightened vascular reactivity within the black population." The key feature of their model is that the heightened vascular reactivity observed in blacks is a function of a wide variety of biological, psychosocial and behavioral, environmental, and sociocultural factors. The contextual model rests on the premise that "race should be viewed as a proxy for effect of differential exposure to chronic social and environmental stressor, rather than as a proxy for the effects of genetic differences" (2). Blacks, as is now well documented, at every level of society are exposed to a larger number of chronic psychosocial stressors than their white counterparts.

Salt plays a key role in the vascular hyperactivity model. Reactivity is generally believed to be autonomic hyperfunction with "beta activity" causing increases in heart rate, stroke volume, and cardiac output, and "alpha activity" causing increased total peripheral resistance. The stressors mediating beta responses are mental arithmetic, competitive reaction time tasks, physical exercise, and preparation for a speech. Those associated with alpha responses are cold pressor tests, mirror tracing, hand grip, and public speaking. High salt intake increases sympathetic nervous system activity, which promotes renal salt retention. Salt in turn, then, plays a potentiating role in the sympathetic nervous system–induced vascular hyperreactivity. The hyperreactivity and hypertension observed in an active-coping lifestyle are associated with greater salt retention. Blacks subjected to heightened psychosocial stressors may also show elevated salt retention.

In Chapter 6, Anderson and McNeilly (2) summarize the evidence to support the contextual model. Race is considered a sociocultural designation that signifies differential exposure to chronic psychosocial stressors. Epidemiological evidence supports the association between increased chronic social stressors and increased prevalence of hypertension. Even in animal studies, chronic stress augments cardiovascular reactivity to acute stress. In the spontaneously hypertensive rat model, the increased reactivity is associated with sodium retention. The physiological mechanisms responsible for cardiovascular manifestation at the cellular (and molecular) level are discussed in Chapter 11. The more recent demonstration that salt sensitivity and salt retention are heightened (whether by genetic or environmental factors) prompts the conclusion that the key element in the contextual model is the observation that chronic psychosocial stressors are more prevalent in blacks with deranged salt metabolism. The deranged salt metabolism superimposed upon (or in consequence of) a long history of chronic social stressors may explain the heightened reactivity because these stressors are biological, behavioral, and psychological risk factors. In other words, altered sodium transport in renal tubular cells and vascular smooth muscle cells may be pathogenetic manifestations of chronic psychosocial stressors. It is this connection (this leap) that distinguishes the contextual model from its competitors. Besides being contextual, it is rigorously physiological in its predictive value.

SALT SENSITIVITY, NUTRITION, INTRACELLULAR IONS, AND RENIN:
PHYSIOLOGICAL CONSIDERATIONS

Recent physiological research has returned to the question of heightened salt sensitivity and the cellular processes involved. The earlier model puts emphasis on a Darwinian strategy whereby blacks in the Western Hemisphere develop hypertension by a salt-sensitive mechanism activated at some step along the slave trade, most probably the middle passage (19). The ultimate implication of this view is that in most Western societies where blacks represent a growing subgroup the reason for the higher prevalence of hypertension is genetic predisposition, dictated most probably by the inability of blacks to metabolize excessive amounts of exogenous sodium chloride. This view leaves open the question of hypertension in black Africans who were not subjected to the slave trade. The fact that some have argued that the colonial period may in some respects be equivalent to the slavery period in terms of salt and psychological stressors remains outside the current debate. Mufunda and Sparks (28) have returned to the question of increased salt sensitivity in native Africans untouched by the whole cadre of factors implicated in the slavery hypothesis (19). Their findings provide a fair number of insights into underlying physiological mechanisms. They allude to the importance of calcium and other dietary factors. The importance of these factors has been under investigation by Sowers et al. (34). The role of intracellular ions and the homeostatic mechanisms which regulate (intra)cellular ions are the primary contributions of Cooper and Borke (5) to the current understanding of the disease. With uncommon rigor and unusual attention to issues of technique, Cooper and Borke present a state-of-the-art coverage of the most salient points and the ramifications of the issues involved. The role of (intra)cellular ions and their regulation is also considered in the context of renal renin secretion in blacks.

The salt-sensitivity hypothesis has been analyzed and extended by Mufunda and Sparks (28). A partial summary of this important issue follows. The epidemiological evidence offers strong support for the view that excess salt is an important factor in contributing to the hypertension observed in blacks, in or out of Africa. The epistemological evidence offers strong support for the conclusion that the ability of some blacks to conserve salt offers a Darwinian evolutionary advantage in salt-deprived environments, especially when such environments provoke excess salt loss. The physiological evidence also supports the hypothesis that Africans in the homeland or in the diaspora are more prone to exhibit an enhanced pressor sensitivity to excess salt. Mufunda and Sparks (28) have concluded, however, that increased salt sensitivity is in itself insufficient to *cause* hypertension in blacks. Their chief line of evidence, mainly from their own studies and experience, is that hypertension is rarely found among indigenous Africans who have remained unacculturated by Western standards. The authors show that the complexities of "Western living habits" play a key role in the disease. Among the Western living habits they cite are increased psychosocial stress, higher alcohol intake, more obesity, increased consumption of simple dietary carbohydrates, and altered dietary electrolytes. Mufunda and Sparks (28) conclude that although salt sensitivity is an important factor in understanding hypertension in blacks, the increased salt sensitivity may have adaptive advantages for retaining sodium in salt-deficient environments and for excreting excess sodium in salt-rich conditions. Psychosocial stressors, as well as other factors, may play a role in disturbing the physiological balance, though the status of salt sensitivity in all blacks remains undefined. Not all blacks exhibit similar predisposition to hypertension despite the long history of selective pressure to render hypertension in blacks a concomitant to survival. The slavery hypothesis has as its central feature the development of increased salt sensitivity as a key survival strategy for blacks in Western societies. Aside from the impact of the psychosocial and sociocultural ramifications of slavery, Mufunda and Sparks (28) suggest that Western influence may also involve an increased sodium to potassium ratio in the diet. In other words, the problem may have started with the slave trade, but it is propagated and maintained by subtle sociocultural pressures that are difficult to detect by straightforward physiological measurements. There appears to be a role for genes and a role for culture and nutrition.

The importance of nutritional factors has been the focus of a long series of studies by Sowers and coworkers (34). In concert with other researchers in the field, they have monitored blood pressure patterns among blacks in terms of changes in dietary calcium, magnesium, potassium, and sodium. They confirm the well-known finding of a higher salt sensitivity among blacks, although a close reading of their report shows, as alluded to earlier by Mufunda and Sparks (28), that the increased salt sensitivity may be insufficient to account for the increased prevalence of the disease in blacks. They suggest a consideration of dietary calcium along with salt sensitivity may better approximate the underlying physiological mechanisms. In addition to dietary calcium, they implicate factors such as parathormone, magnesium, and potassium. The importance of dietary control of hypertension in blacks or whites remains to be fully articulated. They suggest that dopamine may play a role in the mechanism of increased salt sensitivity, though the precise part dopamine plays remains undefined. Sowers et al. (34), however, provided an impressive amount of physiological evidence to implicate profound change in ion metabolism at the subcellular level.

The central role of intracellular ions has been addressed by Cooper and Borke (5). Almost 40 years ago, Page (29) proposed that hypertension is essentially an "ionic" disease whereby the cells of the peripheral blood vessels undergo a disturbance in ionic concentration. It is this disturbance that manifests physiologically as a rise in blood pressure (19). The ions of primary concern are sodium, potassium, and calcium; to study the cellular metabolism of these ions is complicated, mainly because the variables are many and the interactions diverse. Cooper and Borke (5) note that black hypertensives have more enhanced ion metabolism than normotensives, where the strongest evidence for an association may be found in sodium-lithium countertransport. Higher levels of intracellular sodium and calcium are also observed, but their physiological significance is unclear. Cooper and Borke remain speculative about the importance of genetic propensities in altering cellular ion metabolism but are forthright in summarizing the ion transport profiles observed in blacks compared with whites.

A series of conclusions may be drawn, at least tentatively (5), concerning the role of intracellular abnormal ion metabolism in hypertensive blacks. The strongest demonstration for an association between ion transport systems and hypertension in blacks is found in the sodium-lithium countertransport system, an artificial measure of sodium-hydrogen countertransport. A higher level of intracellular sodium is also a characteristic feature of hypertensives in general, although blacks demonstrate a 30% higher intracellular sodium than whites (5). Intracellular calcium is generally higher in hypertensives, but no differences between blacks and whites have been observed. Considering the central role of calcium in the final pathogenetic mechanism of hypertension at the arteriolar level (19), it may not be unreasonable to expect new findings on the cellular regulation of calcium in black hypertensives, particularly subtle changes in calcium pump activity or changes in calcium channel or sodium-calcium exchange transporters (5).

Concerning the influences of underlying genetic differences between the pathogenesis of hypertension in blacks compared with whites, it is not unreasonable to ask whether such differences have been observed at the level of ion metabolism (5). The evolution of a more sensitive salt-retention mechanism appears to be the only pathogenetic difference between blacks and whites, as it relates to hypertension. The higher intracellular sodium in blacks (5) supports the evolution of a hypersensitive sodium-retention system. At the level of the plasma membrane of vascular smooth muscle cells, particularly arterioles, no genetic abnormality in sodium transporting systems of blacks has been identified. At the level of specialized cells involved in hypertension, for example, the renal renin-secreting juxtaglomerular cells, which have been shown to consist of multiple ion transporting systems, there are suggestions of impairment (see Chapter 10, this volume).

Renin profiling has played an important role in defining hypertensive humans (22). More than 25% of all hypertensive humans have a low PRA and a hyporesponsiveness to stimulation (9). Renin profiling has even been used as a diagnostic tool for selecting antihypertensive therapy, which has been fairly successful particularly with regard to calcium. "Varieties" of the disease exist, and the issues of age and sex have some influence, but race has been the most well defined characteristic in assessing and targeting low-renin hypertensives.

Renin status has played a key role in defining black hypertensives (see Chapter 10, this volume). It is generally believed that blacks can be classified as low-renin hypertensives, because this subgroup demonstrates a lower PRA than whites. It is interesting that even normotensive blacks have a lower (generally) PRA than whites (31). Even in children (up to 14 years), PRA may be lower in blacks. Black hypertensives with low PRA also have a lower responsiveness to secrete renin than whites. This hyporesponsiveness occurs also in children. Although some practitioners have called attention to the unwarranted classification of low-renin hypertension in blacks, especially black women (20), others have suggested that low-renin hypertension, like the advanced stage of renal hypertension, is nothing more than a "stage" in the long-term course of essential hypertension (1). Other practitioners have argued that when renin values are adjusted for age and race, low-renin hypertension in blacks and the elderly is less common than previously believed (18). The view of the majority is that low-renin hypertension is a "distinct entity" (4,6,9,35). It should be noted, however, that some workers have found no difference in PRA between blacks and whites (24,25,27,38). The exact reason for the discrepancy is unclear. Whereas some practitioners have argued that the demarcation may be arbitrary (35), others have stressed the importance of measuring technique (32). Nevertheless, low-renin status characterizes blacks in the literature and clinical practice, and several lines of evidence support describing this subgroup as a classic case of low-renin syndrome (11). Several theories (reviewed in Chapter 10, this volume) have been advanced to explain renin impairment in black hypertensives. One theory that has gained general acceptance is that low PRA in blacks is a consequence of volume expansion. But, as reviewed in Chapter 10, this view is unsupported: both blacks and whites have volume expansion and volume contraction; and though volume expansion is more prevalent in the small samples of blacks studied, there is no association between volume status and renin. A similar demonstration has been reported for whites, prompting the conclusion that "reduction of renin in low-renin hypertension is not brought about by sodium retention with volume expansion" (see Chapter 10, this volume).

One possibility that has received support is that the impairment may be in the "release" mechanism (21). Because it is difficult to work with the hyporesponsive mechanism at the cellular level in the human syndrome, some investigators have sought animal models that reflect low PRA status: experimental pheochromocytoma (15), salt loading (13), and hypophysectomy (17). The hypophysectomized rat model has been used successfully to study the mechanism of low PRA because this model has a demonstrable impairment in the release mechanism, very similar to that observed in black hypertensives. In the context of the model, the key question is to account for the low PRA. It was observed that lack of production and storage was not responsible for the impairment, since renin content was in excess of normal (17). Kidneys (and juxtaglomerular cells) from model animals were relatively unresponsive to a variety of stimuli (17), supporting the view that the impairment may be somewhere along the secretory cascade. Since granules from model animals contained substantially more renin than normal, storage mechanism appears intact (33). These model studies show that the impairment in renin hyporesponsiveness was at some point in the exocytic cascade between the storage granules and the extracellular space. Blacks, at least in the prehypertensive stage, store a substantial amount of renin in the granular compartment (see Chapter 10, this volume).

The plasma membrane plays an important role in supergranular exocytosis of renin (11,16). Thus, one interesting possibility is that following supergranular formation the exported renin is trapped in the plasma membrane in renin hyporesponsive states. To test this possibility in model animals, renin activity in the plasma membrane of juxtaglomerular cells was measured under basal and stimulated conditions. Renin in the plasma membrane of model animals was inappropriately high in both conditions (17). Thus, in model studies, renin content and renin storage in granules and plasma membrane are exceedingly high, but renin secretion is inappropriately low. Thus, the reasons for renin hyporesponsivity may not be nonspecific volume expansion (unless this volume is translated intracellularly as inhibition of renin production or supergranular formation), circulating inhibitors of the sodium-potassium pump, extra- or intravascular pressures, or renin production and storage (21), but may be an impairment in the plasma membrane of the juxtaglomerular cells as a step along the renin exocytic cascade (17). This model has been advanced as a useful tool with which to probe the mechanism of low PRA in blacks (17). The observation that the impairment in the low PRA state may be localized to the plasma membrane provides additional evidence to support the view that hypertension may be associated with a generalized membrane pathology.

Techniques such as testing the responsiveness of plasma membrane vesicles to renin secretagogues have prompted a resurgence of interest in the mechanism of action of classical renin secretagogues such as loop diuretics. Loop diuretics (or "high-ceiling" diuretics) such as ethacrynic acid and furosemide are a class of drugs used clinically as antihypertensive agents mainly on account of their salt excretion and renin stimulation. Since drugs of this class inhibit $Na^+/K^+/2Cl^-$ cotransport at the thick limb of Henle's loop close to the macula densa, most workers have interpreted their mechanism of action as macula densa specific (see 37 for review). The view is that their effects may be observable only during tubular fluid flow and not in isolated preparations. Although early work challenged this hypothesis (3,4), the direct effects of loop diuretics in the secretory function of juxtaglomerular cells remain to be identified, but studies in renal cortical slices have provided some clues. The importance of diuretics in the current context stems from the fact that these agents are the only consistently successful therapeutic strategy found to be efficacious in black hypertensives (39).

Loop diuretics such as ethacrynic acid, bumetanide, and furosemide have profound effects on renin secretion. The effect of ethacrynic acid is fast and peaks at about 10 mM (30). The effect is reversible and unaffected by chloride, potassium (or sodium), and calcium (30). The stimulatory effect is blocked by dithiothreitol (DTT), a sulfhydryl protecting agent. In the presence of DTT, ethacrynic acid is ineffective (30). Although studies of renin granules have not excluded an intracellular site of action, the general view is that loop diuretics control renin secretion by attacking the surface membrane of the juxtaglomerular cell (30).

These observations have striking implications for the earlier views on the mechanism of action of loop diuretics. First, the similarity in dose response in vitro and in vivo is striking in itself, suggesting a direct effect. Second, the speed of action (50% maximal activity within 5 min) prompts reconsideration, since these studies were devoid of tubular fluid flow (30). Third, indacrinone, a potent loop diuretic in the ethacrynic acid family but which lacks sulfhydryl reactivity, gives the usual natriuretic effect but fails to affect renin secretion (30). On the other hand, DTT, a sulfhydryl protecting drug that has no specific effect on renin secretion, blocks (and reverses) the effect of ethacrynic acid (30).

Fourth, the nondiuretic but sulfhydryl reagent p-chloromercuriphenylsulfo-nate (PCMS) is a powerful renin secretagogue (30). The additive effect of etha-crynic acid and PCMS reveals a common site of action and provides the first proof of the action of loop diuretics at the level of the plasma membrane of juxtaglomerular cells (30).

THEORY AND THERAPY . . . THE VOLUME-VASOCONSTRICTION SPECTRUM

Unifying theories and successful rational therapies are the most impoverished areas of hypertension research in blacks, although we now have more carefully collected authentic data on this subject than ever before. We have data impli-cating genetic and environmental factors; adaptive and structural mecha-nisms; neural, endocrine, and neuroendocrine pathways; and humoral and hemodynamic alterations. We have essentially all the components of the mo-saic Page (29) described earlier as the basic building block of any thorough understanding of the underlying mechanisms responsible for the pathogenesis of hypertension in any population, black or white. What is lacking is a theo-retical framework and a therapeutic strategy based upon sound experimental facts, not circumstantial evidence. No matter how erudite the symposia and the contributions from distinguished laboratories (hospitals or clinical trials), without a unifying theoretical framework there can be no progress.

Research on hypertension (in black and white) does not lack theories (12). Laragh's "volume-vasoconstriction" approach now giving importance to neph-ron heterogeneity is but a single impressive theory. Guyton's "renal-volume" coupled to "whole-body" autoregulation is another successful theory. But they are only two of the many theories struggling for primacy. There are theories based upon the gene theory; theories implicating calcium, and sodium, and potassium, and chloride, and magnesium; some theories call for special privi-leges granted to salt-losing hormones, others for salt-retaining hormones; the-ories centered on structural alterations, neuroendocrine hypersecretion, and vascular amplification. There are psychological theories, social theories, and cultural theories, but only recently have workers like Dressler, Anderson, James, and Myers come forth with psychosocial theories with sociocultural dimensions to be considered in a contextual framework for the pathogenesis of hypertension in blacks. What research on hypertension in blacks lacks is unifying theories. The contextual model, the interactive approach, the "slave ship" hypothesis, are but a few of the models seeking unifying perspectives. The *equilibrium model* is another (12).

The equilibrium model rests on the fundamental principle that the arter-iole is the focus of cardiovascular regulation. The kidney (and consequently the *afferent arteriole*) is used as the model system as a continuation of the tradition of Bright, Goldblatt, Page, and Barger. The phases in the evolution of renal hypertension may be very similar to those of black hypertensives, although blacks have not been shown to have high prevalence of renovascular hyperten-sion. In blacks the initiating factor(s) may be psychosocial stressors (12). The model also passes privileges to calcium. Several studies have documented three phases in the renal hypertensive process. The first phase is initiated by angiotensin II–mediated vasoconstriction. The angiotensin II results from the renin secreted within seconds of renal artery constriction. Calcium plays a role in both the secretion of renin and the constriction of arterioles. The second phase is represented by a continuation of the first, by a myogenic component, or by salt and water retention, all of which have been shown to involve calcium. The third phase occurs as a continuation of the second phase, in addition to structural remodeling in the blood vessels, resetting of arterial baroreceptors and renal excretory functions, and alteration of responsiveness to vasoactive substances and ion transport systems. Calcium plays a role in most of the third phase processes. The data are compelling that calcium channel blockers may be effective in reversing or preventing any or all three phases of hypertension. The data provide substantial support for the conclusion that the systemic hemodynamic and biochemical patterns of chronic renovascular hypertension are very similar to the patterns of essential hypertension, of which black hypertensives are a clearly defined subgroup. In this regard the equilibrium model may be useful in pointing to the similarities and in identifying the factors involved.

In its most general form, the model holds that stable physical equilibrium will be achieved providing arterioles display the following main features (14): *(1)* the force acting to distend (transmural pressure) must be equal and opposite to the force acting in the wall to constrict the arteriole (wall tension); *(2)* the wall tension consists of at least passive and active components, the latter of which is defined by the level of Ca_i; *(3)* stretch of the arterioles activates the opening of calcium channels in the plasma membrane. This activation leads to increases in Ca_i and thereby to increases in active tension development. The implication, therefore, is that calcium functions as the signal that couples stretch to contraction. This endows calcium with a unique role in the fundamental mechanism for the control of renin secretion, blood flow regulation, and pathogenesis of hypertension (14). Maintenance of the disease is also a function of calcium. The initial event is that Ca_i increases and causes increased resistance. The mechanisms for the increased Ca_i may be increased calcium permeability and decreased calcium pump activity. Both have been documented (12). But mechanisms must be employed to *maintain* the elevated Ca_i. Four mechanisms have been investigated: increased serum or plasma calcium, increased calcium release from intracellular storage sites, generalized increased membrane permeability to calcium, and a defect in the calcium efflux mechanism. The generalized increase in calcium permeability and the defective calcium efflux appear to be the most well supported by available evidence. Regarding the increased permeability to calcium, the decrease can be reversed by calcium channel blockers, most of which are also effective at voltage-sensitive channels. Regarding the calcium efflux, there appears to be a reduced activity of the calcium pump and suppression of the sodium-calcium exchange mechanism. A sodium pump inhibitor is postulated to suppress sodium-calcium exchange by inhibiting the sodium pump (12).

Although the equilibrium model goes far in explaining the fundamental mechanism of these processes and the interrelationships among processes, it goes even further in advancing our understanding of the pathogenesis of hypertension. It provides a theoretical framework for the volume-vasoconstriction approach proposed by Laragh (22,23), for the autoregulation hypothesis advanced by several workers, for the resetting of arterial baroreceptors and renal excretory functions, and for the mosaic approach first proposed by Page (29). The method has an additional implication, which is primarily philosophic, for it challenges us to view circulatory control in a unique way. That is, the physical equilibrium requirement of the arteriole is of importance in any consideration of circulatory control, for it suggests that a particular level of blood pressure is not regulated but is *determined* as a consequence of the circulation's search for stable physical equilibria. This further implies that hypertension may be an "ionic disease" whereby the circulation achieves a new state of stable equilibrium. The equilibrium requirement may be the "something" that Tobian (36) speculated was manifested in hypertension as a change in the "cell membrane of the arterial muscle cells." The model provides logical and physiological explanations for the mechanism whereby calcium channel blockers, β-adrenergic agonists, diuretics, and sodium deprivation reduce blood pressure in hypertensives: by lowering Ca_i and thereby disturbing physical equilibrium in arterioles.

The goal to identify effective therapy underlies most research on black hypertensives. Once it became clear that differences do exist between white and black hypertensives, the objective was to screen (and select) the classical menu and make recommendations for the programs that proved to be efficacious. Wright and Douglas (39) observe that whereas, in general, loop diuretics are effective, the thiazides are more effective in blacks than whites. Blacks are more resistant to increasing renin after antihypertensive therapy, even with potent loop diuretics. But the recent demonstration that loop diuretics stimulate renin, possibly at the level of the juxtaglomerular cell (see above), reopens the issue as to the mechanism of action of antihypertensive therapy such as diuretics. Wright and Douglas (39) examined the evidence concerning *beta blockers* and concluded that, as a group, beta blockers are much less effective in black hypertensives, except when combined with loop diuretics. *Non–beta blockers* and *angiotensin converting enzyme inhibitors* are also reviewed. But the latter, for example, like the beta blockers, are less effective in black hypertensives, probably because renin is generally low in this subgroup and the hypertension is sustained by systems other than RAAS. *Calcium channel blockers* are a new class of drugs shown to be potent in lowering blood pressure in black hypertensives. The data on this line of treatment are still incomplete, but the effects (both experimental and theoretical) are impressive.

SUMMARY AND CHALLENGE

Treatment of hypertension in the black population represents a major two-sided challenge. The first component of the challenge is therapeutic; that is, the ultimate risk to the patient occurs if we fail in assessing the severity of the disease and in accessing the most effective agents. Thiazide diuretics are highly recommended because they lower blood pressure at a low cost, with a long history of safety and low morbidity–mortality rates, but we are still unclear as to their exact mechanism of action in black hypertensives. Research into these mechanisms may uncover potential sites of cellular impairment in blacks that may be involved in pathogenesis of the disorder. Renin production and secretion, kallikrein liberation, and salt-sensitivity induction in the kidney may all be influenced by a mechanism related to the action of thiazide diuretics. It remains a significant challenge to probe and bring to light the exact mechanism whereby one of the most certain drug therapies effectively treats black hypertensives. Calcium channel blockers are next in line, although the field is new and therefore remains unestablished. Except for their effects on predominantly "voltage-sensitive" calcium channels, little is known about the exact site (and mechanism) of action of this class of drugs. It is this paucity of knowledge that renders treatment of black hypertensives, as Wright and Douglas (39) observe, a therapeutic challenge in terms of disease severity, drug efficacy and availability, and risk of failure. The challenge with this population, then, more than any other, is to provide the most economically feasible, biologically tolerable, and therapeutically efficacious treatment (39). The second component of the challenge is theoretical. It is linked to the first in that until we know exactly what mechanisms are responsible for the initiation, development, and maintenance of hypertension in blacks, we may never know with confidence why (or where) a particular therapy is efficacious.

Figure 1.1 summarizes some features of the pathogenesis of hypertension, particularly in blacks, in whom psychosocial stressors have been a key initiating feature and in whom increased total peripheral resistance is the underlying cause of maintaining the disease (12). Psychosocial stressors include low SES, poor and overcrowded schools, community violence, unemployment, John Henryism, and negative interpersonal interactions. Interventions to reduce or eliminate any or all of these stressors should attenuate the physiological stress response, which is characterized by increased serotonin, ACTH, cortisol, epinephrine, β-endorphin, norepinephrine, renin, angiotensin II, aldosterone, ADH, etc. These interventions may be most valuable during the early phases of the disease and for extended periods after the disease is established. Renal impairment in salt and water excretion may be a primary cause of intravascular volume overload. A number of stress response molecules may induce intravascular volume overload by their physiological role in salt and water homeostasis (ACTH, angiotensin II, aldosterone, and ADH), whereas others may induce vasoconstriction directly by increasing Ca_i (norepinephrine, angiotensin, vasopressin). They all, however, induce hypertension by increasing Ca_i. It is here that volume depletion (sodium-deficient intake or diuretic therapy) and calcium channel blockade become effective. Therapeutic agents that selectively inhibit active tension development in vascular smooth muscle are also efficacious, if specificity can be established. Anderson and McNeilly (2) have shown that whereas in whites the cardiac component of the model dominates in raising blood pressure, in blacks it is the vascular constriction that plays a more significant role.

At any juncture along the pathogenetic cascade, genetic predisposition may intervene and dominate pathogenesis. Examples of this are genetically induced increased salt sensitivity or insulin inefficiency to increase volume overload, catecholamine-secreting pheochromocytoma to increase cardiac contractility and vascular smooth muscle active tension development, or abnormal

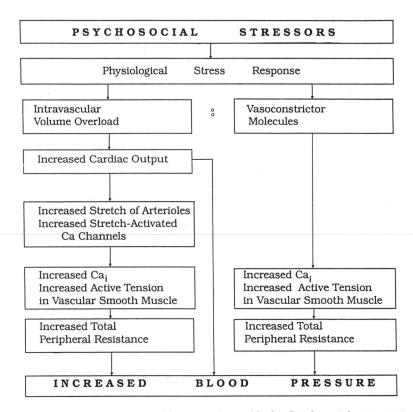

FIGURE 1.1. Pathogenesis of sustained hypertension in blacks. Psychosocial stressors include low SES, poor and overcrowded schools, community violence, unemployment, John Henryism, and negative interpersonal interactions. Physiological stress responses include increases in serotonin, ACTH, cortisol, epinephrine, norepinephrine, renin, angiotensin II, aldosterone, and ADH. Renal impairment in salt and water excretion may be a primary cause of intravascular volume overload. This figure also shows specific sites of action for the *mosaic* of genetic, environmental, anatomical, adaptive, neural, endocrine, humoral, and hemodynamic factors in the pathogenesis of black hypertensives. *Genetic* influence may be important in regulating physiological stress response molecules, intravascular volume overload through renal sodium retentional molecules, and increased Ca_i through calcium transporting molecules. *Environmental* influences may alter psychosocial stressors most profoundly. They also influence the intravascular volume overload component by dietary alterations. *Anatomical* influences are important in intravascular volume overload by structural alteration of renal salt retention mechanisms at the afferent and efferent arterioles and proximal tubule, in decreasing stretch of arterioles, in general due to decreased vascular compliance, and increased total peripheral resistance due to structural remodeling. *Adaptive* influences may affect psychosocial stressors, physiological stress response molecules, intravascular volume overload through renal salt retention molecules, and increased Ca_i and total peripheral resistance through the equilibrium mechanism. *Neural* influences may most profoundly influence liberation of physiological stress response molecules to alter vascular reactivity, increase intravascular volume overload through sympathetic control of renal salt retention, increase cardiac output, and increase total peripheral resistance through an "alpha" response. *Endocrine* influences can be seen in the physiological response molecules, in mediating intravascular volume overload through renal salt and water retention, increasing Ca_i and total peripheral resistance. *Humoral* factors such as ions, sugar, and neuropeptides influence liberation of physiological stress response molecules and subsequently all processes along the pathogenetic cascade. *Hemodynamic* influences such as pressure itself affect cardiac output, alter stretch capabilities of the arterioles and thereby Ca_i, and affect vascular distensibility and structural remodeling to alter total peripheral resistance. Taken together, the model prompts the conclusion that the term "essential" hypertension in blacks should be replaced by the more accurate *psychosocial stressor-induced hypertension*, giving significance to the evidence that in blacks psychosocial stressors are primary initiating factors and assigning the arterioles as the final pathophysiological manifestation of these stressors. Modified from Fray et al. (14).

production of vasoconstrictor molecules. Molecules such as insulin may increase Ca_i directly or indirectly at the cellular level.

Figure 1.2 summarizes the main features of the evidence presented in this book and shows three distinct phases in the pathogenesis of hypertension in blacks when the initial insult is psychosocial stressors. The initial phase (phase I) is characterized by an increase in physiological stress response molecules. The primary role of total peripheral resistance in stress-mediated elevation of blood pressure is well established in blacks (2). Intravascular volume may be normal, but cardiovascular reactivity may be high, thereby potentiating the hypertensive effects of the stress response molecules. Genetic predisposition may also begin to play a role in this early phase. The second phase (phase II) represents a continuation of the first, in addition to increased car-

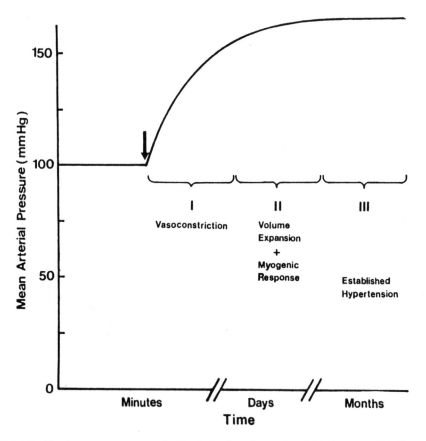

FIGURE 1.2. Blood pressure response in blacks to chronic psychosocial stressors (↓). Response is divided into three phases. Phase I is mediated by one or more of the physiological stress response molecules (serotonin, epinephrine, norepinephrine, renin, angiotensin II, and vasopressin), in addition to genetic predisposition and increased cardiovascular reactivity. Phase II represents a continuation of the first phase, in addition to increased cardiac output as a result of intravascular overload and increased vascular reactivity. Phase III is established hypertension characterized as a chronic stage of the second phase, in addition to elevated intracellular calcium and renin secretory hyporesponsivity. Increased total resistance is the dominant mechanism in Phase III. Modified from Fray et al. (14).

diac output as a result of intravascular volume overload, increased vascular reactivity, and renin hyporesponsivity. Phase II is characterized as the stage at which genetic predisposition begins to have significant effect on Ca_i, vascular reactivity, and salt sensitivity. Impaired renal function and salt excretion may begin to have significant effect in phase II. The final phase (phase III) is established hypertension characterized as a chronic stage of the second phase, in addition to elevated Ca_i, renin hyporesponsivity, and elevated total peripheral resistance. Thus, the pathogenesis of hypertension in blacks, in whom the initial insult is psychosocial stressors, has much in common with experimental renovascular hypertension, where the initial stimulus is partial renal artery occlusion (14). The challenge therefore is to stimulate research to characterize the initiation, development, and maintenance of hypertension in blacks as has been done in renal hypertensives. A positive outcome of the response to this challenge will yield the scientific knowledge on which to base our choice of rational and effective therapies. As a beginning we offer the equilibrium model as a framework within which we may work toward a greater understanding of pathogenesis.

REFERENCES

1. Abe, K., N. Irokawa, H. Aoyagi, M. Seino, M. Yasujima, K. Ritz, K. Ito, T. Chiba, Y. Sakurai, K. Saito, T. Kusaka, Y. Otsuka, S. Miyazaki, and K. Yoshinaga. Low renin hypertension—is it a stage of essential hypertension? *Tohoku J. Exp. Med. 121:* 347–354, 1977.
2. Anderson, N. B., and M. McNeilly. Autonomic reactivity and hypertension in blacks: toward a contextual model. In: *Pathophysiology of Hypertension in Blacks,* edited by J. C. S. Fray and J. G. Douglas. Oxford University Press, New York, 1992.
3. Baumbach, L., P. P. Leyssac, and S. L. Skinner. Studies on renin release from isolated superfused glomeruli: effects of temperature, urea, ouabain and ethacrynic acid. *J. Physiol. (Lond.) 258:* 243–256, 1976.
4. Brunner, H. R., J. E. Sealey, and J. H. Laragh. Renin as a risk factor in essential hypertension: more evidence. *Am. J. Med. 55:* 295–302, 1973.
5. Cooper, R. S., and J. L. Borke. Intracellular ions and hypertension in blacks. In: *Pathophysiology of Hypertension in Blacks,* edited by J. C. S. Fray and J. G. Douglas. Oxford University Press, New York, 1992.
6. Crane, M. G., J. J. Harris, and V. J. Johns. Hyporeninemic hypertension. *Am. J. Med. 52:* 457–466, 1972.
7. Donnison, C. P. Blood pressure in the African native. *Lancet 1:*6–7, 1929.
8. Dressler, W. W. Social and cultural dimensions of hypertension in blacks: underlying mechanisms. In: *Pathophysiology of Hypertension in Blacks,* edited by J. C. S. Fray and J. G. Douglas. Oxford University Press, New York, 1992.
9. Dunn, M. J., and R. L. Tannen. Low-renin hypertension. *Kidney Intl. 5:* 317–325, 1974.
10. Falkner, B. Characteristics of hypertension in black children. In: *Pathophysiology of Hypertension in Blacks,* edited by J. C. S. Fray and J. G. Douglas. Oxford University Press, New York, 1992.
11. Fray, J. C. S. Regulation of renin secretion by calcium and chemiosmotic forces: (patho)physiological considerations. *Biochim. Biophys. Acta 1097:* 243–262, 1991.
12. Fray, J. C. S. Pathogenesis of hypertension in blacks: features of an equilibrium model. In: *Pathophysiology of Hypertension in Blacks,* edited by J. C. S. Fray and J. G. Douglas. Oxford University Press, New York, 1992.
13. Fray, J. C. S. Mechanism of increased renin release during sodium deprivation. *Am. J. Physiol. 234 (Renal Fluid Electrolyte Physiol. 4):* F376–F380, 1978.
14. Fray, J. C. S., D. J. Lush, and C. S. Park. Interrelationship of blood flow, juxtaglomerular cells, and hypertension: role of physical equilibrium and Ca. *Am. J. Physiol. 251 (Regul. Integrative Comp. Physiol. 20):* R643–R662, 1986.
15. Fray, J. C. S., and P. V. H. Mayer. Decreased plasma renin activity and renin release in rats with pheochromocytoma. *Clin. Sci. Mol. Med. 53:* 447–452, 1977.

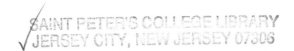

16. Fray, J. C. S., C. S. Park, and A. N. D. Valentine. Calcium and the control of renin secretion. *Endoc. Rev. 8:* 1–42, 1987.
17. Fray, J. C. S., and S. M. Russo. Mechanism for low renin in blacks: studies in hypophysectomized rat model. *J. Hum. Hypertens. 4:* 160–162, 1990.
18. Grim, C. E., F. C. Luft, N. S. Fineberg, and M. H. Weinberger. Responses to volume expansion and contraction in categorized hypertensive and normotensive man. *Hypertension 1:* 476–485, 1979.
19. Grim, C. E., and T. W. Wilson. Salt, slavery and survival: physiological principles underlying the evolutionary hypothesis of salt sensitivity hypertension in Western Hemisphere blacks. In: *Pathophysiology of Hypertension in Blacks,* edited by J. C. S. Fray and J. G. Douglas. Oxford University Press, New York, 1992.
20. Holland, O. B., C. Gomez-Sanchez, C. Fairchild, and N. M. Kaplan. Role of renin classification for diuretic treatment of black hypertensive patients. *Arch. Intern. Med. 139:* 1365–1370, 1979.
21. Jose, A., J. R. Crout, and N. M. Kaplan. Suppressed plasma renin activity in essential hypertension. Roles of plasma volume, blood pressure, and sympathetic nervous system. *Ann. Intern. Med. 72:* 9–16, 1970.
22. Laragh, J. H. Vasoconstriction-volume analysis for understanding and treating hypertension: the use of renin and aldosterone profiles. *Am. J. Med. 55:* 261–274, 1973.
23. Laragh, J. H. Renovascular hypertension: a paradigm for all hypertension. *J. Hypertens. 4* (Suppl. 4): S79–S88, 1986.
24. Levy, S. B., J. J. Lilley, R. P. Frigon, and R. A. Stone. Urinary kallikrein and plasma renin activity as determinants of renal blood flow. The influence of race and dietary sodium intake. *J. Clin. Invest. 60:* 129–138, 1977.
25. Luft, F. C., C. E. Grim, J. T. Higgins, and M. H. Weinberger. Differences in response to sodium administration in normotensive white and black subjects. *J. Lab. Clin. Med.* 90:555–562, 1977.
26. Myers, H. F., and F. H. McClure. Psychosocial factors in hypertension in blacks: the case for an interactional perspective. In: *Pathophysiology of Hypertension in Blacks,* edited by J. C. S. Fray and J. G. Douglas. Oxford University Press, New York, 1992.
27. Mitas, J. A., R. Holle, S. B. Levy, and R. A. Stone. Racial analysis of the volume-renin relationship in human hypertension. *Arch. Intern. Med. 139:* 157–160, 1979.
28. Mufunda, J., and H. V. Sparks, Jr. Salt sensitivity and hypertension in African blacks. In: *Pathophysiology of Hypertension in Blacks,* edited by J. C. S. Fray and J. G. Douglas. Oxford University Press, New York, 1992.
29. Page, I. H. Neural and humoral control of blood vessels. In: *Hypertension,* edited by G. E. W. Wolstenholme and M. P. Cameron. Little, Brown, Boston, 1954, pp. 3–25.
30. Park, C. S., P. S. Doh, R. E. Carraway, G. C. Chung, J. C. S. Fray, and T. B. Miller. Stimulation of renin secretion by ethacrynic acid is independent of $Na^+-K^+-2Cl^-$ cotransport. *Am. J. Physiol. 259: (Renal Fluid Electrolyte Physiol. 28)* F539–F544, 1990.
31. Saunders, E. Hypertension in blacks. *Med. Clin. North Am. 71:* 1013–1029, 1987.
32. Sealey, J. E., and J. H. Laragh. Searching out low renin patients: limitations of some commonly used methods. *Am. J. Med. 55:* 303–313, 1973.
33. Sigmon, D. H., and J. C. S. Fray. Chemiosmotic control of renin release from isolated renin granules of rat kidneys. *J. Physiol. (Lond.) 436:* 237–256, 1991.
34. Sowers, J. R., P. C. Zemel, and M. B. Zemel. Role of nutrition in black hypertensives: calcium and other dietary factors. In: *Pathophysiology of Hypertension in Blacks,* edited by J. C. S. Fray and J. G. Douglas. Oxford University Press, New York, 1992.
35. Thurston, H. J., and J. D. Swales. Low renin hypertension: a distinct entity. *Lancet 2:* 930–932, 1976.
36. Tobian, L. Interrelationship of electrolytes, juxtaglomerular cells and hypertension. *Physiol. Rev. 40:* 280–312, 1960.
37. Vander, A. J. Control of renin release. *Physiol. Rev. 47:* 359–382, 1967.
38. Wisenbaugh, P. E., J. B. Garst, C. Hull, R. J. Freedman, D. N. Matthews, and M. Hadady. Renin, aldosterone, sodium and hypertension. *Am. J. Med. 52:* 175–186, 1972.
39. Wright, J. T., Jr., and J. G. Douglas. Drug therapy in black hypertensives. In: *Pathophysiology of Hypertension in Blacks,* edited by J. C. S. Fray and J. G. Douglas. Oxford University Press, New York, 1992.

II

THE MIDDLE PASSAGE . . . THE EARLY YEARS: GENETIC SHIFTING GROUND

2

Salt, Slavery, and Survival: Physiological Principles Underlying the Evolutionary Hypothesis of Salt-Sensitive Hypertension in Western Hemisphere Blacks

CLARENCE E. GRIM AND THOMAS W. WILSON

The purpose of this chapter is to review the physiological basis of the hypothesis that selective survival for the ability to conserve salt during the African slavery period of Western Hemisphere history resulted in a black population in the Western Hemisphere (142) that has higher blood pressure than black populations born in sub-Saharan Africa. This hypertension is characterized by a low level of activity of the renin–angiotensin–aldosterone system (RAAS) and is directly related to salt intake. This increased "sensitivity" of blood pressure to salt is also associated with an increased sensitivity to the blood pressure–lowering effects of diuretics.

This hypothesis has evolved from the known physiological characteristics of blood pressure in Western Hemisphere blacks, a consideration of the relatively low frequency of hypertension in Africa, and the suggestion that the severe mortality rates during slavery were mediated primarily by excessive sodium depletion from sweating, diarrhea, and vomiting as well as by periods when dietary salt intake was deficient (46).

THEORIES OF SALT SENSITIVITY/CONSERVATION

Compared with U.S. whites and perhaps West African blacks, salt-sensitive blood pressure occurs more frequently in U.S. blacks. This is true in normotensive U.S. blacks (90) fed increasing amounts of dietary sodium. It is also true in hypertensive U.S. blacks treated with diuretics (41). In fact, the prevalence of diuretic-sensitive (and presumably salt-sensitive) blood pressure approaches 75% in U.S. black hypertensives. In contrast, our report of the rarity of hypertension in adult black men in a rural village in Eastern Nigeria who consume as much salt as U.S. blacks suggests that salt-sensitive blood pressure prevalence may be very low in West Africa (143).

U.S. data show there is a continuous Gaussian distribution (70,132) of the "salt handling" trait, which varies from extreme salt resistance to extreme salt sensitivity. We believe this variation in salt handling may have a genetic com-

25

ponent. If Darwinian processes favored the survival of the most "salt-sensitive" of the individuals in a population, one would expect subsequent generations to show a Gaussian distribution shifted toward the salt-sensitive side of the distribution, with a significant shift of the average value and perhaps a narrowing of the width (variance) of the distribution. We have suggested that slavery selected individuals who had an enhanced ability to conserve salt and that the descendants of these individuals are at higher risk for salt-sensitive hypertension. Therefore, there may be a higher proportion of salt-sensitive individuals among Western Hemisphere blacks than among West African blacks.

In our recent review of the literature on the evolution of the salt conservation hypothesis, the hypothesis was summarized as follows: an enhanced genetic-based ability to retain or conserve salt would increase in populations in which reproductive success (fertility) is decreased by high mortality from sodium losses in sweat, stool, or vomit. When such "conservers" are exposed to a high salt intake they may be more likely to have a salt-sensitive increase in blood pressure (144).

It has been speculated that from an evolutionary point of view the ideal salt conserver would minimize sodium losses during times of low sodium intake and would maximize sodium conservation (storing) during a salt load. That is, sodium conservers would have a decided advantage over all others under fluctuating conditions of low and high salt intake. Thus, when salt supplies were limited, a sodium conserver would minimize the time in salt deficit due to a fast-acting renal, sweat gland, gastrointestinal, or other system that evolved to conserve salt. On the other hand, when salt was available in excess, the conserver would retain or even store salt for future protection against salt losses in sweat, stools, or vomit. Thus, in both cases, the sodium conserver should have a considerable survival advantage over others, minimizing a possible sodium deficit in the former case and maximizing a sodium excess in the latter (138).

Three major sodium-conservation mechanisms that would confer protection under severe sodium-depleting conditions that may also be related to the regulation of sodium balance and blood pressure. The first is anatomical differences. It is possible that inherent anatomical differences in the number or function of the sweat glands or renal glomeruli or tubules or in the gastrointestinal tract or in differences in the sympathetic nervous system (SNS) input to these organs or in the RAAS would have allowed better survival under adverse conditions of sodium-depleting stress.

The second is sodium-conserving mechanisms that minimize sodium deficits. "Conserving" mechanisms are those that enable humans to decrease sodium losses in the urine, sweat, or gastrointestinal tract rapidly in an attempt to compensate for losses from any part of the body (32). The most rapid system that would conserve sodium loss is the SNS. The SNS would act by reducing blood flow to the kidneys, the sweat glands, and the gastrointestinal tract. This reduction would be quickly followed by activation of the slower but more effective RAAS, which, by its humoral nature, induces sodium conservation in the urine, sweat, and stool. Renin release is stimulated by sodium and volume depletion (see Chapter 10, this volume). The generated angiotensin II leads to vasoconstriction and decreased flow to sweat glands, the kidney, and the gut.

Angiotensin II also is antinatriuretic in the renal tubule. Over hours to days, angiotensin II stimulates the adrenal to secrete aldosterone. Aldosterone plays a key role in increasing sodium reabsorption from the sweat duct, the distal renal tubule, and from the gastrointestinal tract.

Finally, angiotensin II stimulates thirst and sodium appetite, driving the organism to seek water and salt. Obviously individuals who were very effective at conserving sodium by these mechanisms would be expected to be more likely to survive during periods of severe sodium and water deprivation or losses. While we hypothesize a strong positive correlation between salt conservation and salt sensitivity, the exact relationship between the two remains unclear. It is clear, however, that salt sensitivity in humans (and rats) is an inherited trait and that the trait appears to be more common in black Americans than other ethnic groups. The exact mechanism(s) that result in salt-induced hypertension, however, in either blacks or whites (or rats), is not clear. Current evidence suggests that excess body sodium results in increased peripheral vascular resistance. Guyton (54) has emphasized the overriding dominance of the kidney in salt sensitivity and the "autoregulatory" vasoconstrictive phenomena in the peripheral vascular beds when sodium intake exceeds excretion. deWardner (33) has suggested that increased body sodium stimulates a humoral substance that inhibits sodium, potassium-ATPase, and is natriuretic. It may also increase peripheral vascular resistance by increasing vascular smooth muscle cell calcium as suggested by Blaustein (16). A third sodium-conserving mechanism is "storing" or maximizing a sodium excess. Luft et al. (93) demonstrated that with rapid increases in dietary sodium a positive sodium balance occurs in normal men, which far exceeds the weight gain during the sodium loading. Thus some normal men can, at least acutely, accumulate over 1,000 mM of sodium in a site that does not lead to accompanying water retention and weight gain. The "storing" mechanisms to be considered are those that would enable the organism to store sodium during times of sodium excess. There is little known about this aspect of sodium metabolism and its role in survival. In general, it has been thought that normal individuals can "store" only about 2 liters of extracellular fluid or about 300 mM of sodium. Once this amount is reached, additional salt intake is rapidly excreted and further weight gain does not occur. However, it is also possible to store salt in the bone matrix, and it has been demonstrated that after 3 weeks of a diet containing 1 mM sodium per day a normal man gained about 2 kg of body weight when placed on a 200 mM sodium diet (67). During this weight gain, however, isotopic techniques demonstrated that the body stores of sodium had increased by over 600 mM. Some of this isotopic sodium was still present up to 2.5 years later, suggesting that once laid down in bone, sodium may be very slowly mobilizable. In the standard 70 kg man in balance on a low sodium intake of 1 mM sodium per day, increasing dietary sodium intake to 200 mM/day will result over the next few days in the "storage" of about 240 mM (about 1.5 liters of isotonic fluid) mostly in the extracellular fluid, and about 500 mM of sodium in bone (10,67). In general, it is thought that 46% of total body sodium is found in the bone (111). This amounts to about 2,665 mM. About 45% of this bone sodium (1,200 mM) is rapidly exchangeable. Thus, it appears that bone plays a role in "storing sodium." The mechanisms modulating the storage of sodium in bone in humans are poorly understood but are likely to involve RAAS and plasma pH. It is interesting to note that bone mass tends to be higher in black Americans than whites (11). Unfortunately, possible intraracial differences among blacks have not been examined.

DARWINIAN EVOLUTION: THE ROLE OF SALT

Human physiological control systems are the product of millions of years of adaptation to a hostile physical environment with constant threats of hyperthermia, dehydration, starvation, and sodium depletion. When humans are hot they seek shade; when thirsty, water; when hungry, food; and when sodium depleted, salt. Failure to perceive, avoid, or correct these life-threatening environmental stresses results in death within minutes, hours, days, or weeks. The ability to manipulate the environment to satisfy these physiological warnings has enabled humans to spread more widely over the face of the earth than any other mammal. Physiological, epidemiological, and evolutionary theories are based on the premise that death is rarely, if ever, a random event. When death occurs in a nonrandom fashion it follows that those who survive are more "physiologically fit" for the environment. If this fitness is mediated by inherited factors, Darwinian evolution results.

Neel has coined the term "thrifty" (109) for those genetic traits that have enabled survival during famine and has suggested that some of these genetic traits selected by this survival of the fittest now express themselves in individuals and in whole populations in today's biosocial and nutritional milieu as modern "diseases" such as obesity and diabetes. It is possible that this evolution has produced a variability of salt conservation in the human species and that population differences in this distribution exist today. Thus, it is possible that other "thrifty" genes are related to ability to conserve sodium, though scientific evidence to support this view is lacking.

Denton (32) has suggested that hunger for salt has been a driving force for human evolution and that this drive is linked to the physiological sodium-conserving systems (such as RAAS). He has emphasized that the quest for salt is an innate primal drive activated by inadequate intake of salt or excessive losses of sodium chloride. Other investigators considered the "taste" for salt a luxury and considered "salt to be man's first great addiction of the world" (84).

A review of the literature of salt supplies in pre-twentieth century West Africa (136) suggests that despite well-developed salt trade routes, an average of about 1 g of sodium-based salts per day was available to the inhabitants of West Africa. Significantly, however, this small amount was not distributed evenly to all areas. In the vast interior, sodium salt was very difficult to obtain because of "low salt production, distance from the salt sources, high prices for the mineral, and the use of salt as currency." Unless they lived near a source of sodium salt then, most West Africans consumed very little of the mineral, prompting the conclusion that many tribes simply experienced a permanent "shortage of [sodium] salt" (129). In fact, most West Africans who desired salt-type seasoning had to depend on "salts" produced from the burning of vegetable matter, which was not only the most common type of "salt" available but was also "preferred" by many of the inhabitants (22,114). These vegetable salts were predominantly composed of potassium (of varying quantities), not sodium (129). Although no precise values are available for production, the amount of these potassium salts must have been considerable (45,57,88,102,105,129).

European travelers to West Africa noted the lack of sodium salts in the interior. Their accounts of the salt-deprived areas prompted other Europeans to export substantial amounts of salt to West Africa for trading purposes in the nineteenth century (110). In the late eighteenth century, for example, the Scottish explorer Mungo Park observed the willingness of West Africans to sell human beings to procure salt:

> In the districts of the interior, salt is the greatest of delicacies. It strikes a European very strangely to observe a child sucking a piece of rock salt as if it were sugar. I have frequently seen this done, although the poorer class of inhabitants in the interior are so badly provided with this costly article, that to say that a man eats salt with his meal is equivalent to saying that he is rich. I myself have found the scarcity of this natural product very trying. Constant vegetable food causes a painful longing for salt that is quite indescribable. On the coast of Sierra Leone the desire for salt was so keen among negroes that they gave away wives, children, and everything that was dear to them in return for it (22).

Similarly, as late as 1856, the European traveler Baikie noted on a journey into the Niger delta that "slaves are always purchased with salt, the price of a stout male is from ten to twelve bags of salt ... these are brought up from Nimbe [Nembe] and Bini [Benin river]" (4). In another instance, a traveler to West Africa in 1882 reported that he was offered a young girl for four loaves of salt (17). The lack of salt in West Africa, then, directly influenced the slave trade, as those individuals forced into slavery were frequently bought with the "all important salt" (30). The old Moorish proverb, "The price of a Negro is salt" (20) seems to have been a tragically accurate statement in sub-Saharan Africa.

Helmer was also the first to suggest that selective survival for the ability to conserve sodium in a hot, humid, tropical environment was related to the present-day high prevalence of low renin and high blood pressure in black Americans (60,61). Later, Gleibermann argued that low salt availability in the African past was related to the high blood pressure in U.S. blacks today (44). Denton's view (32) was that Western Hemisphere blacks were descended from "progenitors ... representing twenty to forty thousand or more generations of existence in tropical to subtropical conditions largely in the interior of the continents, and with considerable stress on sodium homeostasis. Greater hedonic liking for salt and less capacity to excrete it could result." After reviewing the history of West African salt availability, Wilson (135–137) suggested that local variations in supplies of salt within ancient West Africa may be important in understanding the striking geographical variability of blood pressure levels within West Africa today. Noting the higher blood pressures among U.S. blacks when compared with West African blacks, Wilson also speculated that the ancestors of U.S. blacks may have migrated from the very low salt areas within West Africa. In general, a common thread running through the work of these authors (and others) (53,85,121,134) relates to physical evolution caused by adaptation to heat and salt supplies within Africa.

Interested in the blood pressure differences between U.S. blacks and African blacks, Waldron et al. (131) in 1982 suggested that the legacy of slavery in the cultural history of U.S. blacks may be partially responsible for their high blood pressure. In 1983 Blackburn and Prineas (13) suggested that the Atlantic passage during the slavery period was characterized by conditions that may be related to a genetic-based salt-sensitive hypertension. In 1988 Grim (46) expanded the thinking on the evolution of salt conservation and salt-sensitive blood pressure in Western Hemisphere blacks by hypothesizing that the *conditions of slavery* (not just the Atlantic passage) favored those with an enhanced ability to conserve salt. He also introduced the selective potential of salt-depletive diseases like diarrheas and fevers besides the influence of excessive sweating from heat and work and low salt supplies. Grim asserted that the descendants of slaves would have a higher prevalence of salt-sensitive blood pressure than the current population of blacks in Africa, and that inheritance played a very important role in these differences (46). Thus, while Helmer, Denton, Gleibermann, Wilson, and others suggested long-term adaptation/evolution of a population adept at conserving salt, Grim suggested an accelerated evolution of salt sensitivity only during the past 450 years. The rapidity of human evolution of other physiological control systems is evident in the development of lactose tolerance in areas that have a long history of dairy cattle domestication (81). The decreasing prevalence of the sickle cell trait in nonmalarial areas of the New World is an example of rapid "relaxed natural selection" (18).

Rapid evolution of salt sensitivity is strongly supported by the observations of Dahl and Shackow (28). They showed that artificial selection of rats could, in three generations, produce one strain with extreme salt sensitivity and another with extreme salt resistance. Dahl and colleagues had noted that an unselected population of Sprague-Dawley rats demonstrated striking variation in the effect of a high salt intake on blood pressure. To test if this was related to genetic factors, the group examined the effect of selective breeding on the blood pressure response to salt. First, the blood pressure response to high dietary salt intake was determined in an unselected group of rats. Matings were produced between a pair with the lowest change in blood pressure with salt loading, the ancestors of the salt-resistant (SR) strain, and another pair with the greatest increase in blood pressure, the ancestors of the salt-sensitive (SS) strain. The first generation of these selective matings demonstrated a significant difference in the blood pressure–raising effects of high salt intake. This process was continued for two more generations, at which time there was no overlap between SS and SR responses to the blood pressure–raising effects of high dietary salt. Importantly, renin levels were significantly lower in the salt-sensitive rats and they died rapidly with severe hypertension on a high salt diet. Studies by Rapp et al. (117) have demonstrated that the salt sensitivity is related to alterations in the renin genotype. The genotype that is associated with low levels of renin is the one associated with salt sensitivity (117). It is important to consider that African Americans have a high prevalence of both low-renin hypertension and salt sensitivity. We suggest that rapid evolution of these traits likely occurred during the slavery period of modern history and will examine the historical and physiological evidence for this argument.

Although slavery existed for centuries within Africa, the expansive transatlantic slave trade began in the early sixteenth century (87) to supply human labor to the mines and plantation economies in the Western Hemisphere. This period of history came to a close in 1888 when slavery was finally abolished in Brazil. The slavery period included both the transatlantic trade in African captives and the institution of slavery in Western Hemisphere economies.

Documents from this time are extant, and the nature of the slave trade and plantation economies resulted in surviving records that are often quantitative. The records that historians have analyzed range from naval surgeons' logs, ships' store records, records from the shipping and receiving ports, sale records, and slave population records in various areas in the Western Hemisphere. Using these extensive records, twentieth century historians have estimated the number of Africans involved in the slave trade (6,27,65). It is estimated that more than 12 million young men and women were imported (31) to North America (especially the West Indies and the United States) or to South America (especially Brazil). Most were imported from either West Africa (from present-day Nigeria to Senegal) or Central Africa (Angola) (27). It has been calculated that the British, French, Dutch, and Danish trade to the Caribbean islands comprised about 39% of the imported Africans. The Brazilian trade comprised about 38%. Sixteen percent were transported into Spanish America and 4% were imported into British North America and the United States (the remaining 2% were imported into the Old World) (27).

In a previous paper (139) we estimated that only 40%–50% of slaves captured in Africa lived for more than 4 years from the point of capture. We may have underestimated. In his 1988 comprehensive study of the Brazilian trade, Miller (104) estimated that fewer than 30 individuals out of 100 captured in Africa survived for more than four years. At each stage of the trade, Miller estimated the proportion who survived. He estimated that 90% survived capture; of those who survived capture 75% lived through the march to the coast; of those who made it to the coast about 87.5% survived being held on the coast for sale; of those loaded on the ships about 90% survived the voyage across the Atlantic (middle passage); 93% of those who arrived in the New World were still alive after holding for quarantine; of those who survived quarantine the probability of surviving the transportation to the final work site was 87.5%. This represents the end of the first year. Of those who arrived at the work site 80% survived the first year of "seasoning," the slave owners' term for the period of adaptation to the plantation economies, 87.5% survived the second year of seasoning, and 91% survived the third year. Because all of these survival probabilities are conditional on each other, to derive a 4 year survival probability we multiply them together. This calculates to a 28% survival probability over a 4 year period (Fig. 2.1). That is, of 100 Africans who were captured in Africa with the intention to be brought to Brazil, only 28 survived beyond 4 years. The survival probabilities presented for the Brazilian trade here may be different from the English, French, or U.S. trade but give an indication of survivability.

Miller and other quantitative historians believe that mortality remained excessive during the postseasoning period as well (72,76). And while mortality rates were extraordinarily high, reproduction success rates were low. Infant mortality rates approached 500 per 1,000 and were partially responsible for

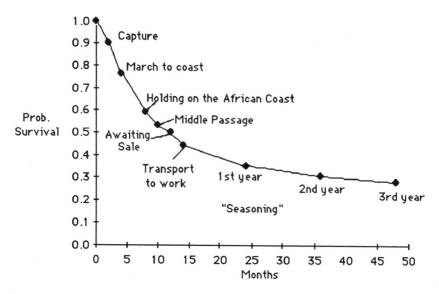

FIGURE 2.1. Four-year survival of sub-Sahara Africans in the transatlantic slave trade: 16th–19th c. Based on Miller (103).

the lack of "natural increase" (i.e., births exceeding deaths) of most populations in the Western Hemisphere (62,126). These high infant and adult death rates and a low fertility rate made it necessary to continue the transatlantic slave trade in most slave societies.

This tragedy was repeated year after year, century after century, and, as we surmise, if a genetic condition was involved and if these deaths did not occur randomly, natural selection was inevitable. Such a "selection" should have a profound effect on the genotypes of future generations of Western Hemisphere blacks. With the abolition of the slave trade, the genetic pool of the survivors was virtually isolated from the original gene pool from which the selection occurred. Thus the concept that it takes an extended period of time for "natural" evolutionary change to occur was likely usurped by the "unnatural" conditions produced by slavery.

MAJOR CAUSES OF DEATH DURING SLAVERY

Slavery has been a major area of interest to quantitative historians (37,38, 42,78,103,104,115,122,127) and a primary interest of biohistorians. The majority of the over 170 sources Kiple cited in his 1986 survey of the literature written on the biological past of blacks were concerned with the slavery era (74). The causes of death during the transatlantic slave trade and of slaves on the plantations reveal that mortality was often due to conditions that ultimately kill by salt and water depletion: sweating, vomiting, and diarrhea. Chroniclers of slave expeditions speak of the effects of heat and excessive sweating on forced marches from inland Africa to the coast, in the confined, unventilated barracoons along the coast, and in the ship holds of the middle passage (23,96). On the slave ships, vomiting due to seasickness was common (39), and the most common causes of death on the middle passage were recorded as diarrheal (the "flux") and febrile diseases, both salt depletors (127). On the plantations, excessive salt losses continued: sweating from hard work in the fields induced a constant salt drain, and a major cause of death in the plantation societies continued to be diarrheal disorders in adults as well as infants (80,120). In the nineteenth century, cholera, a new form of diarrhea, attacked the populations in the Western Hemisphere, and several cholera pandemics swept through the Americas and the Caribbean and killed thousands of blacks (73). Thus, salt-depleting conditions and diseases seemed ubiquitous throughout the slavery period (62,76), favoring those individuals most capable of salt conservation. This continued selection for the salt conservation trait would further enrich the frequency of the trait in the second, third, and subsequent generations of African-Americans than among the first generation of captives.

Over time, some slave societies began going through a kind of epidemiological transition. For example, by 1850 in the United States, respiratory diseases had become the major cause of death of adult slaves but diarrheal diseases were still fourth. Among infants, however, diarrhea remained the leading killer (120). Slave societies differed in their disease and dietary experience, and this variability may be partially responsible for variability in diseases today.

Before reviewing the physiology of sodium-depleting conditions common during slavery, it should be recalled that insufficient water intake and low caloric intake, in addition to inadequate sodium intake, can cause sodium depletion. Inadequate water intake will cause "dehydration natriuresis" (101), and inadequate caloric intake will result in "fasting natriuresis"(128). Inadequate intake of sodium, water, or calories for a period of as short as 8 hours (for water) or 24 hours (for calories) will result in a negative sodium balance (101). Once a negative balance has occurred it can only be restored by dietary sources that exceed these losses.

Overheating and Sweating

> *"An intensely hot and vitiated atmosphere . . . with the thermometer probably ranging between 90° F and 100° F" (124).*

This was reported by an observer below deck in a slave ship in the late 1840s. The ship had its port hold closed as it was attempting to escape from a British antislaver.

The average man produces about 100 kg-cal/h or 2,400 kg-cal of heat each day. To put 2,400 kg-cal into perspective, if this energy were transformed to a cooking stove, enough heat would be generated to bring to a boil 15 liters of water, a normal man's total extracellular fluid volume. This heat must be dissipated by physiological systems. Once the environmental heat equals body heat, 37° C, humans must sweat to cool down. At 100% humidity, the evaporation of sweat cannot occur and the internal temperature of a 70 kg man (42 liters of water) will increase about 2.4° C/h, ending in fatal hyperthermia in 2–4 h.

Besides sweating from heat, sweating may also have been a consequence of the numerous conditions categorized as "fevers." Infectious fevers can also induce salt and water depletion by the induced sweating. As salt and water depletion can increase the risk of heat stroke, which in itself may be associated with diarrhea, it seems likely that heat illness may have been confused with infectious causes of fever.

Survival in the heat requires water, salt, and the ability to sweat under conditions in which the sweat can evaporate and cool the body. The efficacy of man's ability to cool by sweating was first demonstrated in a controlled experiment by Blagden in 1775 (14,15). He reported studies on himself and friends in rooms heated to 126° C for up to three-quarters of an hour. A steak he laid on a platter in the room was thoroughly cooked, but men and a dog survived, although the severe sweating that occurred left them somewhat "giddy." A more recent example of the acute effects of environmental heat on man has been reported by Kuno et al. (82), who studied four young Japanese men under the most severe conditions ever reported (wet bulb temperature of 38°–48° C).

> Sweating was produced immediately after entering the hot chamber. Its amount was moderate during the first five minutes: in the following fifteen minutes it increased enormously so that the sweat secretion seemed to approach its maximum during this period, and later it increased only gradually. Such a copious sweating could last for a considerable period of time, while the subject showed the severe symptoms mentioned above. Just before or at the advent of the stuporous condition, the sweating began to decrease considerably . . . at the time of the suppression, the condition of the subjects became so serious as to compel us to discontinue the experiments.

Thus, rapid increases in temperature, especially below deck during the middle passage, could have rapidly killed those less able to cool effectively. Heat in the confined, unventilated slave ship was comparable to that described above except that the captives were not involved in a voluntary experiment and the heating episode was not time restricted.

The volume of sweat lost in hot conditions can be up to 4 liters/h, which is equivalent to the water contained in the blood volume. Yet with access to water, men can sustain a sweat rate of 3 liters/h for 4 h (36) and or up to 1.5 liters/h for 12 h. Even with a high water intake, this sweating cannot be sustained without the intake of sodium. Ladell (83) reported that men working in a hot environment lost 25 g of sodium chloride in only 162 min. Inadequate replacement of salt and water was manifested by heat cramps, which can be prevented by drinking water that has 10 g of salt per gallon of water. Under hot conditions man does not drink fast enough to replace the losses. As water deficit increases so does body temperature (3); physically fit men hiking at 3–4 mph in an average temperature of 90° F in the desert could not walk longer than 7 h without water. Aside from thirst, the symptoms of dehydration experienced by these men were in large part an indication of impending collapse. Once dehydrated, man does not recover much of his ability to work by resting or by cooling off in a temperate atmosphere. Dehydration thus appears to play a dominant role, and this special category of physical failure has been termed "dehydration exhaustion." When men who had been severely dehydrated were given all the water they wanted to drink, some drank as much as 2 liters in less than 10 min. If rehydration was continued for half an hour, 50%–80% of the incurred deficit was replaced, but they never replaced their entire deficit until they had a meal. Men did not willingly undertake to dehydrate themselves the next day. Only 5% dehydration is required to bring on the first symptoms (3.5 liters in a healthy man). This is distinct from heat exhaustion or heat stroke. Severe dehydration occurs at 10% of body weight (7 liters in a 70 kg man), and man becomes so confused that he will usually not survive unless given intravenous replacement. As dehydration progresses, body temperature rises, at first slowly but then explosively as the ability to dissipate heat declines during volume contraction, and death ensues rapidly when temperature exceeds 41° or 42° C. In the desert without water, 50% of men die in 36 h, 75% by 48 h, and most are dead by 3 days, although an extreme case of survival after 7 days was reported in 1905 by McGee (100) who provided a remarkable description of recovery from extreme dehydration and has provided the best description of death in the desert due to dehydration. On the ocean the temperature is usually more moderate, but humidity approaches 100% at sea level. Studies in Florida on a life raft at 85° F (21) and 75% humidity demonstrated that the sweat loss was 250 ml/h without shade. At 80° F a 10% water deficit (and fatal heat stroke) occurs at about 4 days, assuming that the subject was shaded. These conditions were likely present on many slave ships as well in Western Hemisphere slave populations (4).

The physiological ability to survive when the environmental temperature increases for several days is due to the process called heat adaptation or acclimatization. This physiology is intimately tied to salt and water conservation driven by RAAS. When one is first exposed to heat, vasodilation and the sweat-induced volume depletion activate RAAS, which promotes sodium retention by the acute antinatriuretic effect of angiotensin and by the angiotensin-induced aldosterone secretion from the adrenal. Aldosterone is the major sodium-retaining steroid acting on the colon, the renal tubule, and the sweat gland. In the sweat gland epithelial cells, for example, aldosterone stimulates sodium reabsorption, and sweat sodium concentration falls to as low as 1.7 mM sodium/liter (26). Even when one is heat adapted, sodium excreted through the sweat increases dramatically as the ambient temperature rises or the work load increases. Owing to the high sweat rates, the progress of fluid through the sweat gland is so rapid that there is little time for the sodium to be reabsorbed by the epithelial cells. Regardless of degree of acclimatization, lengthy episodes of this heat dissipation by sweating could be fatal if sodium losses are not replenished. Obviously, an individual with high body sodium stores would have a greater degree of protection against fatal sodium loss through excessive sweating.

We are unaware of studies describing ethnic variation in body sodium stores, except variations in the "sweat system" studied in Israel. Samueloff (119) demonstrated ethnic variations in sweat gland density in the children of parents from two widely diverse Jewish immigrant populations to Israel: Ashkenazi from Europe and Cochin from the Malabar coast of India. The children lived in the same hot, dry area and attended the same school in Israel. The sweating pattern induced by body warming was quite different. The children of European origin produced pulsatile sweating that appeared in large drops that would run down the body. In the Indian children the sweat appeared in miniscule droplets that spread to a fine, even film. The advantages of evaporative cooling of the latter are obvious, and this advantage would be amplified by the darker skin of the Indians heating up faster in the sun to increase evaporation. In studies comparing Bedouins with the Ashkenazi, it was found that although Bedouins had a greater forearm blood flow [an important heat radiation area of the body (133)], the sweating produced by pilocarpine was reduced. In black Africans (97–99) it appears that differences exist in the response to the amount of sweat produced after pilocarpine. However, studies comparing blacks with whites in Africa have not revealed systematic differences once adaptation to working in the heat has occurred. Samueloff (119) concluded that the maximum capacity of the sweat gland activity is genetically determined, and it is less pronounced in natives of hot areas.

Kuno (82) and others have presented evidence that even within the same ethnic group there can be striking anatomical variations in the amount and pattern of sweating. For example, only 16% of Japanese men sweat uniformly over the entire body, 30% sweat everywhere but on the upper extremities, and 40% sweat only on the upper trunk. He also reported striking individual variations in how individuals drink to replace lost sweat while walking and this tendency was stable in an individual, which suggested it was genetic in origin. There is abundant evidence that the sweat control systems are influenced by inherited factors, and twin studies have revealed that both the sweating rate and the pulse rate response to increasing environmental temperature are under significant genetic control (24).

Diarrhea

> "The great mortality appears to arise from a very intractable and offensive form of dysentery" (125).

Basal fecal excretion of sodium is very low (2.5–5.0 mM/day) (40), and modulates down further with decreasing sodium intake, owing to the aldosterone effect on sodium transport in the gastrointestinal tract (86). With diarrhea, however, fecal sodium excretion increases rapidly. Cholera produces the most severe sodium losses, averaging 133 mM sodium/liter in stools, and fatal sodium depletion can occur within a few hours (40). Even noncholera diarrheal stools contain about 97 mM sodium/liter (116). Denton (32) emphasized that with infectious diseases involving electrolyte loss, like diarrhea, "the initial defence for survival must be the regulation of salt and water balance because one needs to withstand the volume depleting impact of the disease for a few days until immunological mechanisms become effective" (32). The rapidity with which diarrhea can kill is best described in Osler's classic description of cholera (112). This nineteenth century description makes it clear that cholera kills by depleting salt and that it can be treated by replenishing with salt and water. Osler notes that there is a great variation in the severity of the diarrhea between individuals; we believe some of this variation is due to genetic factors (although we are not aware of any studies done in this area). The efficacy of "saline solution" is demonstrated in numerous controlled trials in the third world which demonstrated that death in infants and adults can be virtually eliminated by prompt oral administration of a simple sugar and salt solution made by adding to a liter of water 40 grams of sucrose, 3.5 grams of sodium chloride, 2.5 grams of sodium bicarbonate and 1.5 grams of potassium chloride (9). This is given to replace the water volume lost in the stool. Death is rare as long as adequate electrolytes and water are provided.

Vomiting

"(slaves) are far more violently affected by seasickness than the Europeans" (39).

It is estimated that during the first days of any sea voyage more than a quarter of all unaccustomed passengers suffer from seasickness (106), and most captives were unaccustomed to ocean travel. Although ingested sodium is rapidly absorbed in the stomach and upper small bowel, gastric secretions in vomit contain an average of 60 mM Na^+/liter (5). Therefore, acute vomiting can result in severe Na^+ losses. During seasickness it is difficult to replace these losses by the oral route because of the nausea itself. Those who are better able to absorb sodium might tend to have a lower concentration in the gastric juice and vomitus. Thus, a rapid absorber (conserver) would be more likely to be able to store sodium for future needs. We are not aware of studies of ethnic variation in sodium absorption or secretion in the upper gastrointestinal system.

Water Depletion

". . . nobody suffered more intensely from thirst than the poor little slaves, who were crying for water. Exhausted by their sufferings and their lamentations, these unhappy creatures fell on the ground, and seemed to have no power to rise" (23).

Death from water depletion is a result of intracellular dehydration (145) and fatal hyperthermia (fever) (35). In the absence of water humans can survive for 1–5 days depending on the environmental temperature. For detailed descriptions of the clinical manifestations of death from dehydration in man McGee (100) has provided a description of the behavioral and psychological consequences of thirst in man. Studies by McKinley et al. (101) in rats, rabbits, and sheep demonstrated that after 8 h of no access to water a negative sodium balance is evident. In sheep this amounted to 100 mM after 24 h. They suggested that this natriuresis protects against hyperosmolarity that develops due to dehydration. Similar studies have not been done in humans. The dynamic role of ADH and ANF in the response to water depletion and repletion has been studied in rats (68). Dehydration for 72 h produced increases in ADH and decreases in ANF. These changes are almost completely reversed after only 3 min of drinking. As dehydration progresses the renal excretion of sodium increases. We are not aware of ethnic studies comparing water metabolism, but twin studies in whites have shown that the set point for the osmotic release of ADH may be under genetic control (146).

STRATEGIES THAT MAY HAVE LOWERED DEATH RATES FROM SALT DEPLETION

Cooling below Decks

> "That in the year 1753, Ventilators were put into the Vessels in the Slave-
> trade . . . the happy Effect of which was, that instead of the loss of one-
> fourth of those valuable Cargoes in long passages from Africa to the French
> plantations, the loss seldom exceeded a twentieth (55).

> (The ventilators) kept the inside of the ship cool, sweet, dry, and healthy . . .
> (and that) . . . the 340 Negroes were very sensible of the benefits of a con-
> stant ventilation, and were always displeased when it was omitted" (55).

Efforts to keep the captives cool included using sails to direct the air into the
hold and keeping all possible ventilation sources open. However, the most dramatic effects were produced by human-powered "ventilators" invented by
Hales. He believed that "noxious putrid Air" accumulated in ships, mines, and
other confined areas and caused death, and that pumping these places out
would prevent deaths. It is more likely that the cooling effects of Hales's device
would have decreased sweat-induced sodium depletion and thus protected the
captives against heat stroke. Because fever and diarrhea are symptoms of the
condition (79), it seems possible that this cause of death was confused with
infectious febrile illnesses.

Increasing Salt Intake

> "for one-hundred Negroes . . . [load] . . . 4 bushels of salt" (1).

> "I am very sensible, that it's impossible to maintain the Slaves on Board,
> after one quits the Coast, without salt Provision, but then Care might be
> taken to water the Beef and Pork" (8).

To decrease mortality from salt depletion, slave traders could have provided
captives an abundant supply of dietary sodium. Wilson's (138) examination of
over 145 slave ship invoices from Royal African Company between 1682 and
1704 determined that an average of 3.6 bushels of salt were loaded in England
for every 100 captives loaded in Africa. Although there was a very wide range
of the amount of salt per ship, there was about 20 g of salt (340 mM sodium)
per slave per day on a 2-month-long voyage. The fact that this amount of sodium was loaded per slave suggests that it was perceived as an extremely important provision. Of course, salt may not have always been loaded onto the
slave ships, or it may have been sold in Africa, or it may have spoiled on the
journey. This would explain remarks by contemporaries that the captives received only "a little salt sometimes (34)." If raw salt was not available on the
ships, salted fish or beef or pork may have provided captives with the important mineral.

Salt and salted meat were central items in the "hog and hominy" U.S.
slave diet. In his book on antebellum Southern food, the historian Hilliard
remarks that "salt was the only seasoning the slave saw regularly, other con-
diments were unknown," and that slaves received between 2 and 5 pounds of
salt pork per week (63). Similarly, the nutritionist Syckle remarked in her

study of American dietary habits in the nineteenth century that "[a] weekly allowance for each slave of three pounds of pork, a peck of corn, a pint of salt, and molasses became standard for thousands of plantations" (130). In the West Indies salt was an important staple in the diet of displaced West Africans as well. Slaves reportedly received between a quarter and a half pint of salt per week and a weekly allotment of 1 to 4 pounds of salted fish and "eight or nine herrings" (25,56,62). However, salt supplies were not constant. During some periods, the American Revolution, for example, salt was available only intermittently (123).

Water Supplies

> "The . . . company instructed its agents at Benguela to provide double the legally required supply of water, and the reform . . . of 1813 finally brought the required water ration back to a full (2.7 liters) per day, with at least half reserved for drinking and the remainder presumably allotted to cooking purposes" (104).

Adequate water supplies are needed in a hot environment, for without water fatal sodium and water depletion occurs because of sweating. Detailed records of the food, salt, and water provided to the captives are lacking, but some writers note that the captives were fed only twice a day and were given one-half to 1 pint of water twice a day (75).

SUGGESTIONS FOR FURTHER RESEARCH

To test the hypothesis described here we need studies of the key physiological characteristics that we would expect to find in the descendants of the survivors.

Potential Study Populations

We argue that the continuously distributed salt-conservation trait that evolved in Africa was the template on which accelerated Darwinian processes during slavery selected those most adept at conserving salt. In other words, the upper tail of the Gaussian distribution survived the circumstances of slavery. Thus, individuals from that portion of the distribution provided most of the genetic material for subsequent generations. One indication of the truth of this hypothesis are studies that examine admixture between Western Hemisphere blacks and non-African ethnic groups. In one study of the relationship of admixture to blood pressure, McLean (94) presented strong evidence that the greater the dilution of the African gene pool with European genes the lower the blood pressure in African Americans. Similarly, in the Caribbean, Darlu et al. (29) reported that two methods of assessing African genetic heritage—genetic admixture and written family records—reveal a significant effect of African inheritance on blood pressure in the population. U.S. populations with little admixture (such as in the coastal areas of Georgia and South Carolina) will be interesting to compare with West Coast black populations, which have about 20% admixture with European genes (2). Finally, studies on offspring of black individuals with the slavery heritage and those without may be very informative.

Also of interest will be those populations from present-day West Africa that were the major suppliers of captives. We recently completed a study of blood pressure and 24 h urine sodium in a random sample of men in rural Imo State in Nigeria (143). This study revealed that systolic blood pressure did not increase significantly with age despite the fact that the subjects were consuming a diet that contained about 120 mM of sodium per day. This suggests a non-salt-sensitive population in this area or that there is an environmental factor that is protecting against the rise in blood pressure with age. This finding is especially interesting because this part of Africa was a major slave supply region in previous centuries.

Another special population in Africa of interest would be the Ameri-Liberians who are descendants of freed slaves from the United States who migrated to Liberia in the early part of the nineteenth century. Comparative studies in Liberia could thus compare the Ameri-Liberians with the indigenous Liberians. Also many from Sierra Leone are descendants of slaves who were rescued from illegal importers after 1808 and settled back in Africa without having ever made it to the West. Thus these Sierra Leone populations would not have suffered the multigenerational selection process experienced by Western Hemisphere blacks. In addition, recent African American migrants to Africa would be of interest.

Finally, there are many African-born individuals living in the United States today. Testing their salt sensitivity would be of interest. Of particular interest will be our observations that the "normal" nocturnal decline in blood pressure is markedly attenuated in normotensive African American adults (59) and children (58) and hypertensive American-born African Americans (108), whereas hypertensive blacks in South Africa (108), and West African–born blacks living in the United States (141), and black Barbadians living in Barbados (144) have a "normal" nocturnal decline in blood pressure.

Significantly, there has never been a report of a black population in the Western Hemisphere that does not have an increase in blood pressure with age. Thus, we urge a search for such a population, as it should hold important clues to the prevention of hypertension in blacks and other populations. Cross-sectional studies of blood pressure and sodium intake using the INTERSALT protocol (66) would be an efficient method to screen for such populations.

Factors to Look at in These Populations

The physiology of the hypothesis predicts that the survivors would be better at either (1) retaining sodium on a low sodium diet or (2) storing sodium on a high sodium diet. These measures can be obtained by means of careful metabolic analysis. The half-life for urinary sodium excretion coming into sodium balance on both the low salt and the high salt diet should be analyzed for evidence of the ability to conserve sodium rapidly on a low sodium diet and to store sodium on a high sodium diet. Intravenous sodium loading has also been used to study the time course of sodium excretion after sodium loading. It was demonstrated that the amount of sodium retained is increased in first-degree relatives of hypertensives (48), and that the rate of sodium excreted is influenced by age, by the level of activity of RAAS, by genetic factors, and by ethnic factors (50). Similar studies around the world will help to develop an understanding of the endocrinological control systems and blood pressure of black populations today.

The hypothesis predicts that survivors would get a greater increase in blood pressure with sodium loading and a greater decrease in blood pressure with low sodium diet, i.e., they would be more likely to have salt-sensitive hypertension. A number of ways have been developed to test for salt sensitivity. One general method is to place the subject on a low sodium diet for a few days, measure the blood pressure, and then increase sodium intake (70). Twenty-four-hour blood pressures (12) may be a more sensitive method to detect those whose blood pressure increases with salt loading. Those subjects who get a 10% increase in blood pressure when going from a low sodium to a high sodium diet are termed salt sensitive. These methods require a diet kitchen and hospitalization for 8 days. The Saline-Lasix protocol can also be utilized to test for sodium sensitivity (132). Those subjects who had a decrease in blood pressure of >10 mm Hg from the end of sodium loading to the end of sodium depletion were defined as salt sensitive.

The ability to regulate salt loss and perhaps storage resides in RAAS. Studies in twins have shown that this system is under strong genetic control in whites (49) and that American blacks have a lower level of activity RAAS than whites (90). Studies between black groups of differing heritage are lacking. It is also clear that because of the low level of activity in many normotensive blacks it will be necessary to utilize some method to stimulate RAAS in order to increase the range into measurable levels (see Chapter 10, this volume). It is also appropriate to examine the ability of the system to be suppressed. One standardized method is the Saline-Lasix method to diagnose low-renin and other forms of hypertension (51,95), for the investigation of RAAS and sodium metabolism in normotensives and hypertensives (91), in comparative studies of whites and blacks (89), in family members of patients with essential hypertension (48), in genetic studies of blood pressure control systems in white twins (50), in labile hypertension (92), and in defining salt sensitivity (132). This 2-day protocol involves first sodium loading with a 4h infusion of 2 liters of normal saline and then sodium depletion with 1 day of a 10 mM sodium diet combined with 40 mg of Lasix p.o. at 10 A.M., 2 P.M., and 6 P.M. Outpatient methods using intravenous Lasix (69) or oral converting enzyme inhibition (107) may also be useful.

The hypothesis predicts that Western Hemisphere blacks will have a better tolerance to heat than West African blacks. As there are virtually no studies of heat regulation in African Americans or native Africans, recent protocols that quantitate thermal regulation in the heat and examine sweating rates, sweat composition, and hormonal changes during heat acclimatization use treadmill or bicycle exercise (7,77). None of these studies mentions the ethnic group studied. Questions to be asked should include the tolerance to exercise in the heat as evidenced by sweating rates and maintenance of thermal equilibrium. The hypothesis predicts that African Americans who are salt sensitive will acclimatize to heat faster than those who are salt resistant.

The hypothesis predicts also that the survivors would be better able to tolerate water deprivation, be more effective in conserving water during water deprivation and not have as great a dehydration natriuresis. Studies by Phillips et al. (113) using a 24 h water-deprivation test followed by free access to water and then food would seem to be one effective way to test this regulatory system. Quantitation of the natriuresis during dehydration could also be done with this protocol. Another method would be the intravenous infusion of ethanol and hypertonic saline as developed by Robertson et al. (118). Studies in white twins, using Robertson's techniques, have suggested that the osmo-regulatory set point is under genetic control.

What would be the findings today in those who were able to survive de-hydration and high temperatures? Such individuals might be expected to pro-duce less sweat under hot conditions to minimize the risk of fatal dehydration or produce a sweat containing less sodium to minimize the risk of fatal salt and water depletion. This could occur by having anatomically fewer or differ-ent sweat glands to be better able to tolerate increases in body temperature.

Because of the power and economy of twin studies, and because of the greater frequency of twinning in those of African descent, we would strongly recommend that these studies be carried out in twins. For example, twin stud-ies of sweating in blacks from West African and from the Western Hemisphere residing in similar tropical environments would be an efficient method to eval-uate the possibility that these control systems were under genetic control and that selection for this critical mechanism for survival in the heat may have occurred during the slave trade. The economy of the study of twins resides in the fact that twins may be more likely to volunteer for research, even in the Third World (52), and that by studying twins one not only gets the normal data needed for the measurement of interest but also can analyze the data in iden-tical and nonidentical twins to dissect the relative contributions of genes and environment to the physiology. This approach has been used extensively by Grim et al. (49), who have demonstrated, in white twins, that RAAS, the sym-pathetic nervous system, and the ability to retain sodium with sodium loading are under strong genetic control (49). Identical twins raised apart (say one African-born twin raised in Africa and the other raised in the United States) would be ideal for this study, as recently emphasized by Bouchard et al. (19), who found that the systolic blood pressure in adult white twins was as highly correlated in twins raised apart as in twins raised together, strongly suggesting that most of the variation in blood pressure is due to inherited factors.

Historical Research

The major purpose of this chapter was to review the physiological elements in the "natural selection" of salt conservation and salt sensitivity. Thus, we have by necessity given only a brief summary of the historical portion of the hy-pothesis. We are currently collecting information on the demography and epi-demiology of the slavery era with the intention of presenting a comprehensive review of evidence relating to the salt conservation/sensitivity hypothesis from the many Western Hemisphere slavery populations that existed.

What Other Populations Today Might Manifest the Trait of Salt-Sensitive Hypertension

Although we are focusing here on the salt-conserving trait in those of West African descent, it seems likely that this trait may occur as an evolutionary adaptation to salt-depleting "bad times" in the biohistory of any population. Furthermore, populations surviving high mortality based on salt depletive conditions or low salt intake would be expected to have a greater prevalence of salt-sensitive hypertension today. Studies in such unique populations would be of interest. Thus the history of the resettlement of English convicts to Australia on prison ships (some of which were run by previous slaving contractors) reveals that as many as 26% died on this journey and that the conditions on board ship were as severe as on the slave ships (64). Asian Indians were shipped to the Caribbean and South America to supplant slave labor after the abolition of slavery. Little is known of the conditions or mortality of this migration. At the end of the siege and consequent starvation of Leningrad during the Second World War, the most common reason for admission to the hospital was malignant hypertension, which had disappeared during the siege (71). This could have been a consequence of the survival of "salt conservers" who were then suddenly fed highly salted foods brought in to relieve the famine.

The hypothesis predicts that populations who today experience high mortality from salt-depleting conditions, such as famine in Ethiopia or infant diarrhea in Bangladesh, may be expected to have high rates of salt-sensitive hypertension in the future. It also seems likely that studying those populations whose ancestors did and those who did not experience high mortality due to sodium depletion would be one way to test for evidence of selective survival based on the ability to conserve sodium. Future physiological studies should focus on performance in the heat, on water metabolism, and on sodium metabolism including salt sensitivity.

SUMMARY

The historical records of the black diaspora during the slavery period in the Western Hemisphere reveal mortality that approached 70% in the first 4 years of captivity. If a genetic-based salt-conserving mechanism protected some individuals from mortality, then the slave trade may have acted as an evolutionary gate—individuals who survived passage through that gate would possess a different genetic makeup from those who did not. As virtually all sub-Saharan Africans transported to the Western Hemisphere between the sixteenth and nineteenth centuries had to survive conditions of excessive sodium loss, all passed through the same evolutionary gate. The postulated gene(s) for sodium conservation would, therefore, be more frequent in populations descended from African slaves than in populations without this ancestry. Although we are emphasizing the salt survival mechanisms that may have played a role in survival during slavery, it seems equally likely that there may have been selection for other physiological traits that may have increased the likelihood of survival under intense selection pressures. These might include traits that would increase the ability to survive during periods of starvation and therefore increase the risk of obesity and diabetes.

REFERENCES

1. Abstract of Letters Received by the Royal African Company. April 24, 1793 to March 8, 1804. folio 62. 62. T70/28: 62. Held in Public Record Office, Kew Gardens.
2. Adams, J., and R. H. Ward. Admixture studies and the detection of selection. *Science 180:* 1137–1143, 1973.
3. Adolph, E. F., et al. *Physiology of Man in the Desert.* Interscience Publishers, New York, 1947, p. 42.
4. Alagoa, E. J. Long-distance trade and states in the Niger-delta. *J. Afr. Hist. 11:* 319–329, 1970.
5. Anderson, R. J., and S. L. Linas. Sodium depletion states. In: *Sodium and Water Homeostasis,* edited by B. M. Brenner and J. H. Stein. Churchill Livingstone, New York, 1978, pp. 154–177.
6. Anstey, R. The volume and profitability of the British slave trade, 1761–1807. In: *Race and Slavery in the Western hemisphere: Quantitative Studies,* edited by S. L. Engerman and E. D. Genovese. Princeton University Press, Princeton, 1975, pp. 3–31.
7. Armstrong, L. E., D. L. Costill, and W. J. Fink. Changes in body water and electrolytes during heat acclimation: effects of dietary sodium. *Aviat. Space Environ. Med. 58:* 143–148, 1987.
8. Aubrey, T. *The Sea-Surgeon or the Guinea Man's Vade Mecum.* John Clark, London, 1729.
9. Avery, M. E., and J. D. Snyder. Oral therapy for acute diarrhea: the underused simple solution. *N. Engl. J. Med. 323:* 891–894, 1990.
10. Bergstrom, W. H., and W. M. Wallace. Bone as a sodium and potassium reservoir. *J. Clin. Invest. 33:* 867–873, 1954.
11. Birge, S. J., et al. Osteoporosis, intestinal lactase deficiency and low dietary calcium intake. *N. Engl. J. Med. 276:* 445–448, 1967.
12. Bittle, C. C., D. J. Molina, and F. C. Bartter. Salt sensitivity in essential hypertension as determined by the Cosinor method. *Hypertension 7:* 989–994, 1985.
13. Blackburn, H., and R. Prineas. Diet and hypertension: anthropology, epidemiology, and public health implications. *Prog. Biochem. Pharmacol. 19:* 31–79, 1983.
14. Blagden, C. Experiments and observations in a heated room. *Philos. Trans. R. Soc. Lond.* [*Biol.*] *65:* 111–123, 1775.
15. Blagden, C. Further experiments and observations in an heated room. *Philos. Trans. R. Soc. Lond.* [*Biol.*] *65:* 484–494, 1775.
16. Blaustein, M. P. Sodium ions, calcium ions, blood pressure regulation and hypertension: a reassessment and a hypothesis. *Am. J. Physiol. 232 (Cell Physiol. 1):* C165–C173, 1977.
17. Bloch, M. Salt in human history. *Interdisciplinary Sci. Rev. 1:* 336–352.
18. Bodmer, W. F., And L. L. Cavalli-Sforza. *Genetics, Evolution, and Man.* W. H. Freeman, San Francisco, 1976, pp. 405–406.
19. Bouchard, T. J., D. T. Lykken, M. McGue, N. L. Segal, and A. Tellegen. Sources of human psychological differences: the Minnesota study of twins reared apart. *Science 250:* 223–228, 1990.
20. Bovill, E. W. *The Golden Trade of the Moors.* Oxford University Press, London, 1958, p. 140.
21. Brown, A. H., R. E. Gosselin, and E. F. Adolph. Water losses of men on life rafts. In: *Physiology of Man in the Desert,* edited by E. F. Adolph. Interscience Publishers, New York, 1947, pp. 280–314.
22. Bunge, G. *Textbook of Physiological and Pathological Chemistry.* 2nd English ed. trans. by F. H. Starling from the 4th German ed. P. Blakiston's Son & Co., Philadelphia, 1902, p. 95.
23. Buxton, T. F. *African Slave Trade.* American Anti-Slavery Society, New York, 1840, p. 90.
24. Collins, K. J., and J. S. Weiner. Thermoregulation in twins. *Ann. Hum. Biol. 6:* 290–291, 1979.

25. Collins, R. *Practical Rules for the Management and Medical Treatment of Negro Slaves in the Sugar Colonies.* J. Barfield, London, 1811, p. 100.

26. Conn, J. W. The mechanism of acclimatization to heat. *Adv. Intern. Med. 3:* 373–393, 1949.

27. Curtin, P. D. *The Atlantic Slave Trade: A Census.* University of Wisconsin Press, Madison, 1969.

28. Dahl, L. K., and E. Shackow. Effects of chronic excess salt ingestion: experimental hypertension in the rat. *Can. Med. Assoc. J. 90:* 155–160, 1964.

29. Darlu, P., P. P. Sagnier, and E. Bois. Genealogical and genetical African admixture estimations, blood pressure and hypertension in a Caribbean community. *Ann. Hum. Biol. 17:* 387–397, 1990.

30. Davidson, B. *A History of West Africa to the Nineteenth Century.* Doubleday, Garden City, N.Y., 1966, p. 33.

31. Davidson, B. *The African Slave Trade.* Little, Brown, Boston, 1980, pp. 95–101.

32. Denton, D. *The Hunger for Salt: An Anthropological, Physiological and Medical Analysis.* Springer-Verlag, Berlin, 1982.

33. deWardner, H. Kidney, salt intake, and Na^+, K^+-ATPase inhibitors in hypertension. *Hypertension 17:* 830–836, 1991.

34. Donnan, E. *Documents Illustrative of the History of the Slave Trade to America,* Vol II. Octagon Books, New York, 1969.

35. Du Bois, E. F. *Fever and the Regulation of Body Temperature.* C. C. Thomas, Springfield, Ill., 1948.

36. Eichna, L. W., W. F. Ashe, W. B. Bean, and W. B. Shelly. The upper limits of environmental heat and humidity tolerated by acclimatized men working in hot environments. *J. Ind. Hyg. Toxicol. 27:* 59–84, 1945.

37. Eltis, D. Mortality and voyage length in the middle passage, new evidence from the nineteenth century. *J. Econ. Hist. 44:* 301–308, 1984.

38. Eltis, D. Fluctuations in mortality in the last half century of the transatlantic slave trade. *Soc. Sci. Hist. 13:* 315–340, 1989.

39. Falconbridge, A. *An Account of the Slave Trade on the Coast of Africa.* J. Phillips, George Yard, London, 1788, p. 24.

40. Fordtran, J. S., and J. M. Dietschy. Water and electrolyte movement in the intestine. *Gastroenterology 50:* 263–285, 1966.

41. Freis, E. D., D. J. Reda, and B. J. Materson. Volume (weight) loss and blood pressure response following thiazide diuretics. *Hypertension 12:* 244–250, 1988.

42. Galenson, D. W. *Traders, Planters, and Slaves: Market Behavior in English America.* Cambridge University Press, Cambridge, 1986.

43. Gibbs, T. K. Cargill, L. S. Lieberman, and E. Reitz. Nutrition in a slave population: an anthropological examination. *Med. Anthropol. 4:* 175–262, 1980.

44. Gleibermann, L. Blood pressure and dietary salt in human populations. *Ecology Food Nutr. 2:* 143–156, 1973.

45. Gouletquer, P. L. Niger, country of salt. In: *Salt: The Study of an Ancient Industry,* edited by K. W. de Brisay and K. A. Evans University of Essex, Colchester, 1975, pp. 47–51.

46. Grim, C. E. On slavery, salt and the higher blood pressure in Black Americans (abstract). *Clin. Res. 36:* 426A, 1988.

47. Grim, C. E., and T. W. Wilson. The worldwide epidemiology of hypertension in blacks with a note on a new theory for the greater prevalence of hypertension in Western hemisphere blacks. In: *Hypertension in Blacks and Other Minorities,* 1988 Conference Proceeding of the Second Annual Nutrition Workshop, edited by C. O. Enwonwu. Meharry Medical College, Nashville, Tenn., 1989, 57–73.

48. Grim, C. E., F. C. Luft, J. C. Christian, and M. H. Weinberger. Effects of volume expansion and contraction in normotensive first degree relatives of essential hypertensives. *J. Lab. Clin. Med. 94:* 764–771, 1979.

49. Grim, C. E., F. C. Luft, M. H. Weinberger, J. Z. Miller, R. J. Rose, and J. C. Christian. Genetic, familial and racial influences on blood pressure control systems in man. *Aust. N.Z. J. Med 14:* 453–457, 1984.

50. Grim, C. E., J. Z. Miller, F. C. Luft, J. C. Christian, and M. H. Weinberger. Genetic influences on renin, aldosterone, and renal excretion of sodium and potassium following volume expansion and contraction in normal man. *Hypertension 1:* 583–590, 1979.

51. Grim, C. E., M. H. Weinberger, J. T. Higgins, Jr., and N. J. Kramer. Diagnosis of secondary forms of hypertension: a comprehensive protocol. *J.A.M.A. 237:* 1331–1335, 1977.

52. Grim, C. E., T. W. Wilson, G. D. Nicholson, H. S. Fraser, T. A. Hassell, C. M. Grim, and D. M. Wilson. Blood pressure in blacks: twin studies in Barbados. *Hypertension 15:* 803–809, 1990.

53. Grollmann, A. A conjecture about the prevalence of essential hypertension and its high incidence in the black. *Tex. Rep. Biol. Med. 36:* 25–32, 1978.

54. Guyton, A. C. Blood pressure control—special role of the kidneys and body fluids. *Science 252:* 1813–1860, 1991.

55. Hales, S. *A Treatise on Ventilators. Wherein An Account is Given of the Happy Effects of the Several Trials That Have Been Made of Them, in different Ways and for Different Purposes: Which has Occasioned Their Being Received with General Approbation and Applause, on Account of their Utility for the Great Benefit of Mankind.* Part Second. Richard Manby. London, 1758, pp. 82–99.

56. Handler, J. S., and F. W. Lange. *Plantation Slavery in Barbados: An Archeological and Historical Investigation.* Harvard University Press, Cambridge, Mass., 1978, p. 88.

57. Harris, G. D. Rock salt, its origin, geological occurrences and economic importance in the state of Louisiana, together with brief notes and references to all known salt deposits and industries in the world. *Bulletin of the Louisiana Geological Survey 7:* 1–259, 1908.

58. Harshfield, G. A., B. A. Alpert, E. S. Willey, et al. Race and gender influence ambulatory blood pressure of adolescents. *Hypertension 14:* 598–603, 1989.

59. Harshfield, G. A., C. Hwang, and C. E. Grim. Circadian variation of blood pressure during a normal day in normotensive blacks. *Circulation* (Suppl) *78:* 4-II, 188, 1988.

60. Helmer, O. M. Renin-angiotensin system and its relation to hypertension. *Prog. Cardiovasc. Dis. 8:* 117–128, 1965.

61. Helmer, O. M. Hormonal and biochemical factors controlling blood pressure. In: *Les Concepts de Claude Bernard Sur le Milieu Intérieur.* Masson & Cie, Editeurs, Paris, 1967, pp. 115–128.

62. Higman, B. W. *Slave Populations of the British Caribbean: 1807–1834.* Johns Hopkins University Press, Baltimore, 1984, pp. 314–347.

63. Hilliard, S. B. *Hog Meat and Hoecake: Food Supply in the Old South, 1840–1860.* Southern Illinois University Press, Carbondale, Ill., 1972, p. 61.

64. Hughes, R. *The Fatal Shore.* Vintage Books, New York, 1986, p. 145.

65. Inikori, J. E. Measuring the Atlantic slave trade: an assessment of Curtin and Anstey. *J. Afr. Hist. 17:* 197–223, 1976.

66. Intersalt Cooperative Research Group. Intersalt: an international study of electrolyte excretion and blood pressure. Results for 24 hour urinary sodium and potassium excretion. *Br. Med. J. 297:* 319–328, 1988.

67. Jagger, P. I., G. J. Hine, A. J. Cardarelli, B. A. Burrows, and V. Bikerman. Influence of sodium intake on exchangeable sodium in normal human subjects. *J. Clin. Invest. 42:* 1459–1470, 1963.

68. Januszeqicz, P., G. Thibault, J. Gutkowska, R. Garcia, C. Mercure, F. Jolicoeult, J. Genest, and M. Cantin. Atrial natriuretic factor and vasopressin during dehydration and rehydration in rats. *Am. J. Physiol. 251 (Endocrinol. Metab. 14):* E497–E501, 1986.

69. Kaplan, N. M., D. C. Kem, O. B. Holland, N. J. Kramer, J. Higgins, and C. Gomez-Sanchez. The intravenous furosemide test: a simple way to evaluate renin responsiveness. *Ann. Intern. Med. 84:* 639–645, 1976.

70. Kawasaki, T., C. S. Delea, F. C. Bartter, and H. Smith. The effect of high-sodium low-sodium diet on blood pressure and other related variables in human subjects with idiopathic hypertension. *Am. J. Med. 64:* 193–198, 1978.

71. Keys, A., J. Brozek, A. Henschel, O. Miekelsen, and H. L. Taylor. *The Biology of Human Starvation,* Vols. 1 and 2. University of Minnesota Press, Minneapolis, 1950.

72. Kiple, K. F. *The Caribbean Slave: A Biological History.* Cambridge University Press, New York, 1984, pp. 64–65.

73. Kiple, K. F. Cholera and race in the Caribbean. *J. Latin America Studies 17:* 157–177, 1985.

74. Kiple, K. F. A survey of recent literature on the biological past of the black. *Soc. Sci. Hist. 10:* 343–367, 1986.

75. Kiple, K., and B. Higgins. Mortality caused by dehydration during the middle passage. *Soc. Sci. Hist. 13:* 421–437, 1989.

76. Kiple, K. F., and V. H. King. *Another Dimension to the Black Diaspora: Diet, Disease, Racism.* Cambridge University Press, New York, 1981, pp. 114, 147–148.

77. Kirby, C. R., and V. A. Convertino. Plasma aldosterone and sweat sodium concentrations after exercise and heat acclimation. *J. Appl. Physiol. 61:* 967–970, 1986.

78. Klein, H. *The Middle Passage: Comparative Studies in the Atlantic Slave Trade.* Princeton University Press, Princeton, 1978.

79. Knochel, J. P., and G. Reed. Disorders of heat regulation. In: *Clinical Disorders of Fluid and Electrolyte Metabolism,* edited by M. H. Maxwell, C. R. Kleeman, and R. G. Narins. McGraw-Hill, New York, 1987, pp. 1197–1232.

80. Koplan, J. P. Slave mortality in nineteenth century Grenada. *Soc. Sci. Hist. 7:* 311–320, 1983.

81. Kretchmer, N. Food: a selective agent in evolution. In: *Food, Nutrition and Evolution: Food as an Environmental Factor in the Genesis of Human Variability,* edited by D. N. Walcher and N. Kretchmer. Masson Publishing, New York, 1981, pp. 37–48.

82. Kuno, Y. *Human Perspiration.* C. C. Thomas, Springfield, Ill., 1956, pp. 53, 185, 190–211.

83. Ladell, W. S. S. The changes in water and chloride distribution during heavy sweating. *J. Physiol. 108:* 440–450, 1949.

84. Ladell, W. S. S. Disorders due to heat. *Trans. R. Soc. Trop. Med. Hyg. 51:* 189–216, 1957.

85. Lee, M. R. The kidney fault in essential hypertension may be a failure to mobilize renal dopamine adequately when dietary sodium chloride is increased. *Cardiovasc. Rev. Rep. 2:* 785–789, 1981.

86. Levitan, R., and F. J. Ingelfinger. Effect of d-aldosterone on salt and water absorption from the intact human colon. *J. Clin. Invest. 44:* 801–808, 1965.

87. Lovejoy, P. E. *Transformations in Slavery: A History of Slavery in Africa.* Cambridge University Press, Cambridge, England, 1983.

88. Lovejoy, P. E. *Salt of the Desert Sun: A History of Salt Production Trade in the Central Sudan.* Cambridge University Press, Cambridge, England, 1986, pp. 93, 110.

89. Luft, F. C., C. E. Grim, J. T. Higgins, and M. H. Weinberger. Differences in response to sodium administration in normotensive white and black subjects. *J. Lab. Clin. Med. 90:* 555–562, 1977.

90. Luft, F. C., C. E. Grim, and M. H. Weinberger. Electrolyte and volume homeostasis in blacks. In: *Hypertension in Blacks: Epidemiology, Pathophysiology and Treatment,* edited by W. D. Hall, E. Saunders, and N. B. Shulman. Year Book Medical Publishers, Chicago, 1985, pp. 115–131.

91. Luft, F. C., C. E. Grim, L. R. Willis, J. T. Higgins, Jr., and M. H. Weinberger. Natriuretic response to saline infusion in normotensive and hypertensive man. The role of renin suppression in exaggerated natriuresis. *Circulation 55:* 779–784, 1977.

92. Luft, F. C., C. E. Grim, N. S. Fineberg, D. P. Henry, and M. H. Weinberger. Natriuretic responses in labile hypertension. *Am. J. Med. Sci. 283:* 119–128, 1982.

93. Luft, F. C., L. I. Rankin, R. Bloch, A. E. Weyman, L. R. Willis, R. H. Murray, C. E. Grim, and M. H. Weinberger. Cardiovascular and humoral responses to extremes of sodium intake in normal white and black men. *Circulation 60:* 697–706, 1979.

94. Maclean, C. J., M. S. Adams, W. C. Leyshon, et al. Genetic studies on hybrid populations. III. Blood pressure in an American black community. *Am. J. Hum. Genet. 26:* 614–626, 1974.

95. Marshall, S. J., and C. E. Grim. A rapid screening method to detect low renin hypertension. *Clin. Res. 21:* 99, 1973.

96. Martin, B., and M. Spurrell, eds. *The Journal of a Slave Trader (John Newton), 1750–1754.* The Epworth Press, London, 1962.

97. McCance, R. A. Ethnic variations in the response of the sweat glands to pilocarpine: the Sudanese. *J. Physiol. [Lond.] 203:* 61P–62P, 1969.

98. McCance, R. A., and G. Purohit. Ethnic differences in the response of sweat glands to pilocarpine. *Nature 221:* 378–379, 1969.

99. McCance, R. A., J. H. E. Rutishauer, and H. C. Knight. Response of sweat glands to pilocarpine in the Bantu of Uganda. *Lancet 1:* 663–665, 1969.

100. McGee, W. J. Desert thirst as disease. *Interstate Med. J. 13:* 279–300, 1906.

101. McKinley, M. J., D. A. Denton, J. F. Nelson, and R. S. Weisinger. Dehydration induces sodium depletion in rats, rabbits, and sheep. *Am. J. Physiol. 245 (Regulatory Integrative Comp. Physiol. 13):* R287–R292, 1983.

102. Meneely, G. R., and H. D. Battarbee. Sodium and potassium. *Nutr. Rev. 4:* 259–279, 1976.

103. Miller, J. C. Mortality in the Atlantic slave trade: statistical evidence on causality. *J. Interdisciplinary Hist. 11:* 385–423, 1981.

104. Miller, J. C. *Way of Death: Merchant Capitalism and the Angolan Slave Trade, 1730–1830.* University of Wisconsin Press, Madison, 1988, pp. 437–442.

105. Moloney, A. *The Commercial Geography of Yoruba.* Proceedings of the Geographical Section 2: 626–630, 1889.

106. Money, K. E. Motion sickness. *Physiol. Rev. 50:* 1–39, 1970.

107. Muller, F. B., J. E. Sealey, D. B. Case, S. A. Atlas, and T. G. Pickering. The captopril test for identifying renovascular disease in hypertensive patients. *Am. J. Med. 80:* 663–644, 1986.

108. Murphy, M. B., K. S. Nelson, and W. J. Elliott. Racial differences in diurnal blood pressure profile. Abstract, 3rd International Interdisciplinary Conference on Hypertension in Blacks, Baltimore, Md., 1988, p. 21.

109. Neel, J. V. Diabetes mellitus: a "thrifty" genotype rendered detrimental by progress. *Am. J. Hum. Genet. 14:* 353–362, 1962.

110. Newbury, C. W. Prices and profitability in early nineteenth century West African trade. In: *The Development of Indigenous Trade and Markets in West Africa,* edited by C. Meillassoux. Oxford University Press, London, 1971, p. 92.

111. Nichols, G., and N. Nichols. The role of bone in sodium metabolism. *Metabolism 5:* 438–446, 1956.

112. Osler, W. *The Principles and Practice of Medicine.* Birmingham, 1892. reproduced by the Classics of Medicine Library, 1978, pp. 121–122.

113. Phillips, P. A., B. J. Rolls, J. G. G. Ledingham, M. L. Forsling, J. J. Morton, M. J. Crowe, and L. Wollner. Reduced thirst after water deprivation in healthy elderly men. *N. Engl. J. Med. 311:* 753–759, 1984.

114. Porteres, R. *Les Sels Alimentaires.* Direction General de la Sante Publique, Dakar, Senegal 1950, endleaf.

115. Postma, J. Mortality in the Dutch slave trade, 1675–1795. In: *The Uncommon Market: Essays in the Economic History of the Atlantic Slave Trade,* edited by H. A. Gemery and J. S. Hogendorn. Academic Press, New York, 1979, pp. 239–260.

116. Rabbani, G. H. Cholera. *Clin. Gastroenterol. 15:* 507–528, 1986.

117. Rapp, J. P., S. M. Wang, and W. Dene. A genetic polymorphism in the renin gene of Dahl rats co-segregates with blood pressure. *Science 243:* 542–544, 1989.

118. Robertson, G. L., R. L. Shelton, and S. Athar. The osmoregulation of vasopresin. *Kidney Int. 1:* 10, 25–37, 1976.

119. Samueloff, S. Thermoregulatory responses in genetically different ethic groups. In: *Man in Stressful Environments,* edited by K. Shirake and M. K. Yousef. C. C. Thomas, Springfield, Ill., 1987, pp. 23–34.

120. Savitt, T. Medicine and Slavery: The Diseases and Health Care of Blacks in Antebellum Virginia. University of Illinois Press, Urbana, 1978, pp. 121, 143.

121. Schachter, J., and L. H. Kuller. Blood volume expansion among blacks: an hypothesis. *Med. Hypotheses 14:* 1–19, 1984.

122. Sheridan, R. B. Doctors and Slaves: *A Medical Demography of Slavery in the British West Indies 1680–1834.* Cambridge University Press, New York, 1985.

123. Sheriden, R. B. The crises of slave subsistence in the British West Indies during and after the American Revolution. *William and Mary Q. 33:* 615–641, 1976.

124. Slave Trade: Colonial Office Drafts and Letters. July to December, 1849. FO 84/780. Held in Public Record Office, Kew Gardens, United Kingdom: 182.

125. Slave Trade: Colonial Office Drafts and letters. July to December, 1849. FO 84/780: Held in Public Record Office, Kew Gardens, United Kingdom.

126. Steckel, R. A dreadful childhood: excess mortality of American slaves. *Soc. Sci. Hist. 10:* 427–465, 1986.

127. Steckel, R. H., and R. A. Jensen. New evidence on the causes of slave and crew mortality in the Atlantic slave trade. *J. Econ. Hist. 46:* 57–77, 1986.

128. Stinebaugh, B. J., and F. X. Schloeder. Studies on the natriuresis of fasting. I: Effect of prefast intake. *Metabolism 15:* 828–837, 1966.

129. Sundström, L. *The Trade of Guinea.* Uppsala, 1965.

130. Syckle, C. V. Some pictures of food consumption in the United States. Part I. 1630 to 1860. *J. Am. Diet. Assoc. 21:* 508–512, 1945.

131. Waldron, I., M. Nowotarski, M. Freimer, J. P. Henry, N. Post, and C. Witten. Cross-cultural variation in blood pressure: a quantitative analysis of the relationships of blood pressure to cultural characteristics, salt consumption, and body weight. *Soc. Sci. Med. 16:* 419–430, 1982.

132. Weinberger, M. H., J. Z. Miller, F. C. Luft, C. E. Grim, and N. S. Fineberg. Definitions and characteristics of sodium sensitivity and blood pressure resistance. *Hypertension 8:*II, 127–134, 1986.

133. Whittow, G. C. Flow of blood in the forearm of persons acclimatised to heat. *Nature 192:* 759–760, 1961.

134. Williams, R., and P. N. Hopkins. Salt, hypertension, and genetic-environmental interactions. *Prog. Clin. Biol. Res. 32:* 183–194, 1979.

135. Wilson, T. W. History of salt supplies in West Africa and blood pressures today. *Lancet 1:* 784–786, 1986.

136. Wilson, T. W. Ancient environments and modern disease: the case of hypertension among Afro-Americans. University Microfilms, Ann Arbor, 1988.

137. Wilson, T. W. Africa, Afro-Americans, and hypertension: an hypothesis. In: *The African Exchange: Toward a Biological History of Black People,* edited by K. F. Kiple. Duke University Press, Durham, N. C. 1988, pp. 257–274.

138. Wilson, T. W. Salt consumption on British slave ships, 1682–1704: historical evidence on the slavery hypothesis of hypertension in blacks (abstract). *J. Hum. Hypertens.* 4: 790, 1990.

139. Wilson, T. W., and C. E. Grim. The bio-history of slavery and blood pressure differences in blacks today: a hypothesis. *Hypertension 17* (suppl I): I-122–I-128, 1991.

140. Wilson, T. W., and C. E. Grim. The possible relationship between the trans-Atlantic slave trade and blood pressure in blacks today. In: *The Atlantic Slave Trade: Gainers and Losers,* edited by J. E. Inikori and S. E. Engerman. Duke University Press, Durham, N.C. 1991, pp. 339–359.

141. Wilson, T. W., A. C. Egbunike, G. A. Harshfield, N. A. Law, and C. E. Grim. Nocturnal blood pressure is higher in US born blacks than non-US born blacks [abstract]. *J. Hypertens.* 8:S66, 1990.

142. Wilson, T. W., L. H. Hollifield, and C. E. Grim. Systolic blood pressure levels in blacks in sub-Sahara Africa, the West Indies, and the United States: a metaanalysis. *Hypertension* 18:I-87–I-91, 1991.

143. Wilson, T. W., W. Okoroanyanwu, D. Wilson, A. Egbunike, C. G. Hames, and C. E. Grim. Blood pressure does not increase with age in a high sodium intake, rural population in Imo State, Nigeria (abstract). *Circulation 82:* III-21, 1990.

144. Wilson, T. W., D. M. Wilson, C. E. Grim, C. M. Grim, S. A. Garrett, G. D. Nicholson, H. S. Fraser, and T. A. Hassell. The feasibility of twin studies in third world countries: the Barbados experience (abstract). *Acta Genet. Med. Gemellol. 38:* 248, 1989.

145. Winkler, A. W., J. R. Elkinton, J. Hopper, and H. E. Hoff. Experimental hypotonicity: alterations in the distribution of body water and the cause of death. *J. Clin. Invest. 23:* 103–109, 1944.

146. Zerbe, R. L., J. Z. Miller, and G. L. Robertson. Reproducibility and heritability of vasopressin osmoregulation in humans (abstract). *Endocrinology 106:* 78, 1980.

3

Characteristics of Prehypertension in Black Children

BONITA FALKNER

Hypertension is a leading health problem in the United States and in other countries. Epidemiological studies have demonstrated racial and geographical differences in prevalence for essential hypertension (EH). In the United States, blacks have a greater prevalence of EH (10,72). This difference is further accentuated by vital statistics data on mortality. Blacks have a threefold greater mortality from hypertensive disease than whites. This disproportionate mortality rises to more than six times greater in blacks in the age range 35–54 years (87). Thus, the morbid consequences of hypertensive disease are severalfold greater in blacks, particularly in young adulthood and mid-adulthood (35).

It is now accepted that dysregulatory mechanisms, evolving into hypertensive states, have their onset in young children (57,75,96). Investigations in children have characterized levels of blood pressure, identified related parameters (40,89), and provided evidence of hemodynamic changes in children at risk for EH (26,27,79,80,95). However, studies comparing blood pressure levels by race in children have resulted in variable reports (86,88). Epidemiological studies have not consistently detected racial patterns in children to explain the greater prevalence, morbidity, and mortality of EH among blacks. However, physiological and interrelated environmental variations between black and white children have been reported. This chapter discusses biological variations among blacks that are identifiable at a young age and that may characterize those black children who are at risk for EH.

SYMPATHETIC NERVOUS SYSTEM

One line of investigation concerns the sympathetic nervous system (30,39). There is a correlation of stress-induced enhanced sympathetic nervous system activity in adults with EH (3,70) and in children with a family history of EH (23,53,55,60,68,79). Based on the experimental design of these studies, it has been assumed that the cardiovascular hyperresponsivity to sympathetic stimulation has been related to greater β-adrenergic activity. However, many of the clinical studies on neurogenic–cardiovascular interaction have used racially mixed populations. Fredrickson compared racial differences in cardiovascular reactivity with mental stress in adults with EH. Although the black sample was small, he observed that, compared with whites, blacks had fewer cardiac sympathomimetic responses but had greater vascular responses to mental stress (32). Light et al. (56) have investigated the cardiovascular response to active coping stressors in college age males. Blacks were compared with whites in both normotensive and marginally hypertensive groups. Hypertensives demonstrated a greater blood pressure response to the laboratory stress than normotensives. The blood pressure response was greatest in the black hypertensives but without an attendant increase in heart rate (56). These investigators propose that this response reflects a greater peripheral resistance in the marginally hypertensive young blacks, an observation that varies from the more classical description of borderline hypertension. Based on extensive hemodynamic studies, Julius (43) has characterized borderline hypertension as a condition of high blood pressure, high cardiac output, and normal peripheral resistance. The theoretical basis for this model of borderline hypertension is that neurogenic stimulation provokes an enhanced β-adrenergic response, which in turn effects an increased cardiac output (30). However, Light and colleagues have provided preliminary evidence that in blacks, stress-mediated neurogenic stimulation may have a greater effect on peripheral vascular resistance.

We have conducted a series of studies in children on dysregulatory blood pressure mechanisms that contribute to the development of EH. The initial studies concerned the family history of EH, the sympathetic nervous system, and the relationship of cardiovascular response to adrenergic stimulation. We demonstrated that adolescent offspring of parents with EH exhibited a significantly greater heart rate and blood pressure response to the central stress of difficult mental arithmetic compared with offspring of normotensive parents (32). The relationship of family history of EH to stress-induced cardiovascular reactivity has been confirmed by other investigators (54,61). With the known association of environmental stress and EH, the correlation of enhanced cardiovascular reactivity induced by mental stress in adolescents with parental EH suggests a possible model of gene–environment interaction. However, the validity of generalizing from a stress response observed in the laboratory to response occurring during naturalistic environmental experiences remains to be determined. In a 5-year longitudinal study on the predictability of stress-induced reactivity, we found that approximately 50% of the adolescents who exhibited borderline blood pressure elevations progressed to sustained high blood pressure. We also characterized those adolescents who progressed from borderline or variable blood pressure to persistent hypertension. The characteristics of those who exhibited this high risk of EH included parental EH, high resting heart rate, high stress-induced cardiovascular reactivity, and in females, excessive body weight (23). These characteristics were consistent with a neurogenic pattern in the early phase of EH.

The data on cardiovascular reactivity were analyzed further with Fourier analysis and mathematical modeling (48). Figure 3.1A and 1B depict the systolic and diastolic blood pressure response during stress, as percentage change from baseline, for early hypertensive and normotensive adolescents. In the ini-

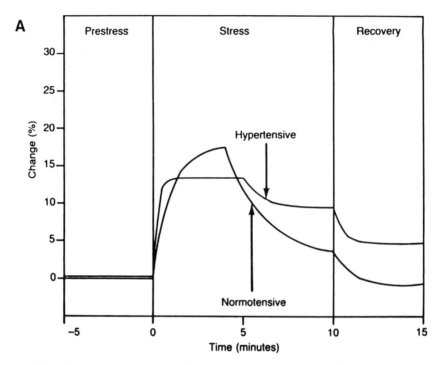

FIGURE 3.1A. The reactivity of systolic blood pressure during stress and recovery for hypertensives and normotensives expressed as percentage of change from baseline or prestress period.
Note that the early response of the normotensive group peaks higher than the early response
of the hypertensive group (though the hypertensives' rate of increase is greater). A "control-
factor" changes the direction of the response. This factor occurs earlier in the normotensives
and is more effective in allowing recovery of normal systolic blood pressure after the cessation
of stress. The hypertensive group remained elevated after the 5-minute recovery period. The
control factor is blunted in the hypertensives.

tial minutes of mental stress, all subjects exhibited an increase in blood pressure. The systolic and diastolic pressure response is quite similar for the two
groups. With continued stress, the normotensives appear to recover or coun-
terregulate the blood pressure toward baseline. However, the hypertensives
display persistence of the blood pressure elevation with limited ability to coun-
terregulate the pressure toward baseline. The statistically significant difference in the stress reactivity between the two groups is most marked in the
later phase of the stress protocol. These data suggested that processes other
than the initial neurogenic-mediated response alone may be operative in the
stress-induced blood pressure differences of the hypertensive versus normotensive.

SODIUM SENSITIVITY

The interrelationship between neurogenic activity and blood volume modified
by sodium intake has been studied in blacks and in whites. In normal humans

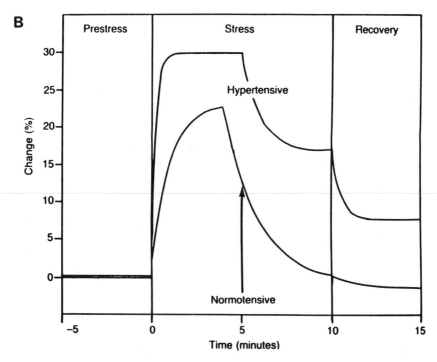

FIGURE 3.1B. The reactivity of diastolic pressure during stress and recovery for normotensives and hypertensives expressed as percentage of change from baseline or prestress period. When diastolic blood pressure is plotted against time, the hypertensive group showed a greater and more rapid rise than the normotensives. A "control-factor" reduces the stress response by about the 5-minute point. The normotensive group was able to approach baseline blood pressure before the end of stress, whereas the hypertensive group did not. The diastolic pressure of the hypertensive group remained elevated after the 5-minute recovery period.

sympathetic activity decreases with increasing sodium intake (39). Higher levels of plasma norepinephrine are reported in essential hypertension than in normal control subjects at each level of dietary sodium intake (62,86). In response to sodium load, blacks excrete less sodium and potassium than whites, and blacks also experience greater suppression of plasma renin activity (58). These studies delineate a relationship between sympathetic activity and sodium balance.

Dimsdale et al. (20) investigated vascular sensitivity to infused norepinephrine in adult blacks and whites under conditions of low and high dietary salt intake. During the infusion, hypertensives had a higher blood pressure at each norepinephrine dosage, but the slopes of the dose-response curve were the same for normotensives and hypertensives. However, on high salt intake, black hypertensives had an augmented blood pressure response to infused norepinephrine, whereas white hypertensives had a reduced dose-response to the same infusion. This report, which demonstrates augmented alpha receptor sensitivity in blacks, also delineates a peripheral vascular variation in black hypertension that emerges under a high salt condition.

We hypothesized that the differences in neurogenic-mediated cardiovas-

cular response patterns may be related to altered vascular tone relative to
sodium and volume balance. A study was conducted to investigate the interaction of blood pressure sensitivity to a sodium load with stress-induced cardiovascular reactivity. Young adult (18–22 years of age) blacks were compared
with whites in their blood pressure response to chronic oral sodium loading.
The sodium load consisted of adding 10 g of sodium chloride to the usual diet
for 14 days. The cardiovascular reactivity to stress was studied before and after
sodium loading. In this study, we again replicated our earlier finding that
stress-induced reactivity was greater in offspring of hypertensives than in offspring of normotensives. However, we also found that normotensive whites
exhibited greater central stress reactivity than normotensive blacks (21). The
prevalence of blood pressure sensitivity to a sodium load was greater in young
blacks (39%) than in young whites (18%) (27). In sodium-sensitive subjects,
the sodium load raised baseline blood pressure, and sodium excretion was
blunted compared with sodium-insensitive subjects (both normotensive and
borderline hypertensive). However, stress-induced cardiovascular reactivity
was not altered by the sodium load (23). Subsequently, we used the same design to study the effect of potassium loading on central stress-induced reactivity in blacks. Following chronic potassium load, potassium-sensitive subjects
had a reduction in baseline blood pressure. However, the mental stress–induced cardiovascular reactivity was not altered by the potassium load. Data
from these investigations indicate that shifts in sodium or potassium balance
do not interact with the β-adrenergic-mediated cardiovascular reactivity. In
blacks, the baseline blood pressure change induced by the shifts in sodium and
potassium balance may be related to functional changes in peripheral vascular
resistance. Light et al. (56) and Dimsdale et al. (20) reported data that are
consistent with this concept. Several studies have now reported greater β-mediated cardiac responsivity in whites and greater α-mediated adrenergic activity in blacks (2,32). These reports are also consistent with our findings on racial differences in reactivity (22).

GROWTH

Epidemiological investigations on blood pressure in childhood have characterized levels of blood pressure and have delineated related parameters such as
body weight, height, and maturation (11,18,40,72,89). The recent blood pressure distribution curves published by the Second Task Force Report on Blood
Pressure Control in Childhood (86) demonstrate a progressive increase in blood
pressure throughout childhood. In females the curves flatten with no further
increase at age 13–14 years. In males the blood pressure rise continues
through age 18 years. These blood pressure patterns correspond to normal
growth patterns in adolescents. In females adult stature is reached by age 13–
14 years, but growth continues through age 18 years in males. Longitudinal
studies also indicate that blood pressure tracking occurs throughout childhood
and adolescence (51,52,91). Eight years of longitudinal investigation in the
Bogalusa Heart Study have yielded data that demonstrate that repeated childhood blood pressure measurements in the upper quartile predict upper quartile blood pressure 9 years later.

In these longitudinal studies of blood pressure and growth throughout childhood, a consistent significant correlate of blood pressure is body weight and height (45,52,73). Analysis of data in the Muscatine Study also demonstrate the importance of relative growth rate in the rank order of childhood blood pressure, where the trend in body size correlates with the trend in blood pressure (50). Relative fatness, obesity, and changes in obesity also correlate with blood pressure in childhood (8). These studies indicate that blood pressure correlates with body size and tracks with body growth. The data also indicate that obesity is a risk factor for EH. However, in an investigation of body composition and blood pressure in adolescents, Wilson et al. (94) demonstrated that boys with persistently elevated blood pressure (> 95th percentile) were characterized by early maturation and excess size for age in the absence of obesity. Girls with elevated blood pressure had decreased physical fitness and obesity.

Family history of EH has been demonstrated to be a significant risk factor for EH. In the Bogalusa study, family history of hypertension was shown to predict, independently, later systolic blood pressure status (82). The predictive value of family history of hypertension on later blood pressure status in children was also reported in the Minneapolis children's blood pressure study (68). The relative greater growth rates of children with higher blood pressure may be related to familial patterns of blood pressure and also to familial patterns of weight or adiposity. Rosenbaum et al. (77) reported a significant relationship between familial patterns of body composition, blood pressure, and childhood risk factors.

The association of relative fatness with blood pressure in children does not exclude the contribution of other factors. As cited previously, Wilson et al. (94) described lean males with significant hypertension. Burke et al. (6) also described a group of lean children with persistent high diastolic pressure in the Bogalusa Study. Similarly, Katz et al. (46) described a group of lean black adolescent males and fatter black females with higher blood pressure. The available literature demonstrates the importance of growth and growth rates as determinants in the risk for EH. It is possible that the somatic growth correlates for blood pressure may be only a surrogate measurement of cardiovascular growth. Therefore, other biological factors contributing to cardiovascular growth on the basis of genetic and racial variations may also contribute to high blood pressure in late childhood.

The predisposition to EH, or the prehypertensive state in childhood, is regulated through genetic factors. Culpepper et al. (13) proposed that the genetic predisposition in children may facilitate the development of cardiovascular changes at pressure loads that are mildly elevated and of relatively short duration. These investigators and others have demonstrated that adolescents with blood pressure in the highest quartile have greater left ventricular mass and myocardial posterior wall thickness (12,36,49,80). Schieken et al. (81) also demonstrated that adolescents in the upper blood pressure quartile had increasing vascular resistance after adjusting for body size. These data concur with a study by Mahoney et al. who demonstrated greater forearm vascular resistance at maximal vasodilatation in adolescents at the upper blood pressure quartile (59). This report suggests the presence of changes in vascular structure in the high blood pressure group. A biracial study of echocardiographic function and blood pressure in children and young adults in Bogalusa demonstrated a correlation of cardiac output with body size, and an increase in cardiac output with age and blood pressure quartile. Following adjustment for body size, white males had greater cardiac output than black males. Black males had higher peripheral vascular resistance than whites. Of further interest was the finding that peripheral vascular resistance was greater in black males than in white males even at lower blood pressure quartiles (85).

In addition to racial differences in cardiovascular function in children, there are racial and familial differences in adrenergic-mediated cardiovascular reactivity (22,69) and also in sodium sensitivity (93). With our studies on cardiovascular reactivity, we have demonstrated that the cardiovascular reactivity response to a central neurogenic stimulus is reproducible within individuals over time and is consistently greater in borderline hypertensives and in offspring of hypertensive parents. Therefore, centrally induced reactivity appears to be useful as a predictor of hypertension. However, this model alone is limited within clinical investigations to explain the mechanism of developing EH. Data indicated that in young blacks, functional and possibly structural changes occur in the peripheral vasculature that may mediate the hypertensive process. The relationship of these physiological changes in the context of growth biology needs further exploration.

METABOLISM AND GROWTH

The biologic growth factor that has a demonstrated correlation with blood pressure is insulin. An association of plasma insulin with blood pressure in children (9–12 yr) was first reported by Florey et al. (29). They found a weak relationship of insulin with blood pressure and a stronger relationship between plasma glucose and blood pressure in childhood (29). Voors compared childhood blood pressure strata with an index of peripheral insulin resistance. The product of the one-hour glucose and insulin level following a glucose load was greatest in white males in the highest blood pressure stratum. They also found a correlation of one-hour insulin with body weight in all blood pressure strata for blacks and whites (90). In children, Smoak et al. (84) reported a relationship of obesity and the clustering of systolic blood pressure, fasting insulin, and plasma lipids. In another report from the Bogalusa Heart Study, fasting insulin levels in older children (9–14 yr) correlate with blood pressure and ponderosity, and are significantly higher in black children (7). Rocchini et al. (76) studied the effect of diet, exercise, and weight loss on blood pressure and plasma insulin levels in obese adolescents. Although weight loss resulted in a decrease in plasma insulin and blood pressure, in the group with added exercise the decrease in blood pressure was related to the decrease in fasting insulin independent of the changes in body weight or body fat. This report suggests that the effect of insulin on blood pressure may be mediated by factors other than adiposity.

Insulin may contribute to the pathogenesis of EH (44,47) by its trophic effect on vascular smooth muscle. Elevated plasma insulin levels or abnormalities in insulin-stimulated glucose metabolism could induce variations in cardiovascular growth patterns owing to the anabolic effect of insulin. Although its acute metabolic effects have been studied more extensively than its anabolic effects, insulin is one of the longest established growth factors. Higher levels of insulin in childhood could stimulate growth as a primary event or in association with insulin-like growth factors.

Two hyperinsulinemic childhood disorders support a direct relationship between insulin and growth stimulation: infants of diabetic mothers and a subset of growth hormone–deficient children with craniopharyngiomas manifest excessive growth and increased insulin levels (5).

Higher insulin levels could be associated with increased levels of insulin-like growth factor I (IGF-I). The insulin-like growth factors are thought to be related to growth in childhood, and their levels are influenced by insulin, growth hormone, and nutritional states (33). Perfusion of rat livers with insulin results in an increased IGF-I concentration in the medium, suggesting a direct effect of insulin on the generation of IGF-I by the liver (14). Of further relevance is that IGF-I has been demonstrated to stimulate aortic smooth muscle cell replication in vitro (9).

Several clinical and animal studies support the direct relationship between IGF-I levels and growth. Acromegaly is associated with gigantism, growth hormone excess, elevated insulin levels, and overproduction of IGF-I. African pygmies, who have short stature, are small despite normal nutritional and normal growth hormone levels. They have decreased IGF-I levels and lack of a pubertal growth spurt (63,64). Toy poodles are an animal pygmy model that, in contrast to standard poodles, have almost unmeasurable levels of IGF-I (21). However, the contribution of IGF-I to insulin resistance and to cardiovascular growth in children remains to be investigated.

The consideration of insulin as a mediator of somatic growth and also of cardiovascular growth is relevant in light of the recent attention to the issues of insulin resistance. Insulin resistance, defined as a suboptimal metabolic effect of a given amount of insulin, is generally expressed as relative hyperinsulinemia. Hyperinsulinemia or insulin resistance is commonly observed in obesity and non-insulin-dependent diabetes mellitus (NIDDM) (2–6).

Data have also emerged that indicate that hyperinsulinemia, or insulin resistance correlates with hypertension independent of NIDDM or obesity. Manicardi et al. (60) compared the insulin response to an oral glucose load in obese hypertensive and obese normotensive males. Obese hypertensives achieved plasma insulin levels twice as high as the obese normotensives, indicating more severe insulin resistance. Fournier et al. (31) demonstrated a correlation of fasting insulin with blood pressure in nondiabetic subjects that existed after adjusting for adiposity. Modan et al. (65) investigated EH and glucose intolerance in a large Israeli population. Their analysis revealed a significant independent effect of insulin levels on blood pressure when adjusted for body mass index, age, sex, and glucose intolerance.

In a rigorous experimental study, Ferrannini et al. (28) utilized a euglycemic hyperinsulinemic clamp technique to study lean middle-aged hypertensives with normal glucose tolerance. Compared with age- and weight-matched normotensive controls, the hypertensives exhibited marked impairment of glucose uptake in response to the insulin infusion. Their data provide substantial evidence that EH is associated with insulin resistance independent of obesity or carbohydrate tolerance. The concurrent metabolic studies in their protocol indicate that the insulin resistance of EH is located in the peripheral tissues.

The physiologic effects of insulin may also affect other blood pressure regulatory systems. DeFronzo (15,16) demonstrated by closed clamp technique in dogs that small increments in insulin levels stimulated an increase in renal tubular sodium reabsorption. Thus, as demonstrated by Feranninni et al. (28), higher insulin levels, or insulin resistance in the peripheral tissues, in hypertensive men, would result in higher plasma insulin levels. These higher levels could direct increased sodium reabsorption and a volume-dependent increase in blood pressure.

Chronic insulin release has been shown to be altered by β-mediated sympathetic activity (which is regarded to be higher in EH). It has been suggested that the peripheral uptake of glucose decreases with increasing β-mediated sympathetic activity, resulting in increasing resistance to insulin (4). In vitro studies have demonstrated an inhibitory action of epinephrine on insulin-mediated glucose metabolism (1,83,92). With in vivo studies of hyperinsulinemic euglycemia in man, Diebert and DeFronzo (19) showed that simultaneously infused epinephrine blocked the inhibitory effect of insulin on hepatic glucose production. Thus, stress-associated levels of epinephrine augmented hepatic glucose production in the face of hyperinsulinemia. However, there was a total reduction in insulin-stimulated glucose metabolism, which indicates that epinephrine also induces peripheral tissue resistance to the effects of insulin. This effect of epinephrine was prevented by simultaneous administration of the beta blocker propranolol. However, Rowe et al. (78) showed that there was a significant increase in plasma norepinephrine levels in response to euglycemic hyperinsulinemia, indicating that elevated levels of plasma insulin may increase sympathetic nervous system activity in the absence of decreases in blood glucose. There is ample evidence of augmented adrenergic activity in EH, including elevated plasma catecholamines (37,38) and greater stress-induced blood pressure responses (54,61).

The role of insulin resistance in the pathophysiology of EH may also be mediated through its effect on cell membrane cation transport. Abnormalities of sodium transport have been demonstrated in EH (34,42) and obesity (17,67). Despite the emphasis on sodium transport in EH, there is obligatory linkage of sodium efflux with potassium influx, and there is evidence that indicates that insulin is involved in internal potassium balance in humans (65,66).

It has been proposed that abnormalities in insulin metabolism play a role in the etiology and in the clinical course of EH (74). Variation in insulin action, or insulin resistance, was also a hypothetical mechanism that could account for the variations in adrenergic activity, sodium sensitivity, and cation transport, which we have described in a young black population. It was also hypothesized that the anabolic effects of insulin could affect growth, both somatic growth and growth of the peripheral vasculature.

We subsequently performed a study on a subgroup of young adult black males who had been subjects in our previous investigations. The purpose of this study was to determine if insulin resistance could be detected at an early phase of EH. The confounding effects of obesity and carbohydrate intolerance were excluded by enrolling lean males (body mass index [BMI] < 27 kg/m^2) who had a normal oral glucose tolerance test. Subjects were classified as normotensive (systolic < 135, diastolic < 85 mm Hg) or marginal hypertensive (systolic ≥ 135 and/or diastolic ≥ 85 mm Hg). Hypertensives (diastolic > 95 mm Hg) were excluded. Insulin-stimulated glucose uptake was studied using the euglycemic hyperinsulinemic clamp technique ("clamp"). The two groups were matched for age, BMI, and triceps skinfold thickness. Weight was greater in the marginal hypertensives ($p < .05$) as was height. Blood pressures were significantly greater in the marginal hypertensives. The "clamp" method establishes hyperinsulinemia with a steady-state insulin infusion. The primed insulin infusion was calculated to raise the fasting insulin to 100 µU/ml above fasting. Euglycemia was maintained during hyperinsulinemia by a simultaneous glucose infusion. The rate of glucose infusion then becomes an index of sensitivity (or resistance) to the action of insulin. A high glucose infusion rate indicates sensitivity to insulin. A lower glucose infusion rate indicates less sensitivity or resistance to insulin.

Data from these studies are as follows: Fasting glucose was the same in both groups. The "clamped" glucose was also the same and indicated the euglycemia was maintained in both groups. Fasting insulin, although within normal clinical range, was significantly greater in the hypertensives ($p < .05$), despite the small sample size. Insulin-stimulated glucose metabolism (calculated from the glucose infusion rate) at the same degree of steady-state hyperinsulinemia was significantly lower in the marginal hypertensives ($p < .02$). Plasma samples were assayed for catecholamines before insulin infusion and at the completion of the "clamp" period. There was no change in epinephrine or norepinephrine during hyperinsulinemia in either group, and there were no differences between groups. These data provide evidence that the "clamp" procedure did not provoke a stress response in the subjects to confound the results. The catecholamine data also indicate that plasma catecholamine levels alone do not adequately explain the interrelationship between insulin resistance and adrenergic activity. We analyzed the relationship of blood pressure with glucose infusion rate (M) for the entire population (Fig. 3.2) and found a significant negative correlation between M and systolic blood pressure ($p < .01$). Additionally, previous data from each subject on their cardiovascular response to stress were related to the index of insulin-stimulated glucose metabolism. Despite a small sample size, significant correlations again emerged. There was a significant inverse correlation of M with stress systolic pressure ($r = -.685$, $p < 0.01$) and stress diastolic pressure ($r = -.613, p < 0.01$). Therefore, these data do demonstrate a functional relationship of adrenergic activity and insulin resistance.

This preliminary study demonstrated a significantly greater fasting insulin and a significantly reduced insulin-stimulated glucose uptake in young adult males with marginal blood pressure elevation. It provides evidence of insulin resistance at marginal blood pressure elevation in the absence of adiposity and in the absence of carbohydrate intolerance. Although our subjects were all lean, we evaluated further the greater weight in hypertensives. A regression analysis of body weight versus M showed no correlation. BMI and triceps skinfold thickness were not different. The greater weight appeared to

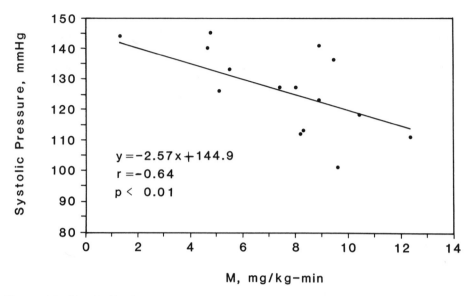

FIGURE 3.2. Systolic blood pressure is correlated with M (insulin-stimulated glucose uptake) for all subjects. Regression analysis demonstrates a significant negative correlation; $p < 0.01$.

be due to greater height rather than greater adipose mass. Each subject had participated in a series of studies beginning at birth and continuing with child and adolescent blood pressure studies. From anthropometric data on each subject at age 20–22 years, percentage muscle mass was calculated (41). This analysis resulted in mean values that were no different between normotensives (38.6 ± 5.2%) and marginal hypertensives (41.7 ± 4.4%). Percentage body fat was also determined (95), resulting in a mean of 13.0 ± 1.8 for the normotensives and 15.5 ± 2.5% for the marginal hypertensives, which was also not different. Therefore, the difference in insulin resistance identified in the marginal hypertensives was not confounded by adipose mass. Our preliminary data have provided evidence of an association of insulin resistance, higher fasting insulin, greater somatic growth rates, and elevated blood pressure in young blacks.

SUMMARY

Longitudinal epidemiological studies have begun to provide some descriptive characterization of children at risk for EH. The genetic effect expressed clinically as a positive family history of EH is a consistent characteristic in children at risk for EH. With the known greater prevalence of EH in adults, it is expected that black children will have a greater risk rate on the basis of family history.

The available data in childhood also indicate that body size and growth rates are major determinants of blood pressure. Children achieving greater stature or greater adiposity have higher blood pressure. Of greater relevance is the question of differential rates of cardiovascular growth. There is now evidence that there may be differences in the peripheral vascular structure in black children. While this evidence is to some degree inferred from studies that have shown high peripheral vascular resistance in black children, the data are consistent with greater vascular reactivity in young blacks.

The role of insulin as a mediator in developmental vascular biology is currently an attractive explanation for the progressive changes in vascular structure and increasing vascular resistance in blacks. It is hypothesized that there exists a primary genetic defect in insulin-stimulated glucose uptake resulting in hyperinsulinemia. Resistance to insulin-stimulated glucose uptake and hyperinsulinemia have been identified in patients with EH and in young adults with borderline hypertension. Hyperinsulinemia may contribute to EH by interacting with the adrenergic nervous system or affecting sodium transport by the kidney or vascular cells. Hyperinsulinemia may also directly affect cardiovascular growth through an anabolic effect of insulin of IGF-I, resulting in structural vascular changes. While this hypothetical pathway may not be unique to blacks, there are sufficient data to suggest that this pathway may play a major role in EH among blacks. Further investigations involving multiple disciplines will be necessary to test this hypothesis.

REFERENCES

1. Abramson, E. A., and R. A. Arky. Role of beta adrenergic receptors in counter regulation to insulin-induced hyperglycemia. *Diabetes 17:* 141–146, 1968.
2. Anderson, N. B., J. D. Lane, M. Muranka, R. B. Williams, and S. J. Houseworth. Racial differences in blood pressure and forearm vascular responses to the cold face stimulus. *Psychosom. Med. 50:* 57–63, 1988.
3. Baumann, R., H. Ziprian, W. Godicke, W. Hartrodt, E. Naumann, and J. Lauter. The influence of acute psychic stress situations and vegetative parameters of essential hypertensives at the early stage of the disease. *Psychother. Psychosom. 22:* 131–137, 1973.
4. Berglund, G., B. Larsson, O. Anderson, O. Larsson, K. Svardsudd, P. Bjorntorp, and L. Wilhelmsen. Body composition and glucose metabolism in hypertensive middle-aged males. *Acta Med. Scand. 200:* 163–169, 1976.
5. Bucher, H., J. Zapf, T. Torresani, A. Prader, E. R. Froesch, and R. Illig. Insulin-like growth factors I and II, prolactin, and insulin in 19 growth hormone-deficient children with excessive, normal, or decreased growth after operation for craniopharyngioma. *N. Engl. J. Med. 309:* 1142–1146, 1983.
6. Burke, G. L., D. S. Freedman, L. S. Webber, and G. S. Berenson. Persistence of high diastolic blood pressure in thin children. The Bogalusa Heart Study. *Hypertension 8:* 24–29, 1986.
7. Burke, G. L., L. S. Webber, S. R. Srinivasan, B. Radhakrishnamurthy, D. S. Freedman, and G. S. Berenson. Fasting plasma glucose and insulin levels and their relationship to cardiovascular risk factors in children: the Bogalusa Heart Study. *Metabolism 35:* 441–446, 1986.
8. Clarke, W. R., R. F. Woolson, and R. M. Lauer. Changes in ponderosity and blood pressure in childhood: the Muscatine Study. *Am. J. Epidemiol. 124:* 195–206, 1986.
9. Clemmon, D. R., and J. J. Van Wyk. Evidence for a functional role of endogenously produced somatomedin-like peptides in the regulation of DNA synthesis in cultured human fibroblasts and porcine smooth muscle cells. *J. Clin. Invest. 75:* 1914–1918, 1985.
10. Comstock, G. W. An epidemiologic study of blood pressure levels in a bi-racial community in the Southern United States. *Am. J. Hyg. 65:* 271–278, 1957.
11. Cornoni-Huntley, J., W. R. Harlan, and P. E. Leaverton. Blood pressure in adolescence. The U.S. Health Examination Survey. *Hypertension 1:* 566–573, 1979.
12. Culpepper, W. S. Cardiac anatomy and function in juvenile hypertension. *Am. J. Med. Sept.:* 57–59, 1983.
13. Culpepper, W. S., P. C. Sodt, F. H. Messerli, D. C. Ruschhaupt, and R. A. Arcilla. Cardiac status in juvenile borderline hypertension. *Ann. Intern. Med. 98:* 1, 1983.
14. Daughaday, W. H., L. S. Phillips, and M. L. Mueller. The effects of insulin and growth

hormone on the release of somatomedin by the isolated rat liver. *Endocrinology 98:* 1214–1219, 1976.

15. DeFronzo, R. A. The effect of insulin on renal sodium metabolism. *Diabetologia 21:* 165–171, 1981.

16. DeFronzo, R. A., M. Goldberg, and Z. S. Agus. The effects of glucose and insulin on renal electrolyte transport. *J. Clin. Invest. 58:* 83–90, 1976.

17. DeLuise, M., G. L. Blackburn, and J. S. Flier. Reduced activity of the red cell sodium-potassium pump in human obesity. *N. Engl. J. Med. 303:* 1017–1022, 1980.

18. DeSweit, M., P. M. Fayers, and E. A. Shineburne. Blood pressure in four and five year old children. The effects of environmental and other factors in its measurement—the Brompton Study. *Hypertension 2:* 501–505, 1984.

19. Diebert, D. C., and R. A. DeFronzo. Epinephrine-induced insulin resistance in man. *J. Clin. Invest. 65:* 717–721, 1980.

20. Dimsdale, J. E., R. Grahm, M. G. Ziegler, R. Zusman, and C. C. Berry. Age, race, diagnosis, and sodium effects on the pressor response to infused norepinephrine. *Hypertension 10:* 564–569, 1987.

21. Eigenmann, J. E., J. Patterson, J. Zapf, and E. R. Froesch. Insulin-like growth factor I in the dog: a study of different dog breeds and in dogs with growth hormone elevation. *Acta Endocrinol. (Copenh.) 105:* 294–301, 1984.

22. Falkner, B., and H. Kushner. Race differences in stress induced reactivity in young adults. *Health Psychol. 8(5):* 613–627, 1989.

23. Falkner, B., and H. Kushner. The effect of chronic sodium loading on the cardiovascular response to stress in young blacks and whites. *Hypertension 15:* 36–43, 1990.

24. Falkner, B., G. Onesti, E. T. Angelakos, M. Fernandez, and C. Langman. Cardiovascular response to mental stress in normal adolescence with hypertensive parents. *Hypertension 1:* 23–29, 1979.

25. Falkner, B., H. Kushner, G. Onesti, and E. T. Angelakos. Cardiovascular characteristics in adolescents who develop essential hypertension. *Hypertension 3:* 251–256, 1981.

26. Falkner, B., D. T. Lowenthal, M. B. Affrime, and B. Hamstra. R wave amplitude during aerobic exercise in hypertensive adolescents following treatment. *Am. J. Cardiol. 51:* 459–463, 1983.

27. Falkner, B., D. T. Lowenthal, M. B. Affrime, and B. Hamstra. R wave amplitude changes in hypertensive children. *Am. J. Cardiol. 50:* 152–156, 1982.

28. Ferrannini, E., G. Buzzigoli, R. Bonadonna, M. A. Giorico, M. Oleggini, L. Graziadei, R. Pedrinelli, L. Brandi, and S. Bevilacqua. Insulin resistance in essential hypertension. *N. Engl. J. Med. 317:* 350–357, 1987.

29. Florey, C. V., S. Uppal, and S. Lowy. Relation between blood pressure, weight, and plasma sugar and serum insulin levels in school children aged 9–12 years in Westland Holland. *Br. Med. J. 1:* 1368–1371, 1976.

30. Folkow, B. Physiological aspects of primary hypertension. *Physiol. Rev. 62:* 347–504, 1982.

31. Fournier, A. M., M. T. Gadia, D. B. Kubrusly, J. S. Skyler, and J. M. Sosenko. Blood pressure, insulin, and glycemia in non diabetic subjects. *Am. J. Med. 80:* 861–864, 1986.

32. Fredrickson, M. Racial differences in cardiovascular reactivity to mental stress in essential hypertension. *J. Hypertens. 4:* 325–331, 1986.

33. Froesch, E. R., and J. Zapf. Insulin-like growth factors and insulin: comparative aspects. *Diabetologia 28:* 485–493, 1985.

34. Garay, R. P., C. Nazaret, P. Hannaert, and M. Price. Abnormal Na, K cotransport function in a group of patients with essential hypertension. *Eur. J. Clin. Invest. 13:* 311–320, 1983.

35. Gillum, R. F. Pathophysiology of hypertension in blacks and whites. *Hypertension 1:* 468–475, 1979.

36. Goldring, D., A. Hernandez, S. Choi, J. Y. Lee, S. Londe, F. T. Lindgren, and R. M. Barton. Blood pressure in a high school population. II. *Clin. J. Pediatr. 95:* 298–303, 1979.

37. Goldstein, D. S. Plasma catecholamines and essential hypertension: an analytical review. *Hypertension 5:* 86–90, 1983.

38. Goldstein, D. S., C. R. Lake, B. Chernow, M. G. Ziegler, M. D. Coleman, A. A. Taylor, J. R. Mitchell, I. J. Kopin, and H. R. Keiser. Age dependence of hypertensive-normotensive differences in plasma norepinephrine. *Hypertension 5:* 100–104, 1983.

39. Hallbach, M. Interaction of central autonomic hypersensitivity and environmental stimuli: importance for development of spontaneously hypertensive rats. In: Regulation of Blood Pressure by the Central Nervous System, edited by G. Onesti, M. Fernandez, and K. Kim. Grune & Stratton, New York, 1976, p. 129.

40. Harlan, W. R., J. Cornoni-Huntley, and P. E. Leaverton. Blood pressure in childhood. The National Health Examination Survey. *Hypertension 1:* 599–604, 1979.

41. Heymsfield, S. B., C. McManus, V. Stevens, and J. Smith. Muscle mass as a reliable indication of protein-energy malnutrition severity and outcome. *Am. J. Clin. Nutr. 35:* 1192–1199, 1982.

42. Hilton, P. J. Cellular sodium transport in essential hypertension. *N. Engl. J. Med. 314:* 222–229, 1986.

43. Julius, S. Borderline hypertension: an overview. *Med. Clin. North Am. 61:* 595–605, 1977.

44. Kaiser, N., A. Tur-Sinai, M. Hasin, and E. Cerasi. Binding, degradation and biological activity of insulin in vascular smooth muscle cells. *Am. J. Physiol. 249* (Endocrinol. Metab. 12): E292–E298, 1985.

45. Katz, S. H., M. C. Hediger, J. I. Schall, E. J. Bowers, W. F. Barker, S. Aurand, P. B. Ebelith, A. B. Gruskin, and J. S. Parks. Blood pressure, growth and maturation from childhood to adolescence. *Hypertension 2*(Suppl): I-55–61, 1980.

46. Katz, S. L., M. L. Hediger, B. S. Zemel, and J. S. Parks. Blood pressure, body fat, and dehydroepiandrosterone sulfate variation in adolescence. *Hypertension 8:* 277–284, 1986.

47. King, G. L., D. Goodman, S. Buzney, A. Moses, and C. R. Kahn. Receptors and growth-promoting effects of insulin and insulin-like growth factors on cells from bovine retinal capillaries and aorta. *J. Clin. Invest. 75:* 1028–1036, 1985.

48. Kushner, H., and B. Falkner. A harmonic analysis of cardiac response of normotensive and hypertensive adolescents during stress. *J. Hum. Stress 7:* 21–27, 1981.

49. Laird, W. P., and D. E. Fixler. Left ventricular hypertrophy in adolescents with elevated blood pressure: assessment by chest roentgenography, electrocardiography, and echocardiography. *Pediatrics 67:* 255–259, 1981.

50. Lauer, R. M., and W. R. Clark. A longitudinal view of blood pressure during childhood: the Muscatine Study. *Stat. Med. 7:* 47–57, 1988.

51. Lauer, R. M., A. R. Anderson, R. Beaglehole, and T. L. Burns. Factors related to tracking of blood pressure in children. U.S. National Center for Health Statistics Health Examination Surveys Cycles II and III. *Hypertension 6:* 307–314, 1984.

52. Lauer, R. M., W. R. Clarke, and R. Beaglehole. Level, trend and variability of blood pressure during childhood: the Muscatine Study. *Circulation 69:* 242–249, 1984.

53. Lawler, K. A., and M. T. Allen. Risk factors for hypertension in children: their relationship to psychophysiologic responses. *J. Psychosom. Res. 23:* 199–204, 1981.

54. Light, K. C., and P. A. Obrist. Cardiovascular reactivity to behavioral stress in young males with and without marginally elevated causal systolic pressures: comparison of clinic, home, and laboratory measures. *Hypertension 2:* 802–809, 1980.

55. Light, K. C., and P. A. Obrist. Cardiovascular reactivity to behavioral stress in young males with and without marginally elevated casual systolic pressure: a comparison of clinic, home, and laboratory measures. *Psychophysiology 19:* 481–489, 1982.

56. Light, K. C., P. A. Obrist, A. Sherwood, S. A. James, and D. S. Strogatz. Effects of race and marginally elevated blood pressure on responses to stress. *Hypertension 10:* 555–563, 1987.

57. Londe, S., J. J. Bourgoignie, A. M. Robson, and D. Goldring. Hypertension in apparently normal children. *J. Pediatr. 78:* 569–573, 1971.

58. Luft, F. C., C. E. Grim, J. T. Higgins, Jr., and M. H. Weinberger. Differences in response to sodium administration in normotensive white and black subjects. *J. Lab. Clin. Med. 90:* 555–562, 1977.

59. Mahoney, L. T., W. R. Clarke, A. L. Mark, and R. M. Lauer. Forearm vascular resistance in the upper and lower quartiles of blood pressure in adolescent boys. *Pediatr. Res. 16:* 163–166, 1982.

60. Manicardi, V., L. Camellini, G. Bellodi, C. Caselli, and E. Ferrannini. Evidence for an association of high blood pressure and hyperinsulinemia in obese man. *J. Clin. Endocrinol. Metab. 62:* 1302–1304, 1986.

61. Manuck, S. B., and J. M. Proietti. Parental hypertension and cardiovascular response to cognitive and isometric challenge. *Psychophysiology 19:* 481–489, 1982.

62. Masuo, K., T. Ogihara, Y. Kumahara, A. Yamatodani, and H. Wada. Increased plasma norepinephrine in young patients with essential hypertension under three sodium intakes. *Hypertension 6:* 315–321, 1984.

63. Merimee, T. J., J. Zapf, and E. R. Froesch. Insulin-like growth factors (IGFs) in pygmies and subjects with the pygmy trait: characterization of the metabolic actions of IGF-I and IGF-II in man. *J. Clin. Endocrinol. Metab. 55:* 1081–1087, 1982.

64. Merimee, T. J., J. Zapf, B. Hewlett, and L. L. Cavalli-Forza. Insulin-like growth factors in pygmies. *N. Engl. J. Med. 316:* 906–911, 1987.

65. Modan, M., H. Halkin, S. Almog, A. Lusky, A. Eshkol, M. Shefi, A. Shitrit, and Z. Fuehs. Hyperinsulinemia: a link between hypertension, obesity and glucose intolerance. *J. Clin. Invest. 75:* 809–817, 1985.

66. Moore, R. D. Effects of insulin ion transport. *Biochim. Biophys. Acta 737:* 1–49, 1983.
67. Mott, D. M., R. L. Clark, W. J. Andrews, and J. E. Foley. Insulin resistant Na pump activity in adipocytes from obese humans. *Am. J. Physiol. 249 (Endocrinol. Metab. 12):* E160–164, 1985.
68. Munger, R. G., R. J. Prineas, and O. Gomez-Marin. Persistent elevation of blood pressure among children with a family history of hypertension: the Minneapolis Children's Blood Pressure Study. *J. Hypertens. 6:* 647–653, 1988.
69. Murphy, J. K., B. S. Alpert, D. M. Moes, and G. W. Somes. Race and cardiovascular reactivity, a neglected relationship. *Hypertension 8:* 1075–1083, 1986.
70. National Health Survey, Blood pressure of adults by race and area in the United States, 1960–1962, National Center for Health Statistics Series II, No. 5, Washington, D.C., U.S. Department of Health, Education and Welfare, 1964.
71. National Health Survey, Blood pressure of persons 18–74 years in the United States, 1971–1972, National Center for Health Statistics Series II, No. 150, Washington, D.C., U.S. Department of Health, Education and Welfare, 1975.
72. Nestle, P. J. Blood pressure and catecholamine excretion after mental stress in labile hypertension. *Lancet 1:* 692–698, 1969.
73. Prineas, R. J., R. S. Gillum, H. Horibe, and P. F. Hannan. Minneapolis Children's Blood Pressure Study. Part II. Multiple determinants of blood pressure. *Hypertension 2*(Suppl): I-24–31, 1980.
74. Reaven, G. M., and B. B. Hoffman. A role for insulin in the aetiology and course of hypertension. *Lancet 2:* 435–436, 1987.
75. Report of the Task Force on Blood Pressure Control in Children. *Pediatrics 58*(Suppl): 797–810, 1977.
76. Rocchini, A. P., Katch, A. Schork, and R. P. Kelch. Insulin and blood pressure during weight loss in obese adolescents. *Hypertension 10:* 267–273, 1987.
77. Rosenbaum, P. A., R. C. Elston, S. R. Srinivasan, L. S. Weber, and G. S. Berenson. Cardiovascular risk factors from birth to 7 years of age: the Bogalusa Heart Study. Predictive value of parental measures in determining cardiovascular risk factor variables in early life. *Pediatrics 80:* 807–816, 1987.
78. Rowe, J. W., J. B. Young, K. L. Minaker, A. L. Stevens, J. Pallotta, and L. Landsberg. *Diabetes 30:* 219–225, 1981.
79. Safar, M. E., Y. A. Weiss, J. A. Levenson, G. M. London, and P. L. Milliez. Hemodynamic study of 85 patients with borderline hypertension. *Am. J. Cardiol. 31:* 315–322, 1973.
80. Schieken, R. M., W. R. Clarke, and R. M. Lauer. Left ventricular hypertrophy in children with blood pressure in the upper quartiles of distribution. The Muscatine Study. *Hypertension 3:* 669–675, 1981.
81. Schieken, R. M., W. R. Clarke, and R. M. Lauer. The cardiovascular response to exercise in children across the blood pressure distribution. The Muscatine Study. *Hypertension 5:* 71–79, 1983.
82. Shear, C. L., G. L. Burke, D. S. Freedman, and G. S. Berenson. Value of childhood blood pressure measurements and family history in predicting future blood pressure status: results from 8 years of follow-up in the Bogalusa Heart Study. *Pediatrics 77:* 862–869, 1986.
83. Sloan, I., P. Saul, and I. Bihler. Influence of adrenalin or sugar transport in soleus, a red skeletal muscle. *Mol. Cell. Endocrinol. 10:* 3–12, 1978.
84. Smoak, C. G., G. L. Burke, L. S. Webber, D. W. Harsha, S. R. Srinivasan, and G. S. Berenson. Relation of obesity to clustering of cardiovascular disease risk factors in children and young adults. *Am. J. Epidemiol. 125:* 364–372, 1987.
85. Soto, L. F., D. A. Kitcuchi, R. A. Arcilla, D. D. Savage, and G. S. Berenson. Echocardiographic functions and blood pressure levels in children and young adults from a biracial population. The Bogalusa Heart Study. *Am. J. Med. Sci. 297:* 271–279, 1989.
86. Task Force on Blood Pressure Control in Children. Report of the Second Task Force on Blood Pressure Control in Children, 1987. *Pediatrics 79:* 1–25, 1987.
87. Vital Statistics of the United States, 1973, Vol. II. Mortality Pathology U.S. Department of Health, Education and Welfare. Public Health Service, National Center for Health Statistics, 1977.
88. Voors, A. W., T. A. Foster, R. R. Frerichs, L. S. Weber, and G. S. Berenson. Studies of blood pressure in children ages 5–14 years in a total bi-racial community. *Circulation 54:* 319–347, 1976.
89. Voors, A. W., L. S. Webber, D. H. Harsha, and G. S. Berenson. Racial differences in cardiovascular risk factors of youth. Bogalusa Heart Study. Abstracts of 18th Annual Conference on Cardiovascular Disease, Epidemiology. Dallas, Am. Heart Assoc., 1978.
90. Voors, A. W., B. Radhakrishnamurthy, S. R. Srinivasan, L. S. Webber, and G. S. Berenson.

Plasma glucose level related to blood pressure in 272 children ages 7–15 years sampled from a total biracial population. *Am. J. Epidemiol. 113:* 347–356, 1981.

91. Voors, A. W., L. S. Webber, and G. S. Berenson. Time cost study of blood pressure in children over a three year period. *Hypertension 2*(Suppl): I-102–108, 1980.

92. Walass, O., and E. Walass. Effects of epinephrine on rat diaphragm. *J. Biol. Chem. 187:* 769–776, 1950.

93. Weinberger, M. H., J. Z. Miller, F. C. Luft, C. E. Grim, and N. S. Fineberg. Definitions and characteristics of sodium sensitivity and blood pressure resistance. *Hypertension 8*(Suppl II): II-127–II-134, 1986.

94. Wilson, S. L., A. Gaffney, W. P. Laird, and D. E. Fixler. Body size, composition, and fitness in adolescents with elevated blood pressure. *Hypertension 7:* 417–422, 1985.

95. Wormsley, J., and J. V. Durnin. A comparison of the skinfold method with extent of over-weight and various height-weight relationships in assessment of obesity. *Br. J. Nutr. 38:* 271–284, 1977.

96. Zinner, S. A., P. S. Levy, and E. H. Kass. Family aggregation of blood pressure in childhood. *N. Engl. J. Med. 283:* 461, 1971.

III

THE CONTEXTUAL MODEL . . .
SOCIOCULTURAL AND
PSYCHOSOCIAL DIMENSIONS

4

Social and Cultural Dimensions of Hypertension in Blacks: Underlying Mechanisms

WILLIAM W. DRESSLER

The role of social and psychosocial factors in the etiology of essential hypertension has been seriously entertained for over 50 years. In the initial volume of the journal *Psychosomatic Medicine,* Alexander (2) first formulated the hypothesis that a neurotic coping style characterized by chronic suppression of hostile feelings could be a precursor of hypertension. Since then, a host of psychological and personality variables have been investigated as potential hypertension risk factors (44). More recently there has been a resurgence of interest in suppressed, or, as it has come to be referred to, "cynical" hostility, and elevated blood pressure (42). The consistency and weight of these empirical findings leaves little doubt that there is an underlying mechanism in essential hypertension that is bound up in the behavior and emotion of the individual; at the same time, however, research has largely proceeded in piecemeal fashion, investigating this or that psychological trait in small clinical samples and ignoring the social profile of blood pressure within and between larger social groups.

The social patterning of blood pressure was observed at about the same time as Alexander's suppressed hostility hypothesis emerged. Donnison (discussed by Henry and Cassel [28]) worked as a physician in East Africa during the 1920s. He was struck by the fact that he could find no cases of hypertension among early 2,000 hospital admissions. The tribal groups among whom he worked had not yet been seriously affected by culture change accompanying colonialism, and he attributed the lack of hypertension to these stable social patterns. In modern society, on the other hand, the rapid rate of culture change results in dramatic changes in patterns of social relationships, changes to which people as they age find it increasingly difficult to adapt. It was to this difficulty in social adjustment that Donnison attributed the rise of blood pressure with age in industrial societies, and hence the incidence of hypertension.

Any model of the pathophysiology of hypertension must link the broad social profile of blood pressure to individual-level processes that result in sustained disease. The aim of this chapter is to review a program of research that was developed in the study of hypertension and culture change, and that helps to account for both social profile and individual response. Furthermore, because of the specific nature of the model, it helps to account for the problem to

69

which this volume is centrally addressed: the increased risk of hypertension within black populations. This model will be referred to as a "sociocultural model of hypertension." At the outset, basic observations on the social patterning of blood pressure that serve as a background to the model will be reviewed. Next, this sociocultural model of hypertension will be reviewed, first in terms of its development and second in application to understanding hypertension in a black community. The possible intervening physiological mechanisms that link social relationships, individual behavior, and cardiovascular response will then be discussed. Finally, the chapter concludes with a discussion of the implications of these ideas for future research.

SOCIAL PROFILING OF BLOOD PRESSURE: BASIC OBSERVATIONS

Henry and Cassel (28) provided an extensive review of research on blood pressure in societies outside North America and Europe. They found that societies maintaining a traditional way of life had population average blood pressures that were lower than those observed in industrial societies. Furthermore, in societies in which a traditional way of life was maintained there was little or no correlation between age and blood pressure within the population.

Waldron and her associates (46) further systematized these observations by merging data on population average blood pressures with data on societal characteristics from the Human Relations Area Files (HRAF). HRAF is a data bank with information on over 3,000 societies throughout the world. Available data include technological, economic, social structural, political, and belief-system characteristics. There was a total of 84 studies of blood pressure in non-Western societies for which HRAF data were available. The most important test performed on these data was the correlation of population average blood pressure with subsistence technology/economy. Ratings on the latter ranged from hunting and gathering at the most basic level, to an industrial technology/economy at the most elaborate level. It was found that as the technological/economic base of the societies became more complicated and elaborate, population average blood pressure increased. Also, the slope of the regression of blood pressure on age was coded for each of the 84 studies. This also increased with elaboration of the societies' technology/economy.

This research serves as a striking confirmation of one component of the epidemiological transition. It shows that as societies develop or modernize, the risk of chronic disease, especially cardiovascular disease, becomes greater. Several other findings of note emerged from the study by Waldron et al. (46). First, these findings were observed for both males and females, and for different age groups. Second, where it was possible, population average body mass indices and sodium intake were coded; controlling for these factors made no difference. Third, the increase in blood pressure was not constant over the levels of social development. Rather, there was a sharp increase in blood pressure between societies with economies based primarily on extensive but still nonmarket agriculture, and those societies with extensive, unmechanized, market-oriented agricultural technologies. It is within these latter societies, where social class differences begin to emerge most clearly, that Waldron et al. (46) found a significant correlation between degree of economic competition between classes and blood pressure.

This cross-cultural survey converges with the well-known epidemiological observation of an inverse relationship between "socioeconomic status" and cardiovascular disease in industrial societies. This relationship is most evident in prospective studies of coronary heart disease mortality, in which there is an increased risk of mortality among those persons in the lowest socioeconomic strata (34). This relationship has also been observed in epidemiological studies of hypertension, especially in relation to one indicator of socioeconomic status, education. Those persons with less than a high school education have significantly higher rates of hypertension and higher average blood pressures than persons with some college education or more (29).

Profiling blood pressure by culture and social class is directly relevant to understanding black–white differences in blood pressure. Average blood pressures and rates of hypertension are lower in black communities in Africa in rural areas or areas in which a more traditional way of life is maintained (10). In urban areas in Africa, and in most black communities in the Western Hemisphere, blood pressures and rates of hypertension are substantially higher, such that rates of hypertension in urban North American black communities are the highest in the world (26).

Within African-American samples, there is an inverse relationship between socioeconomic status and blood pressure, with socioeconomic status measured both as education and as a composite of education and occupation (29–31). This inverse relationship is of the same magnitude as that observed in white samples, although at any given socioeconomic level, blacks have higher rates of hypertension than whites. Also, this inverse relationship is still observed when age, sex, and the body mass index are statistically controlled.

The relationship of socioeconomic status and blood pressure has also been examined in communities in Africa and the West Indies, with some surprising results. In some studies the familiar inverse relationship is observed, whereas in others there is a direct relationship between socioeconomic status and blood pressure (10,15). A similar confusing pattern of results has emerged in studies of skin color and blood pressure within black communities. In some studies, controlling for socioeconomic status reduces to insignificance the blood pressure differences between darker and lighter-skinned black people (30,31); in other studies, controlling for socioeconomic status makes no difference, and darker-skinned blacks have significantly higher blood pressures than lighter-skinned blacks (5,27).

In general, these findings suggest that social and cultural factors contribute substantially to variation in blood pressure and rates of hypertension within and between populations. Specifically, blood pressures vary considerably by indices of social class or socioeconomic status. At the same time, however, this relationship is not nearly as straightforward as it is usually supposed to be. This is evident in the way in which the blood pressure–social class relationship varies between different societies. Therefore, there is a phenomenon awaiting explanation, but the way in which the problem is currently conceptualized, the ways in which variables are measured, and the specification of models, all need refinement.

What is it about social class that influences the population pattern of hypertension? Conventional wisdom would have it that lower-class individuals smoke and drink more, and consume a more imprudent diet both with respect to caloric intake and the intake of specific food items (e.g., salt), which in turn leads to higher blood pressure (25). When blood pressure is adjusted for these factors, however, social class differences persist, although these differences are attenuated (39). Similarly, an increase in alcohol and tobacco consumption and the intake of sodium and fat accompanies social development or modernization, but where these factors have been controlled for, societal differences in blood pressure persist (10,46).

Another alternative is that the lower class has unequal (less) access to medical care compared with the upper class, which in turn results in poor health (25). One could also account for the emergence of cardiovascular disease in the process of modernization if it were argued that this situation is primarily a reflection of social inequalities; that is, the higher rates of cardiovascular disease in industrial societies might be a function of higher rates in lower-class groups who lack access to health care. If, however, societies are compared in which health care is made available to the lower class through national health care schemes, the socioeconomic gradient in hypertension is still observed (34,39).

This finding has led some to argue that sociocultural and class differences in "psychological stress" are the cause of the social profile of blood pressure. It has been argued that life in modern society, and especially within lower social classes, is inherently more stressful than life in traditional society or upper classes. There are two main difficulties with this argument. First, although it is assumed that life in less complex societies is less stressful, there is ample "stress" in traditional society (36). Second, "stress" is a problematic concept in a number of ways. Although the problems with the concept have been discussed extensively (35,49), one important difficulty involves the leap of inference required to go from the concept of social class to any concept of stress. The leap here requires that we focus on only one hypothetical correlate of class—namely, psychological stress—in the broad array of social and behavioral factors that are entailed by class differences and that might be implicated in the etiology of hypertension. Furthermore, it requires that this one factor be an intrapsychic factor that is notoriously difficult to measure reliably.

In general, then, current approaches to explaining cultural and class differences in hypertension or average blood pressure have either proven to be inadequate empirically (conventional risk factors, access to medical care), or to be problematic conceptually (psychological stress). New approaches are needed. Haan and colleagues (25) suggest that a useful starting point would be a more thorough investigation of the demands placed on individuals in lower classes or developing societies and the resources that persons can bring to bear in meeting those demands. This is, in short, a call for the direct investigation of the dimensions of social class and class-related behaviors, rather than to assume that social class or modernization is a proxy variable for some other etiologic factor.

This has in fact been the approach taken in a series of studies of blood pressure in developing societies, one that has been extended to the investigation of hypertension within the black community in the United States. Two assumptions guided this research. First, it was assumed that social change and modernization placed specific social and behavioral demands on individuals, and that those demands could be identified and quantified. Second, it was assumed that in part those demands, and the resources individuals have to meet those demands, would be a function of the specific cultural context in which social change took place. These assumptions provided an orientation for the development of a sociocultural model of hypertension. The derivation and empirical evaluation of this model will be reviewed.

SOCIOCULTURAL MODEL OF HYPERTENSION

The investigation of blood pressure within societies undergoing culture change or modernization, or of migrants from traditional to more modernized communities, has been seen as a potentially useful research design for discovering factors of etiologic significance for hypertension (10). Most such studies have approached modernization as though there was a single continuum between traditional, tribal societies, on the one hand, and modern, industrial societies, on the other. In terms of the social epidemiology of hypertension, the task of the researcher was to discover what social or behavioral characteristics were "added on" to communities or individuals as the trajectory of modernization proceeded; hence, this model has been referred to as an "accretion model" of modernization (21). In general, the use of this model has shown that as individuals become more involved in a wage labor economy; as they receive more Western education; as they gain fluency in nonlocal languages; and, as they come to interact socially less in the context of traditional family and kinship and more in the context of nonkin, nontraditional relationships, blood pressure tends to rise (10,37). These variables can be measured on individuals, or they can be used to contrast communities and average blood pressures between communities. The correlations of modernization and blood pressure persist when age, gender, and obesity are controlled; however, the magnitude of the association tends to be small.

It has become increasingly clear that this unidimensional model fails to account adequately for what is occurring in contemporary developing societies. Many societies have been unable to develop any sort of meaningful industrial economy. In societies that have developed substantial industrial economies (e.g., Brazil), there have also developed staggering foreign debts and high rates of unemployment and inflation. This has led some to emphasize the "dependency" of developing societies on fully industrialized nations, and the interlocking, systemic nature of development and underdevelopment (48). Any research attempting to examine characteristics and behaviors that are related to the risk of cardiovascular disease must do so from a perspective that acknowledges that individual modernization occurs in these contexts of social and economic change. A research approach that treats particular traits as "modern," and that distinguishes among individuals as having few or many of these traits, is unlikely to identify accurately more than a small portion of individual variability in blood pressure.

Another difficulty with a unidimensional perspective is that it fails to take account of the cultural factors or social relationships within traditional society that might counterbalance the disruptive effects of culture change. In many respects the process of modernization or development can be seen as the penetration of Western, market-oriented values into local communities organized along more traditional lines, which means that within local communities there will be a variety of responses to these changes, responses that may alter the nature of the change and hence the disease risk.

CULTURAL CHANGE AND HYPERTENSION RISK

Adopting the perspective outlined here, research on modernization and blood pressure was undertaken in St. Lucia, an island in the eastern Caribbean (8,9). St. Lucia is one of the smaller islands of the Lesser Antilles and, like its neighbors, is quite mountainous. Originally settled by the French, it came under British colonial domination in the early nineteenth century, becoming fully independent in 1978. The majority of St. Lucia's population is African Caribbean, descended from slaves brought there to work on sugar plantations. As in other Western Hemisphere black societies, hypertension and its sequelae are becoming significant health problems in St. Lucia.

The effective conditions of the plantation economy persisted in St. Lucia until very recently. Basically this meant a system of two social classes organized society. On the one hand, there was a small upper class of land owners, businessmen, professionals, and civil servants who controlled the economic and political life of the island. On the other hand, there was a vast lower class of unskilled laborers and domestic servants who supplied the human labor to run the economic system. Upward social mobility was essentially unheard of, and with the exception of a very few small-scale businessmen, there was no middle class.

Around the time of the Second World War, these conditions began to change as a result of the confluence of a variety of factors. Most important among these was the introduction of a new cash crop (bananas) that did not require the large-scale capital investment of sugar cane. This meant that laborers, if they had access to a piece of land, could personally participate in the national economy. Coupled with other innovations in the economy and postwar foreign aid, there was an expansion of opportunities for upward social mobility, relative to the complete lack of opportunity that existed before.

Aspirations for a new way of life expanded within the population, but at a rate higher than it was possible for the economy to absorb. Smith, writing of Puerto Rico, described the nature of these new aspirations:

> "Modernization" is closely bound up with "Americanization;" this is the case for most Caribbean societies, even in the absence of direct political ties. . . . The image of the "admirable man" toward which everyone strives each in his own way, is increasingly the man who lives the good life of mass consumption society in the way depicted by advertising agencies. Commercial television, films, and newspaper and magazine advertising all try to give a local cast to "the image" but it comes out basically North American (40).

In other words, higher social status or prestige came to be associated with the accumulation of consumer goods and the adoption of behaviors perceived to be associated with the middle classes in industrial societies, as these are depicted in the media. The importance of these behaviors as indicators of social status have been long recognized in the sociological literature (45,47), and the term "lifestyle" was originally coined (nearly a century ago) to describe this dimension of class behavior. What is striking about the process in a developing society like St. Lucia is that persons' aspirations for a high status lifestyle can expand very quickly, and their struggle to attain such a lifestyle can begin; however, the slowly expanding economy of a developing society is unlikely to provide the real opportunities for upward mobility in the occupational class system that can provide the economic resources to sustain those aspirations. Therefore, it is inevitable that some persons will be attempting to maintain a high status lifestyle in the context of low occupational class, and the resulting conflict may lead to higher blood pressure.

The hypothesis was tested on a sample (n = 100) of 40–49 year olds from a community in St. Lucia. Lifestyle was measured with a 12-item index assessing acquisition of consumer culture, including owning a radio, a stereo, an automobile, imported furniture, and similar items. Occupational class was assessed with a six-category ranking from unskilled laborer (lower class) to professional (e.g., teacher, higher class). When the two factors were dichotomized and cross-tabulated, those persons with a higher lifestyle and lower occupational class had the highest systolic and diastolic blood pressure, adjusted for age, sex, and the body mass index ($p < .03$), as shown in Table 4.1. This test provided initial support for the hypothesis that an incongruity between lifestyle and occupational class is a risk factor for elevated blood pressure in the context of a society undergoing modernization.

The next study in which this hypothesis was examined was carried out in a town in central Mexico, approximately 100 miles northwest of Mexico City (21). In this study the measurement of lifestyle and occupational class was considerably improved. The lifestyle scale was expanded to a total of 38 items, 26 of which assessed ownership of material goods. An additional 12 items were respondent reports of behaviors such as reading magazines, watching television, and attending the cinema; in short, items that increase individual expo-

TABLE 4.1. Blood Pressure and Occupational Class and Material Lifestyle in St. Lucia

Class/lifestyle	Blood pressure	
	Systolic	Diastolic
Low occupational class/ low material lifestyle	135.3	86.3
Low occupational class/ high material lifestyle	142.5[a]	90.5[a]
High occupational class/ low material lifestyle	130.0	80.3
High occupational class/ high material lifestyle	132.6	85.7

[a]Significantly different from other categories ($p < .03$).
From Dressler (8).

sure to messages reinforcing the link between lifestyle and prestige. The measurement of occupational class was also refined, taking into account that within developing societies the achievement of a higher occupational class usually entails having multiple persons employed in the home and the pooling of economic resources. Therefore a household measure of occupational class was developed.

The statistical model for testing the hypothesis was also refined. The hypothesis states that as the attempt to maintain a high status lifestyle exceeds occupational class (or available economic resources), blood pressure will be higher. Operationally, this can be measured as a difference score between lifestyle and occupational class, taking direction into account. In the refined measurement, both lifestyle and occupational class could be treated as metric variables and standardized to the same scale; then, occupational class could simply be subtracted from lifestyle. The resulting difference score had a mean of zero, a standard deviation of 10, and was normally distributed. Positive scores were indicative of lifestyle exceeding occupational class; negative scores were indicative of occupational class exceeding lifestyle.

The measurement of blood pressure was also refined in this study. In St. Lucia, the auscultatory method of measurement of blood pressure was used (although all blood pressures were measured by a single observer), and three readings were averaged for each individual. In Mexico, an automated device (Dinamap Model 845XT) was used. This device eliminated many of the problems associated with the auscultatory method, and again, three readings were averaged. In a sample of 147 persons, lifestyle incongruity was associated with higher systolic and diastolic blood pressure, and this association was independent of age, sex, and the body mass index.

The hypothesis was investigated next in a study conducted in Brazil (22). There are several aspects of this study that are of special interest. First, it was carried out in an urban center (population of over 400,000 persons) in one of the more economically successful states (Sao Paulo), in one of the most developed among developing countries. Second, all of the methodological improvements from the study in Mexico were carried over to the study in Brazil. Third, data on dietary intake were collected in Brazil. Specifically, four 24-hour dietary recalls were obtained from each person in the sample (n = 129). These were converted to nutrient intake using standard procedures, and then the nutrient intakes were averaged for each individual. This method helps to reduce the problem of intraindividual variability in estimating nutrient intake. And fourth, a variety of social and psychological variables were included in the analysis to see if these might compromise the effect of lifestyle incongruity. Some were self-explanatory (e.g., education, family income, level of debt); one was a measure of relative deprivation, or the degree to which the respondent perceived himself or herself to be relatively worse off financially at the time of the data collection than 5 years earlier.

In a multiple regression analysis, age, sex, and the body mass index were forced into the equation first. Lifestyle incongruity, the social–psychological variables, and a variety of nutritional variables were then allowed to enter on a stepwise basis. No variables entered the equation for systolic blood pressure. For diastolic blood pressure the following variables entered in the following order: lifestyle incongruity, perceived stress, calcium intake, and total fat intake. Again, the lifestyle incongruity hypothesis was confirmed, this time controlling for dietary variables measured in a technically sophisticated way. Therefore, however the effect of incongruity is mediated, it is not a result of differences in dietary intake.

These observations do not suggest that dietary patterns are unrelated to lifestyle or occupational class. In the Brazilian sample, calcium intake is associated with higher occupational class ($r = .27, p < .01$) and higher lifestyle ($r = .34, p < .002$). Fat intake is associated with lifestyle incongruity ($r = .17, p < .05$). This latter finding is not unanticipated in the sense that the consumption of certain kinds of high fat and processed foods is a component of a high status lifestyle. What one eats is a measure of one's status just as a car or any other material item can be. But while diet and lifestyle are related in the same social process, these factors have independent effects on blood pressure.

Perhaps even more striking is the independence of the effects of lifestyle incongruity from other social and psychological factors. The only psychosocial variable with a significant effect on blood pressure is perceived stress. This is a unidimensional scale in which the respondent rates the amount of change in daily life perceived to be associated with a variety of common life events, such as marriage, getting or losing a job, death of a spouse, and others. It is a measure of perceived sensitivity to change and personal efficacy, and it is independent of lifestyle incongruity. (Subsequent analyses of the St. Lucian data (11) also demonstrated independence of incongruity and perceived stress.) Other social–psychological variables, including income, education, and relative deprivation, failed to enter the analysis, either on their own or after other variables were entered and controlled. The failure of the relative deprivation scale to enter the analysis is particularly instructive, because conventional notions of "stress" would suggest that persons who are struggling to maintain a high status lifestyle in a lower class context would *feel* deprived, frustrated, and pessimistic about the future. In fact, there is an inverse relationship between lifestyle incongruity and relative deprivation ($r = -.21, p < .01$); that is, persons with larger incongruities *feel* less deprived but actually have higher blood pressure. Therefore, the effect of lifestyle incongruity is mediated in a way that is out of the conscious awareness of the individual.

PROTECTIVE DIMENSIONS OF CULTURE

The notion that social and cultural factors may protect individuals from developing high blood pressure or other health problems has been discussed by a number of authors, notably Cassel (3). A major protective dimension suggested by Cassel was social support. This factor has been defined in a variety of ways, but for our purposes social support will be defined as the perception or belief that there are persons to whom an individual can turn for help or assistance in times of felt need. At times, the operational definition of social support may consist simply of the presence or absence (or number) of significant social relationships reported by an individual; this is more appropriately thought of as social integration. In some studies social support or social integration has been found to lower the risk of cardiovascular disease directly; in others it has been found to be significant only among persons exposed to a risk-enhancing situation or event (4).

This cultural dimension was investigated within each of the studies discussed here. It was also assumed that the salient dimensions of social support would vary considerably across different cultural contexts. In St. Lucia, unique features of the West Indian family were investigated (7,8). Students of West Indian kinship have pointed out that marriage, child-bearing, and household formation are separate events that follow a distinctive cultural trajectory. A typical developmental sequence involves mating and child-bearing preceding either marriage or the establishment of a separate household. Males and females may have children with two or more persons during this initial stage; however, it is essential to realize that this is a normative social process in which paternity is openly and proudly recognized, and that one's responsibilities for financial and emotional support of one's children are clear, no matter where or with whom they reside. A second stage involves the establishment of an independent household and cohabitation of a man and woman with their common children, along with the woman's children from other relationships. This specific union may or may not persist, but the third stage involves formal Christian marriage of a man and woman, who live with their common children and the woman's other children. A husband will thus have responsibilities to his own household, as well as to those in which his "outside" children reside.

To Western, middle-class eyes this may seem an odd arrangement. But under conditions of extreme economic marginality, this system of marriage and the family has the virtue of spreading resources around through networks of households linked by common children. Not surprisingly, persons who have children with more than one person have lower blood pressures (7). In St. Lucia there is also a strong value placed on mutual solidarity among adult siblings, and a person with one or more sibs resident in the community has lower blood pressure (8). Both multiple matings and presence of adult siblings are indicators of an individual's integration into a network of mutual support.

The nature of social supports in the Mexican community are quite different (20). The ideal family type in traditional Mexican culture is an extended family consisting of a father and mother, and one or more married sons and their wives. There is a strong patrilineal bias not only in residence but in power and authority within the family. Women, in terms of cultural ideals, are expected to be self-effacing and submissive; their world is within the household and their life's purpose is to care for and protect the honor of the family. Men, on the other hand, are free to move out of the household and to establish their place in the wider social world. One important system of nonkin social relationships is the system of *compadrazgo*. Ostensibly, in this system one's *compadres* are godparents to one's children; in reality, relationships among *compadres* are used to establish formal, quasi-kinship networks of individuals upon whom one can rely for support.

In the Mexico study of social support, respondents were asked to whom they would turn for help in response to a set of six hypothetical problems (e.g., borrowing money, illness, job problems, etc.). Each question was repeated for each of four potential sources of social support: relatives, friends, neighbors, and *compadres*. Four measures of social support were formed by counting the number of problems for which an individual would turn to each of the four potential sources of support. For men, each of the social support measures was related to lower blood pressure, with the inverse correlation being greatest for support from *compadres* ($r = .39$, $p < .01$ for systolic blood pressure and $r = -.26$, $p < .05$ for diastolic blood pressure). For women, there were no significant correlations for the sample as a whole. Older (over 40) women had lower blood pressure if they perceived more support from relatives. Younger (under 40) women had *higher* blood pressure if they perceived more support from friends.

These results are consistent with traditional Mexican culture. Men, given their social dominance, benefit from social supports of all kinds. Older women benefit from social support from relatives or, in other words, support within the family. As they age, their own children grow and provide support, and their age gives them a leadership role within the family. Younger women have the least power and authority within the family; they are expected to be self-effacing. Therefore, if they seek support outside the family from friends, it is potentially socially disruptive and hence related to higher blood pressure.

The reseach in both St. Lucia and Mexico shows that the kinds of social support systems that function to protect individuals from the risk of elevated arterial pressure are extraordinarily sensitive to local nuance and meaning in social relationships. The research from Mexico also shows that the effects of social support may vary considerably within a society. This latter finding was confirmed in Brazil (12). The traditional cultural ideal of the family in Brazil is very similar to traditional Mexican culture; however, the research site in Brazil was a major city, and not surprisingly, family and social structure had undergone substantial change. For example, *compadres* served little more than a ceremonial function in Brazil, as opposed to the "networking" function in Mexico. Also, women in Brazil have undergone a substantial change in status. No longer are they limited in their social and career opportunities as they would have been in a more traditional setting.

The same measures of social support were used in Brazil as had been used in Mexico. Because of the less traditional nature of the social system in Brazil, it was found that the source of support dimension could be collapsed to kin (relative support) versus nonkin (friends, neighbors, *compadres*) support. When this was done, higher kin support was related to lower blood pressure for males, and higher nonkin support was related to lower blood pressure for females, controlling for age and the body mass index. Again, these results are consistent with a model of social and cultural dimensions of hypertension in which the protective effects of social support are specific to the meaning of social relationships within specific cultures. The risk of elevated blood pressure associated with lifestyle incongruity, on the other hand, appears to be invariant across different cultures (15,17).

A SOCIOCULTURAL MODEL OF HYPERTENSION IN AN AFRICAN-AMERICAN COMMUNITY

A recent study of hypertension was carried out in the black community of a small city in the southern United States, guided by the theoretical orientation described in this chapter. A major aim of the research was to determine if this model had any utility for understanding hypertension in an African-American community, a community rarely thought of as undergoing social change of the kind described for developing countries. A secondary aim was to expand the model in several ways. First, this would test the model under conditions in which there was at least potential access for more persons to more economic resources. Second, measures of perceived psychological stressors were obtained that allowed for further evaluation of the rather surprising finding that the effect of lifestyle incongruity was independent of perceived stressors. And third, the potential modulating effect of social support on hypertension risk would be explored further.

Within an earlier study of depressive symptoms carried out in this community (16), the socioeconomic parameters of the population had been examined. Using these data as a frame of reference, a sampling strategy was designed that would sample middle-income neighborhoods in order to increase representation of more affluent households. Also, sampling was limited to an age range of 25–55-year-olds, the range within which the slope of blood pressure on age is greatest. A total of 186 households in the community was surveyed; blood pressures and covariates (e.g., body mass index) were obtained using standard techniques (13).

Lifestyle was measured as before, with a scale incorporating the ownership of material goods and exposure to mass media information resources. Occupational class was measured with a standard ranking and was calculated on the household level. A measure of chronic social role stressors was included to assess psychological stress. This Likert-response format scale included items on which the respondents rated the frequency with which they experienced problems in major social roles, such as marriage and work. When systolic and diastolic blood pressure were regressed on lifestyle incongruity, chronic social role stressors, and covariates, incongruity was related to higher blood pressure, independently from age, sex, the body mass index, or stressors. Age and lifestyle incongruity interacted such that the effect of incongruity was exacerbated among older (40–55 year olds) persons. Chronic social role stressors appeared to have an effect on systolic blood pressure among older persons, but this was found to be among persons who had been diagnosed as hypertensive and hence probably secondary to labeling effects (2). The effect of incongruity was independent of diagnosis. Therefore, the hypothesis was supported for an African-American sample in which sampling was designed to include more affluent households; the effect of incongruity was found to be independent of psychological stress and diagnosis (13).

The lifestyle incongruity hypothesis was expanded by recent developments in social class theory. It has been argued that the true importance of factors such as occupation is the way in which these factors are used to exclude persons from competition for scarce resources. It is further argued that any convenient social criterion can be used as a criterion of exclusion. If, as it has been argued, the true importance of lifestyle is as a claim to a higher prestige or social status, then a discrepancy between lifestyle and other exclusionary criteria should be associated with blood pressure as well. In industrial societies, a lack of educational credentials often excludes persons from higher status. Using the data from the Southern black community, it was found that the degree to which lifestyle exceeded years of education was related to higher systolic and diastolic blood pressure, independently from age, sex, the body mass index, chronic social role stressors, family income, and Type A behavior (14).

This confirmation of the hypothesis led to a consideration of other factors used to exclude individuals from higher status. In many societies, skin color is just such a criterion of social exclusion. In skin color–conscious societies, like Brazil and the United States, the darker skin color associated with African-descent ethnicity is used to deny individuals higher social status. It is this special case of social exclusion that we call "discrimination" or "racism." Therefore, the hypothesis was formulated that those individuals who were attempting to maintain a higher status lifestyle, but who had darker skin, would have higher blood pressure. Data from Brazil and the United States confirmed this hypothesis (18).

The most accurate specification of the lifestyle incongruity hypothesis would thus be one in which all three criteria of social exclusion (occupational class, education, and skin color) would be combined with lifestyle to define the discrepancy. This is illustrated in Table 4.2. In this categorical measure, "class rank" refers to the combination of occupation, education, and skin color. Individuals whose class rank exceeds their lifestyles are in the upper 20% of the occupational and educational distribution, or who have lighter skin color, but whose lifestyle score is below the upper 20% of that distribution. Persons whose class rank equals their lifestyle tend to fall along the middle of the distributions of all variables. Persons whose lifestyle exceeds their class rank tend to fall into the middle third of the lifestyle score distribution, but also fall into the bottom 20% of the occupational and educational distribution, or who have the darkest skin color. The risk of hypertension among persons whose lifestyles exceed their class rank is nearly eight times that of the risk among persons whose class rank exceeds their lifestyle.

The degree of lifestyle incongruity is likely to be exacerbated in the black community. First, despite large initial shifts in the occupational structure of the black community in the early stages of the Civil Rights Movement, there have been few gains, or little upward mobility, of black people in the occupational structure (16). Second, the proportion of African Americans receiving a college education or more has increased steadily over the past 40 years, but still this proportion is about half of the corresponding proportion for whites

TABLE 4.2. Prevalence of "Hypertension" by Categories of Lifestyle Incongruity[a] and Risk Odds Ratio

Lifestyle incongruity	% hypertensive	ROR[b]
Class rank > lifestyle (n = 21)	9.5	1.00
Class rank = lifestyle (n = 96)	11.5	2.80
Lifestyle > class rank (n = 60)	26.7	7.89
		(p = .01)

[a]Defined by multivariate measure.
[b]Risk odds ratio, adjusted for age, sex, and the body mass index.
From Dressler (18).

(16). And third, the use of skin color as a criterion of social exclusion differentially affects African Americans. At the same time, however, the cultural messages that define a particular lifestyle as a salient criterion of success in industrial society are no less significant in their influence in the black community. These factors combine virtually to insure that the degree of incongruity between lifestyle and class will be exacerbated in the black community, and hence the risk of hypertension associated with that incongruity.

At the same time, there are social supports within the black community that help to ameliorate this risk. Traditionally, the extended family has functioned as the major source of social support within the black community, and, especially for older segments of the community, this emphasis on extended kin support continues (16). But the process of social change within the black community has also altered the definition of social support systems. The extended family provided unqualified support under conditions of social and economic marginality. Under contemporary social conditions, where there has been some amelioration of the extent of marginality, younger blacks have found themselves to be thrust into situations in occupational and educational settings to which many of their family members, especially older family members, have had little exposure. This has led to an increased salience of peer or nonkin social support systems among younger blacks, in order that support can be sought from individuals who share similar experiences. It has not, however, diminished the overall frequency of interaction of younger black persons within their kin groups (16).

In the research on hypertension in a Southern black community, it was hypothesized, based on this reasoning, that nonkin social support would be related to a lower risk of hypertension among 25–39 year olds, and that kin social support would be related to a lower risk of hypertension among 40–55-

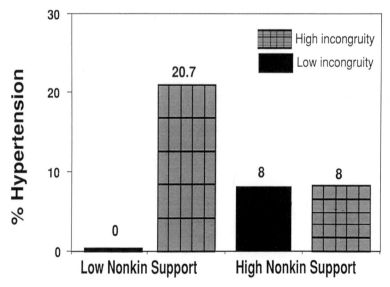

FIGURE 4.1. Prevalence of hypertension by lifestyle incongruity and nonkin support for 25–39 year olds in a Southern black community (19).

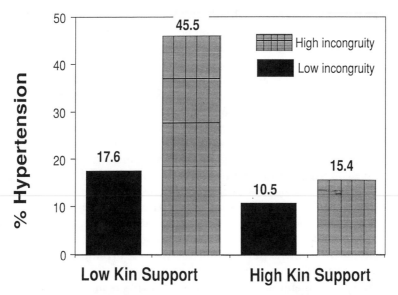

FIGURE 4.2. Prevalence of hypertension by lifestyle incongruity and kin support for 40–55 year olds in a Southern black community (19).

year-olds. Social supports were measured using an expanded scale as described for research in Mexico and Brazil. Unlike previous studies, no main effect of social supports was observed in the study in the black community; rather, within each age group, there was an interaction between lifestyle incongruity and the specific social support scale predicted to be salient for that particular age group. The pattern of these results is shown in Figures 4.1 and 4.2. In the younger age group, the individuals at the greatest risk of hypertension have higher lifestyle incongruity and lower nonkin social support. In the older age group, the individuals at the greatest risk of hypertension have higher lifestyle incongruity and lower kin social support. Within each age group, high social support effectively blunts the risk associated with incongruity. These effects are highly statistically significant, and are observed after controlling for age, sex, the body mass index, social role stressors, and diet (19).

SOCIAL FACTORS AND HYPERTENSION: INTERVENING MECHANISMS

Taken together, these studies provide consistent support for a sociocultural model of hypertension. In this model, risk of hypertension is created by the confluence of three factors: a higher lifestyle, lower class rank, and perception of little access to social support. This can be thought of as describing a particular point in three-dimensional space occupied by an individual, with the dimensions of that space defined behaviorally (by lifestyle), socially (by class rank), and culturally (by belief about social support). Although these three dimensions can be used to locate persons who are (or are not) hypertensive, it remains a static description. There still is little indication of the process or of the mechanisms by which an individual who comes to occupy a certain point in this three-dimensional space also comes to have elevated blood pressure.

When the issue of "intervening mechanism" is addressed in social–medical research, the implicit meaning of the phrase is intervening "physiological" mechanisms. It must be emphasized, however, that the location of the individual in the three-dimensional sociocultural model of hypertension, as it has been tested thus far, tells us as little about intervening social and psychological mechanisms as it does about intervening physiological mechanisms. Therefore, each of these must be discussed in turn.

With respect to social mechanisms, as it was argued earlier, a particular style of life is fundamentally a projection of the social identity. In Western industrial societies, a model of pecuniary success has come to dominate cultural images of the person. The evidence of this pecuniary success is in the form of the material goods that one can accumulate, as well as the "information goods" one can control (e.g., knowledge of trends in style advertised in the media). The individual who pursues such a lifestyle attempts to live up to this ideal, and to receive the esteem of others as a result.

It is important to emphasize, however, that this is not a crass, purely materialistic drive, for the most part. Veblen (45) pointed out the moral component to this process; that is, lifestyles come to be regarded as "conventional standards of decency." Those who seek to maintain such a conventional decency must live up to this cultural ideal, at least in appearance, or risk forfeiting their good name and self-respect (45). This perspective on lifestyle is essential to understanding the results reported before. For example, the individual scoring the highest on the lifestyle scale in the Southern black community study owns a home, car, typical consumer goods (stereo, refrigerator), and reports reading many magazines and watching television regularly—in short, a thoroughly typical American lifestyle. Yet, if that person is also of low occupational class standing, has little education, or has darker skin, he or she is likely to be hypertensive. Therefore, it is unlikely that it is the struggle to live a grand lifestyle that is at issue here; more likely it is being *denied* the status associated with a conventional middle-class lifestyle.

There is some direct evidence that this occurs. In a study of perceptions of racism and discrimination, conducted in this same black community, it was found that one of three dimensions of perceived racism pertained to common social interactions such as being poorly served in a store or restaurant by a white clerk, or having to deal with an unhelpful white secretary (1). Lifestyle incongruity has a small but significant ($r = .22, p < .01$) correlation with self-reports that these kinds of mundane interactions are upsetting. This result is striking, because in all the studies of incongruity this is the only correlation of incongruity with an attitudinal/psychological variable. This indicates that individuals who are incongruous are sensitive about their presentation of self in mundane interactions and to a perceived lack of regard shown them. It is especially significant that this perception of social interaction is observed, given that there is no correlation of incongruity with psychological stress. Therefore, the available evidence is consistent with the presentation of self in social interaction, and a perceived lack of confirmation of that presentation of self, as an intervening social mechanism in this model.

This perspective also accounts for the modulating role of social support on

the risk associated with lifestyle incongruity. It is highly unlikely that a perceived availability of social support could play an objective role in reducing
incongruity. Such a reduction would require the individual to enhance his or
her occupational or educational status, and while one's social network certainly could facilitate this enhancement on an individual basis, it seems unlikely that this process would underlie the overall social pattern.

It is more likely that social support helps to enhance the social identity of
the individual. The individual who strives to maintain a middle-class sense of
identity, but who is denied confirmation of that identity in social interaction
owing to inappropriately low class rank, may still maintain a valid sense of
social identity because he or she "knows" that there are other people to whom
he or she can turn, to whom he or she is important. This sense of social support
may thus round out an otherwise fragmented sense of social identity.

This emphasis on social intervening mechanisms does not preclude the
operation of psychological intervening mechanisms. While the research to date
on the sociocultural model leads to a clear rejection that psychological stress
is an intervening mechanism, the possibility that other emotional states play
a role is large. Most likely among these is suppressed hostility (2,42,44). It
seems plausible that lifestyle incongruity and the related sense of being denied
social status would lead to frustration and anger. Simultaneously, however, it
would be counterproductive for the individual seeking positive recognition
from others to display that frustration and anger openly. The incongruent individual may thus be hypervigilant in social interaction, continually scanning
the social milieu for clues that he or she is (or is not) being confirmed in status.
If that confirmation is not forthcoming, this might lead to anger and frustration, which in turn must be suppressed at the risk of alienating others and
thus reducing the likelihood of positive social feedback. A cycle of social presentation, vigilant scanning, anger–frustration, and suppression would then
lead to elevated blood pressure.

Social support could also play an ameliorating function in this process.
One virtue of the measurement of perceived social support in this research is
that the major dimension of support assessed is a truly social (as opposed to
instrumental or material) support (16). A prominent form of social support is
feedback (4), or simply the reassurance that one is functioning appropriately.
This kind of positive feedback helps to assuage the anger and tension usually
thought of as "stress." Furthermore, it could effectively counter the particularly damaging dimension of anger suppression that has been termed "cynical
hostility" (42). It is this dimension of hostility, in which other individuals are
viewed with distrust and suspicion, that appears to be particularly pathogenic.
Regularly receiving benign and reassuring feedback in a system of social support may help to moderate the cynical hostility that could be regularly elicited
in the social interactions of persons caught in incongruity.

Finally, we consider the physiological mechanisms that intervene between
social interaction and sustained hypertension. There are at least two possible
pathways that might link sociocultural factors and blood pressure elevation.
The first is that the incongruous individual who lacks a sense of social support
is in a more-or-less continuous state of hypervigilant coping, a state in which
the psychosocial stressors are activated to trigger physiological stress response
molecules (see Chapter 11, this volume). The individual not only scans the

social environment for cues regarding status confirmation, he or she also monitors his or her own internal emotional state to maintain anger and frustration at a suppressed state. Finally, there is no respite through social support. Laboratory research has shown that this state of hypervigilant coping is associated with higher circulating levels of neuromuscular transmitters, which in turn would lead to increased peripheral resistance and higher blood pressure (23). In this particular formulation of the model, it is unnecessary to postulate any underlying structural remodeling to account for sustained elevated blood pressure, although if blood pressure is sustained at a level inconsistent with metabolic needs for extended periods, structural remodeling will occur (28).

A second pathway may be stress reactivity (24,33,38). A variety of studies have shown that, compared with normotensives, hypertensives (or borderline hypertensives) show greater transient blood pressure elevation in response to environmental stimuli, including especially laboratory stressors. It has been proposed that these transient elevations of blood pressure occur more frequently in the real world to individuals who develop sustained hypertension, and that this relationship is mediated by vascular structural remodeling (23). Furthermore, there is some experimental evidence to provide plausible links between the sociocultural model of hypertension and blood pressure reactivity. Consistent elevations of blood pressure have been observed while an individual is speaking (32). This reaction is enhanced when an individual is speaking to an experimenter who is dressed in such a way as to project high status. On the other hand, when the subject is speaking to a lower status person, the blood pressure increase is smaller. In addition, transient blood pressure elevations are enhanced by placing the experimental subject in a situation in which he or she is expected to convince another individual of the correctness of some idea (41,43). This reaction is not dependent on the chronic hostility level of the subject. Finally, it has been shown that subjects exposed to a laboratory stressor show a larger blood pressure response if they did not receive social approval following the stressor (6).

These lines of experimental evidence are consistent with the social and psychological intervening mechanisms for the sociocultural model of hypertension in blacks. Furthermore, these laboratory studies demonstrate the link between these factors and blood pressure reactivity. The individual with high lifestyle incongruity and low social support may be consistently projecting a sense of self in social interaction that fails to be confirmed. Cardiovascular reactivity may be enhanced in these frustrating and unsatisfying interactions. When repeated over a period of years, sustained hypertension may result (see Chapter 11, this volume). The specific variables in the sociocultural model of hypertension outlined in this paper can be plausibly linked to disease through a set of social, psychological, and physiological mechanisms. The precise pathway of the physiological mechanism has been developed further in Chapter 11.

CONCLUSIONS AND IMPLICATIONS

The aim of this chapter has been to present a model of social and cultural influences in hypertension that can link broad social profiles of hypertension, such as differences in population average blood pressure by type of society, with individual-level processes, such as the presentation of self in mundane social interaction and the physiological responses that might accompany that interaction. Although certain parts of the model have been more adequately supported than others, the overall coherence of the results suggest that these dimensions are significant. Here it may be useful to consider some of the more general implications of the present model.

One general conclusion is that research in hypertension ignores features of the social environment in model construction. This failure results in poorly specified causal models and biased estimation of the risk associated with other variables. Furthermore, there are various features of social structure and culture associated with hypertension, features that are rarely captured by the inclusion of some single "stress" parameter. A refined understanding of hypertension requires that the full range of relevant parameters be included.

One implication of these results is that the interpretation of the effects of certain variables is not as straightforward as is sometimes assumed. Take, for example, skin color. The color of skin is obviously influenced heavily by heredity, and so it seems "natural" to interpret any association of skin color and blood pressure as resulting from this genetic factor (or at least as being a marker of some biological process). But the color of skin has been a contentious and divisive issue in Western culture for centuries; the color of skin has led to markedly different experiences for different segments of the population. It therefore seems just as "natural" to look to the social implications of differences in skin color as the mediating influence on blood pressure. When appropriately specified, such a model is empirically useful. (The same argument can be made for simple demographic variables like education; understanding the role of these variables requires that they be incorporated into appropriate social models. The effects of these seemingly simple variables cannot be unambiguously interpreted.)

It should be noted that the sociocultural model of hypertension is itself in considerable need of further refinement. The sociocultural model needs to be replicated in more populations, in research designs that include other, more conventional risk factors (the notion of bias in the estimation of model parameters cuts both ways). It also needs to be replicated using a prospective study design. The consistency of the results from these cross-sectional studies stimulates this further work.

One useful aspect of this model is its convergence with laboratory studies of physiological parameters and cardiovascular reactivity (32,42,43). Too often the correspondence between what goes on in the laboratory and what is measured in the field is obscure. But the emphasis in the sociocultural model of hypertension on mundane social interaction mediating the association of blood pressure and the measured variables links this model very directly with recent laboratory research. This link could be enhanced in three ways. First, laboratory analogs of the behavioral factors hypothesized to mediate effects in the sociocultural model could be developed. Second, parameters of the sociocultural model could be used as guides in sampling subjects for laboratory studies (i.e., how do individuals who are high incongruity/low social support react to laboratory stressors versus individuals who are high incongruity/high social support?). And third, more innovative research designs (such as ambulatory monitoring) could be used to study more intensively what behaviors and emotional parameters distinguish individuals who vary on dimensions of the sociocultural model. Through the extension of knowledge of hypertension, using novel theories and methods, a more refined understanding of human biology and its intersection with human behavior can be obtained.

REFERENCES

1. Adams, J. P., and W. W. Dressler. Perceptions of injustice in a black community: dimensions and variation. *Hum. Relations 41:* 753–767, 1988.
2. Alexander, F. Emotional factors in essential hypertension. *Psychosom. Med. 1:* 173–179, 1939.
3. Cassel, J. The contribution of the social environment to host resistance. *Am. J. Epidemiol. 104:* 107–123, 1976.
4. Cohen, S. Psychosocial models of the role of social support in the etiology of physical disease. *Health Psychol. 7:* 269–297, 1988.
5. Costas, R., M. R. Garcia-Palmieri, P. Sorlie, et al. Coronary heart disease risk factors in men with light and dark skin in Puerto Rico. *Am. J. Public Health 71:* 614–619, 1981.
6. Cumes-Rayner, D. P., and J. Price. Understanding hypertensives' behavior. II. Perceived social approval and blood pressure reactivity. *J. Psychosom. Res. 34:* 141–152, 1990.
7. Dressler, W. W. "Disorganization," adaptation, and arterial blood pressure. *Med. Anthropol. 3:* 225–248, 1979.
8. Dressler, W. W. *Hypertension and Culture Change: Acculturation and Disease in the West Indies.* Redgrave Publishing Company, South Salem, N.Y., 1982.
9. Dressler, W. W. Hypertension and culture change in the Caribbean. In: *Health Care in the Caribbean and Central America,* edited by F. McGlynn. Studies in Third World Societies, Publication No. 30. College of William and Mary, Williamsburg, Va., 1984, pp. 69–93.
10. Dressler, W. W. Social and cultural influences in cardiovascular disease: a review. *Transcultural Psychiatr. Res. Rev. 21:* 5–42, 1984.
11. Dressler, W. W. Psychosomatic symptoms, stress, and modernization: a model. *Cult. Med. Psychiatry 9:* 257–286, 1985.
12. Dressler, W. W. Blood pressure, sex roles, and social support. Abstracts of the 85th Annual Meeting of the American Anthropological Association. Philadelphia, Pa., 1986.
13. Dressler, W. W. Lifestyle, stress, and blood pressure in a Southern black community. *Psychosom. Med. 52:* 182–198, 1990.
14. Dressler, W. W. Education, lifestyle, and arterial blood pressure. *J. Psychosom. Res. 34:* 515–523, 1990.
15. Dressler, W. W. Culture, stress, and disease. In: *Medical Anthropology: A Handbook of Theory and Method,* edited by T. M. Johnson and C. F. Sargent. Greenwood Press, Westport, Ct., 1990, pp. 248–267.
16. Dressler, W. W. *Stress and Adaptation in the Contest of Culture: Depression in a Southern Black Community.* State University of New York Press, Albany, 1990.
17. Dressler, W. W. Cross-cultural differences and social influences in social support and cardiovascular disease. In: *Social Support and Cardiovascular Disease,* edited by S. A. Shumaker and S. M. Czajkowski. Plenum Publishing, New York, 1992 (in press).
18. Dressler, W. W. Social class, skin color, and blood pressure in two societies. *Ethnicity and Disease 1:* 60–77, 1991.
19. Dressler, W. W. Social support and arterial pressure in a Southern black community. MS.
20. Dressler, W. W., A. Mata, A. Chavez, F. E. Viteri, and P. N. Gallagher. Social support and arterial blood pressure in a central Mexican community. *Psychosom. Med. 48:* 338–350, 1986.
21. Dressler, W. W., A. Mata, A. Chavez, and F. E. Viteri. Arterial blood pressure and individual modernization in a Mexican community. *Soc. Sci. Med. 24:* 679–687, 1987.
22. Dressler, W. W., J. E. D. Santos, P. N. Gallagher, Jr., and F. E. Viteri. Arterial blood pressure and modernization in Brazil. *Am. Anthropol. 89:* 389–409, 1987.
23. Folkow, B. Stress and blood pressure. In: *Adrenergic Blood Pressure Regulation,* edited by W. H. Birkenhager, B. Folkow, and H. A. J. Struyker Boudier. Excerpta Medica, Amsterdam, 1985, pp. 87–93.

24. Fredrikson, M., and K. A. Matthews. Cardiovascular responses to behavioral stress and hypertension: a meta-analytic review. *Ann. Behav. Med. 12:* 30–39, 1990.
25. Haan, M. N., G. A. Kaplan, and S. L. Syme. Old observations and new thoughts. In: *Pathways to Health: The Role of Social Factors,* edited by J. P. Bunker, D. S. Gomby, and B. H. Kehrer. The Henry J. Kaiser Family Foundation, Menlo Park, Ca., 1989, pp. 76–135.
26. Hall, W. D., E. Saunders, and N. Shulman, eds. *Hypertension in Blacks: Epidemiology, Pathophysiology, and Treatment.* Year Book Medical Publishers, Chicago, 1985.
27. Harburg, E., L. Glieberman, P. Roeper, M. A. Schork, and W. J. Schull. Skin color, ethnicity, and blood pressure. I. Detroit blacks. *Am. J. Public Health 68:* 1177–1183, 1978.
28. Henry, J. P., and J. C. Cassel. Psychosocial factors in essential hypertension. *Am. J. Epidemiol. 90:* 171–200, 1978.
29. Hypertension Detection and Follow-up Program Cooperative Group. Race, education, and prevalence of hypertension. *Am. J. Epidemiol. 106:* 351–361, 1977.
30. Keil, J. E., H. A. Tyroler, S. H. Sandifer, and E. Boyle. Hypertension: effects of social class and racial mixture. *Am. J. Public Health 67:* 634–639, 1977.
31. Keil, J. E., S. H. Sandifer, C. B. Loadholt, and E. Boyle. Skin color and education effects on blood pressure. *Am. J. Public Health 71:* 532–534, 1981.
32. Long, J. M., J. J. Lynch, N. M. Machiron, S. A. Thomas, and K. L. Malinow. The effect of status on blood pressure during verbal communication. *J. Behav. Med. 5:* 165–172, 1982.
33. Manuck, S. B., A. L. Kasprowicz, and M. F. Muldoon. Behaviorally-evoked cardiovascular reactivity and hypertension: conceptual issues and potential associations. *Ann. Behav. Med. 12:* 17–29, 1990.
34. Marmot, M. G. Socio-economic and cultural factors in ischaemic heart disease. *Adv. Cardiol. 29:* 68–76, 1982.
35. Mason, J. W. A historical view of the stress field. *J. Hum. Stress 1:* 6–12, 22–36, 1975.
36. Murphy, H. B. M. Blood pressure and culture: the contribution of cross-cultural comparisons to psychosomatics. *Psychother. Psychosom. 38:* 244–255, 1982.
37. Patrick, R. C., I. M. Prior, J. C. Smith, et al. Relationship between blood pressure and modernity among Panopeans. *Int. J. Epidemiol. 12:* 36–44, 1983.
38. Pickering, T. G., and W. Gerin. Cardiovascular reactivity in the laboratory and the role of behavioral factors in hypertension: a critical review. *Ann. Behav. Med. 12:* 3–26, 1990.
39. Shaper, A. G., S. J. Pocock, M. Walker, N. M. Cohen, C. J. Wale, and A. G. Thomson. British Regional Heart Study: cardiovascular risk factors in middle-aged men in 24 towns. *Br. Med. J. 283:* 179–186, 1981.
40. Smith, R. T. Social stratification in the Caribbean. In: *Essays in Comparative Social Stratification,* edited by L. Plotnikov and A. Tuden. University of Pittsburgh Press, Pittsburgh, Pa., 1970, pp. 43–76.
41. Smith, T. W., and K. D. Allred. Blood pressure responses during social interaction in high- and low-cynically hostile males. *J. Behav. Med. 12:* 135–143, 1989.
42. Smith, T. W., and K. D. Frohm. What's so unhealthy about hostility? Construct validity and psychosocial correlates of the Cook and Medley Ho scale. *Health Psychol. 4:* 503–520, 1985.
43. Smith, T. W., K. D. Allred, C. A. Morrison, and S. D. Carlson. Cardiovascular reactivity and interpersonal influence: active coping in a social context. *J. Pers. Soc. Psychol. 56:* 209–218, 1989.
44. Sommers-Flanagan, J., and R. P. Greenberg. Psychosocial variables and hypertension: a new look at an old controversy. *J. Nerv. Ment. Dis. 177:* 15–24, 1989.
45. Veblen, T. *The Theory of the Leisure Class.* New edition. B. W. Huebsch, New York, 1918.
46. Waldron, I., M. Nowotakski, M. Freimer, et al. Cross-cultural variation in blood pressure: a quantitative analysis of the relationships of blood pressure to cultural characteristics, salt consumption, and body weight. *Soc. Sci. Med. 16:* 419–430, 1982.
47. Weber, M. Class, status, party. In: *From Max Weber: Essays in Sociology,* edited by H. H. Gerth and C. W. Mills. Oxford University Press, New York, 1946, pp. 180–195.
48. Worsley, P. Social class and development. In: *Social Inequality: Comparative and Developmental Approaches,* edited by G. D. Berreman. Academic Press, New York, 1981, pp. 221–255.
49. Young, A. The discourse on stress and the reproduction of conventional knowledge. *Soc. Sci. Med. 14B:* 133–146, 1980.

5

Psychosocial Factors in Hypertension in Blacks: The Case for an Interactional Perspective

HECTOR F. MYERS AND FAITH   H. MCCLURE

Blacks are at greatest risk for hypertensive disease. The available epidemiological evidence overwhelmingly identifies blacks[1] as running a disproportionate risk of morbidity from essential hypertension, of suffering disproportionately from the sequelae of this disease, and of running the greatest risk of early mortality from this disease and its sequelae compared with other U.S. population groups (43,73,75–77). These racial differences are also observed in urbanized areas of Africa (2), in the West Indies (7,8), in South America (88), and in Central America (81).

There are several reasons that these racial differences have interested researchers over the past several decades. There is growing evidence that several biological and psychosocial factors are implicated in the observed pattern of racial differences in vulnerability to hypertension (4). Unfortunately, however, differences in the questions asked, in the presumed causal mechanisms studied, and in the methodologies used have resulted in a piecemeal approach to the problem. Therefore, as noted by Myers et al. (70), the absence of an integrated, multidisciplinary perspective that considers multiple contributors is a major obstacle in advancing our understanding of the pathogenesis of hypertension in different population groups.

This chapter reviews and discusses the available evidence on the contribution of psychosocial factors in essential hypertension. We argue for a move away from studies that investigate the independent contributions of subsets of psychosocial factors (e.g., socioeconomic status [SES], life stresses, diet, etc.) and a move toward a multidimensional and interactional perspective that tests the joint effects of the most salient contributors. Such an approach would be targeted at identifying the major contributors in each of several domains (e.g., behavioral and lifestyle contributors, individual personality characteristics, family context attributes, socioecological factors, etc.) and testing how these

---

1. The terms *blacks* and *whites* are used in this manuscript to denote ethnocultural groups that differ in cultural, social, and psychological roots. These groups also differ in their biological attributes, but, as noted by Cooper (17) and others, the genetic heterogeneity of these groups (especially among blacks) makes comparisons of biological differences between them scientifically questionable. Nevertheless, the field continues to treat these groups as distinct biological entities and to investigate biological and genetic factors that might account for the observed group differences in risk for hypertension.

contributors interact to confer additional risk for hypertension. How, for example, does a high sodium/low potassium diet and low SES interact with high life stress *and* an anger-reactive coping style to enhance risk?

A multidimensional model is offered that starts with the premise that essential hypertension develops in individuals who possess an underlying biological vulnerability or diathesis for the disease. Psychosocial factors, including socioeconomic status, behavioral or lifestyle factors, psychological attributes, and family dynamics, are viewed as contributing, either singly or in interaction, to the timing of the onset of the disease, to disease course, and ultimately to disease morbidity and mortality. This model has been variously referred to as a diathesis-stress model, or, more recently, as a biobehavioral or biopsychosocial model (4,70). Specific attention is placed here on discussing the evidence linking four psychosocial factors for which there is strong empirical support: two are socioecological factors: *(1)* socioeconomic status, and *(2)* socioecological stresses; and two are psychological factors; *(3)* the predisposition toward active effortful coping with stress (i.e., John Henryism), and *(4)* styles of coping with anger and hostility. We also argue for greater attention to be paid to *(5)* the patterns of interpersonal interactions within families as the primary setting in which psychosocial factors are mediated and expressed.

SOCIOECONOMIC STATUS

There is substantial evidence that lower socioeconomic status, whether measured by education, income, or occupation, or some combination of these variables, is associated with greater morbidity and mortality from essential hypertension and its sequelae in all ethnic and gender groups (25,43,44,75–77). For example, the Hypertension Detection and Follow-up Cooperative Group (43) found that lower education was associated with significantly higher resting blood pressures and a higher prevalence of hypertension. This study also noted that blacks were twice as likely to be hypertensive than whites, and this racial imbalance was evident in all age groups and in both genders. However, the magnitude of the racial difference in prevalence was reduced proportionate to increases in SES.

There is also evidence that lower SES appears to be particularly pathogenic for blacks (i.e., poverty results in greater negative consequences for blacks than for other ethnic groups) (53). It has been argued that this is partly because race and social class interact to increase levels of psychological distress, and because lower socioeconomic status exposes blacks to greater social and economic oppression and discrimination than that experienced by whites or other groups. This consequence is also attributable to the confluence of debilitating social context deficits and high-risk behaviors and lifestyles found in poverty-stricken communities. Low SES blacks are more likely to reside in high socioecological stress neighborhoods (i.e., high crime, high unemployment, low income, high marital and family instability), to consume diets high in sodium and saturated fats but low in calcium and potassium, to be overweight (especially black women), and to consume excessive amounts of alcohol, tobacco, and illegal drugs. All of these aspects of a poverty-stricken lifestyle interact to enhance substantially the risk for hypertension and other diseases above and beyond that which is attributable simply to low education or low income.

SOCIOECOLOGICAL STRESS AND SOCIAL DISORGANIZATION

The psychosocial variable that is consistently associated with enhanced risk for essential hypertension is living in high socioecological stress areas. The studies by Harburg et al. (36–38,45,71) showed that for both males and females, black and white, those who lived in communities characterized by high crime, high unemployment, low income, high social instability, and disorganization were significantly more likely to evidence higher resting blood pressures and a higher prevalence of essential hypertension than their ethnic and gender counterparts living in more socioecologically wholesome communities. The highest resting blood pressures were observed in those communities that were both low in SES and high in social instability.

These socioecological effects had the greatest impact on young black males, who were two and a half times more likely to have elevated diastolic blood pressures (i.e., DBP > 95 mm Hg) than their cohorts in socioecologically less stressful areas. This effect may be age-related, since among older black males (i.e., age > 40 years), stress areas did not predict the prevalence of either borderline or established hypertension. Syme (86) suggested that these results reflect the efforts of younger black men to gain control over difficult and uncontrollable circumstances (e.g., the availability of meaningful employment opportunities in their communities), and the associated greater feelings of anger and frustration.

Thus, all of the available evidence seems to indicate that environments that are psychologically oppressive, because of low economic and social resources, low access to the critical social pathways of opportunity, high threat to personal safety, or unstable social structures, enhance the risk for developing hypertension. This contextual risk is further enhanced by the development of a variety of high-risk behaviors and lifestyles including poor diets, obesity, and substance use and abuse. These studies also point to the potentially important role that individual psychological predisposition or coping styles may play in mediating the effects of both the contextual and personal risk factors.

JOHN HENRYISM

James and colleagues (46–48) hypothesized that persons with "a strong personality predisposition to cope actively with psychosocial stressors in [their] environment" but with few resources for successful coping (e.g., low educaton) would be at greater risk for hypertension than either their counterparts without this predisposition or those similarly disposed but who possessed the requisite resources (48, p. 665). This coping style has been labeled "John Henryism" after the legendary black folk hero John Henry, who epitomized the value of hard work as a means of overcoming even overwhelming odds. This hypothesis was first tested in a study of rural black men (46,47) and later on a community sample of black and white men and women (48). The results of the first study confirmed the hypothesis: black men who were high on John Henryism but with low educational attainment had the highest mean blood pressures (46). This relationship was further enhanced by perceptions among the more successful blacks that race had interfered with their success (47). In a more recent study (48), these investigators tested this hypothesis across races and gender groups and found confirmation of greater prevalence of hypertension in high John Henryism (JH), low SES black men and women, but not in whites. However, the JH × SES interaction effect was not obtained when mean resting systolic and diastolic blood pressures were tested in each of the ethnic groups. The authors noted that differences in the meaning of SES among blacks may have mitigated against confirming the association between SES, JH, and blood pressure. Also, the attenuated SES range among whites may have precluded finding any significant association between SES, JH, and blood pressure or any differences in the prevalence of hypertension.

In any event, these studies support the suggestion that young blacks who are striving to achieve some modicum of social mobility and are predisposed to compensate for their limited educational resources by active, effortful coping (i.e., hard work and determination) run substantially higher risk of becoming hypertensive than other blacks (86). This evidence may also be congruent with Dressler's social incongruity hypothesis, which posits enhanced risk for hypertension in blacks whose lifestyles exceed their occupational status (see Chapter 4, this volume). However, none of this evidence should be interpreted as suggesting that effortful coping is unhealthy for blacks (e.g., that laziness and surrender is healthier that continuing to struggle). Rather, the evidence underscores the importance of a balance between educational and other resources and one's aspirations, on the one hand, and the demands and obstacles one faces in the pursuit of these aspirations, on the other. Without the requisite resources, compensating with increased effort or living beyond one's psychological and social means may incur the additional cost of a compromised cardiovascular system.

COPING WITH ANGER AND HOSTILITY

For the past half century the elusive link between specific personality traits and elevated blood pressure has been pursued. This research was prompted by Alexander's (3) hypothesis that hypertensives experience conflict over the expression of hostility, aggression, and other strong emotions. After many failed attempts to identify a specific hypertensive personality (40), investigators have begun to focus attention on the specific contribution that the experience and expression of anger and hostility might play in the pathogenesis of this disease. Studies have yielded results that indicate that suppressed anger, unexpressed hostility, and inhibited power motivation are associated with elevated blood pressure (21,30,34,36). This was true for both blacks and whites, but was especially evident among younger black males. It is not clear, however, whether suppressed anger in part of the core psychodynamics of all hypertensives or is only relevant to a subset, or whether suppressed anger operates as a psychological risk enhancer that interacts with other biological vulnerabilities (e.g., a sodium-retention trait) to accelerate the dysregulation of the blood pressure control mechanisms. If the former is true, then we would expect that an anger-suppression style would be evident in a substantial majority of essential hypertensives. On the other hand, if the latter is true, then we would expect that this coping style would manifest its effect *only* in the presence of some other underlying vulnerability.

The major lines of evidence on diverse populations and from both prospective and cross-sectional studies indicate that the odds of being diagnosed hypertensive are significantly higher for those with a tendency to suppress anger than for those who more openly express it (31). For example, Harburg and associates (35,36) found that individuals who habitually suppressed anger when provoked had higher resting blood pressures and were more likely to be diagnosed as hypertensive than those who expressed their anger when provoked. This anger-suppressing style was shown to enhance the risk for hypertension attributable to known risk factors such as race, gender, and neighborhood socioecological stress, and appears to confer additional risk in both adolescents and adults (18,22,31,34,36,49,50).

Studies using behavioral observations and experimental manipulations suggested that the anger-suppressing style found in many hypertensives may be part of a psychological profile that includes a lack of appropriate assertiveness and a tendency toward greater interpersonal self-consciousness, anxiety, and submissiveness (41,74). Two reports indicated that hypertensives evidenced a greater preference not to self-disclose, but would increase their level of self-disclosure if the situation required it (19,20). This responsiveness to situational demands, however, was associated with potent dysregulatory effects on their blood pressures. Normotensives, on the other hand, were more self-disclosing regardless of contextual demands and showed no associated blood pressure dysregulation (19). In the second study, the researchers investigated the impact of perceived social approval and disapproval on the level of self-disclosure and blood pressure reactivity in normotensives and borderlines and found that self-disclosure under conditions of perceived mild social disapproval produced marked blood pressure reactivity only in the borderlines (20). This evidence was partially confirmed by the results obtained by Winkleby et al. (90), who found evidence in a large sample of San Francisco bus drivers that suggested that hypertensives may deny the subjective experience of stress even in high stress jobs. Together, these findings indicate that there is at least a subset of essential hypertensives who evidence a pattern of hypersensitivity to social exposure/social judgment, and have difficulty acknowledging stress and expressing anger and hostility without guilt or conflict.

It is also noteworthy that although most published studies report an association between increased blood pressure and inhibited anger, other studies have either failed to find this association (52,54) or have found it only in subgroups, e.g., white men but not black men or women of either race (22). Still others have found an apparently contradictory association between anger directed outward and increased blood pressure (38,80). For example, Harburg et al. (38) found that blacks who reported a tendency to express anger outwardly to an angry boss had higher diastolic blood pressures than those who reported a tendency to suppress anger or to use a more reflective coping style. Some researchers have also observed greater hostility and aggressiveness in hypertensive compared with normotensive subjects (79).

In an effort to account for these apparently contradictory findings, several investigators have suggested that both habitual anger-in and habitual anger-out coping styles, i.e., reflexive rather than reflective anger-coping, are associated with elevated blood pressure, and that the relationship between anger-coping style and blood pressure is mediated by a variety of personal and environmental characteristics. For example, Manuck et al. (60) and others explain the apparent contradictory findings by suggesting that lack of "appropriate assertiveness" may be the psychological Achilles heel in a subset of hypertensives. This group of hypertensives may respond to provocation with either inappropriate submissiveness or with heightened hostility and aggressiveness. In one study, Manuck et al. (60) subjected borderline hypertensives and normotensives to a challenging role-play task and also asked their significant other to rate their level of social competence. Their results indicated that compared with normotensives, there were at least two distinct subgroups of hypertensives: one subgroup exhibited high levels of hostility and aggressiveness and significant increases in systolic blood pressure and heart rate during the role play, while a second subgroup behaved less assertively during the role play, were rated as socially less competent by their significant other, and exhibited somewhat higher diastolic blood pressures. Thus, these results suggest that enhanced risk for hypertension may not be associated with one anger-coping style but: (1) by how the anger stimulus is perceived and (2) by the degree of arousal and conflict that is experienced in that setting and in response to the provocation. In appropriately assertive persons, both psychological and physiological arousal would be appropriate to the provocation regardless of how the anger was expressed. In less appropriately assertive persons, however, provocation may result in excessive psychological and physiological arousal and a struggle over how to cope with the anger. The resultant behavioral response could be either excessive aggressiveness or inappropriate submissiveness along with excessive physiological arousal.

Also, while several studies report an association between anger expression and resting blood pressure levels in both hypertensives and normotensives, it is unclear whether pattern of anger expression and assertiveness mediate cardiovascular stress reactivity only in individuals already diagnosed as hypertensive or who are biologically at risk for the disease. For example, a study by Perini et al. (72) found evidence that anger suppression mediated cardiovascular stress response in hypertensives only. Similarly, in a study in which black hypertensive and normotensive women were asked to discuss a family conflict while being filmed, McClure (63) found that anger expression style mediated the blood pressure responses only in the hypertensives. Smith and Houston (82) also failed to find a relationship between measures of anger expression and blood pressure responses in normotensive males who were presented with two challenging tasks.

A recent study by Durel et al. (24) further complicates this picture by reporting gender and race differences in the patterns of association between anger trait, anger expression style, and blood pressure at rest and during active-coping stress. These differences may be more evident in response to some types of stresses but not to others. They reported that white women evidenced a strong positive association between state-trait anger (STAI-T), systolic blood pressure (SBP), and diastolic blood pressure (DBP) at rest and under active interpersonal conflict stress; while black women evidenced strong associations between STAI-T anger, SBP, and DBP at rest, work, and in response to cold pressor stress. On the other hand, among black men, only cognitive anger was associated with DBP at rest, while among white men there was a negative association between hostility (Ho scale) and SBP at rest and during a video game task, and a negative association between somatic anger and SBP and DBP reactivity to the cold pressor task.

These results further underscore the fact that hypertension is not a single disease that develops from one source or through a single psychosocial or biological pathway, but is rather a complex disease that develops through multiple interacting pathways. Clearly, anger-coping is a complex issue, and the available evidence seems to suggest that one pathway worth further investigation involves whether a reflexive style of coping with anger (i.e., habitual anger-in or habitual anger-out) confers additional risk for this disease above and beyond that attributable to race, age, gender, ponderosity, SES, socioecological stress, and biological predisposition (e.g., a positive family history of hypertension, sodium sensitivity, etc.). It is also worth noting that different measures of anger and different contexts in which anger is elicited and blood pressure is measured may yield different results, and that these differences may be mediated by gender and race.

THE EFFECT OF RACISM AND DISCRIMINATION ON HYPERTENSION IN BLACKS

Scholars have speculated that the disproportionate morbidity and mortality from essential hypertension and related psychosomatic disorders in blacks is at least in part attributable to conflicts related to the experience of racism and discrimination (5,31,39,44,54,67,68). These investigators have argued that a major developmental task for blacks, and especially for black males, is to develop ways of coping with the ego-deflating experiences and the resulting anger and frustration they are likely to face throughout their lives because of their race. Empirical support for this hypothesis is provided by Gentry (31), who found in the Detroit blood pressure study that blacks evidenced significantly higher interracial hostility than whites, and that those blacks who also possessed the tendency to suppress anger were most likely to evidence the highest mean diastolic blood pressures. In an effort to explore further this question, Harrell (39) proposed six cognitive styles or philosophical perspectives that blacks have developed to cope with racism. These include: (1) an apathetic style characterized by passivity and accommodation to social demands and expectations, (2) a "piece of the action" style in which efforts are continuously made to succeed and to gain socially valued resources despite obstacles, (3) countercultural solutions to racism that transcend the problems of life rather than confronting them directly (e.g., developing nonmainstream lifestyles), *(4)* an activist, Black Nationalist style with a strong commitment to confront racism in all of its various forms and faces, *(5)* an authoritarian style in which rules are used to remove ambiguity by prescribing specific ways of responding "appropriately" to racial conflicts, and *(6)* a style characterized by cognitive flexibility, historical awareness, and open-mindedness. Efforts by Clark and Harrell (15) to investigate whether a particular racial coping style would be associated with enhanced cardiovascular reactivity to an active coping stressor (i.e., mental arithmetic) failed to support their expectations that an apathetic/submissive style would be associated with lower blood pressures. The only coping style that was consistently associated with any pattern of blood pressure reactivity when other risk factors were controlled was a cognitively flexible style, which was associated unexpectedly with higher resting SBP and higher recovery DBP.

In a subsequent study utilizing more emotionally involving stimuli (i.e., fearful, neutral versus racist stimuli), Sutherland and Harrell (85) found that black undergraduate females evidenced more reactive heart rates and electromyocardiograms (EMGs) to both the racist and fearful imagery. These studies yielded somewhat contradictory results, although only the second study actually tested the impact of exposure to racism on cardiovascular function. In a more recent study, Armstead et al. (6) tested the hypothesis that exposure to racially provocative stimuli would elicit consistently stronger cardiovascular reactivity in blacks than anger-provoking but nonracist stimuli and neutral stimuli. Their results indicated, consistent with the hypothesis, that blacks exhibited higher cardiovascular reactivity to the racist stimuli than to either the anger-provoking/nonracist stimuli or the neutral stimuli. However, self-reported anger arousal (i.e., state anger) was obtained in response to both the racist and the anger-provoking/nonracist stimuli.

This is the first concrete experimental evidence supporting the hypothesis that anger elicited by racist experiences or by racially loaded encounters results in marked cardiovascular reactivity in blacks above and beyond that which is observed in response to racially neutral anger provocation. However, this evidence does not prove that racially triggered anger is more pathogenic to cardiovascular function than anger elicited by any other stimulus, or that this type of anger is more deleterious to blacks than to others. It cannot be assumed, for example, that whites would not also evidence cardiovascular reactivity to racist stimuli (although the emotional content of that arousal might be different from blacks) or that women would be any less angry and reactive to sexist stimuli. What this study does show, however, is that by virtue of greater exposure to racist and discriminatory encounters, blacks may run a greater risk than whites of exposure to anger-eliciting stimuli that provoke very strong, conflicted emotions with commensurate cardiovascular hyperreactivity. Evidence from the work by James et al. (46–48) suggests that this greater exposure to racially induced stresses should result in even greater risk for hypertension in those blacks who respond with increased effort and determination but lack adequate instrumental resources (i.e., high John Henryism and low education).

Future studies will need to pursue this question about the role of racism-induced anger and reactivity in hypertension, and to investigate how individual anger-coping styles might mediate this additional stress burden. We might hypothesize, consistent with previous evidence on anger-coping, that greater cardiovascular reactivity and slower recovery should be observed in blacks who are *reflexive* anger responders (i.e., both habitual suppressors and habitual overexpressors), while lower reactivity and faster recovery should be observed in those who have developed more *reflective* coping strategies.

FAMILY FACTORS IN HYPERTENSION

The evidence discussed thus far has focused on testing hypotheses about various psychosocial stressors in individuals as a function of their blood pressure status, SES, neighborhood socioecological stress, and coping styles. However, there is substantial justification for taking a family rather than an individual perspective in the study of illnesses such as essential hypertension (33). For example, there is ample documentation of familial clustering of blood pressure and the risk factors associated with hypertension in the United States (65,83,91,92), in populations from diverse geographical and cultural backgrounds (87), and in children, adolescents, and adults (12,66,92).

The data showing moderate concordance of blood pressures in families (91,92) and increased disease risk in persons with a family history of hypertension (26,42) have generally been interpreted as evidence of a biologically inherited vulnerability to hypertension. Nonetheless, there is growing interest and support in the field for exploring a "family psychosomatic" hypothesis of hypertension, i.e., investigating what proportion of attributable familial risk for this disease is due to nongenetic familial processes (69).

The moderate levels of concordance observed between family members and genetically unrelated individuals living together (e.g., married couples) cannot be attributed to genetics but to attributes of the shared environment, including diet, nutrition, life stresses, the development of complementary styles of managing stresses, etc. (33,83). In a study involving 233 families, Connor et al. (16) provided evidence of a strong link between family dietary habits, familial metabolic aggregation (e.g., familial aggregation for urinary sodium, potassium, and creatinine excretion), and mean familial systolic blood pressure. This supports the view that families contribute to risk for hypertension in its members through the socialization of high-risk behavioral and social practices and not simply through genetic endowment.

In the case of blacks, there is ample evidence that their diets are lower in potassium and calcium, and have higher sodium to potassium and sodium to calcium ratios than those reported for whites (29,32,56–58,62). The issue of disparities in nutrition in general is covered in greater detail in Chapter 8, this volume. Myers et al. (68) argued that these black–white differences in electrolyte intake probably reflect socioeconomic and sociocultural differences, and that these differences are established and maintained through family and community processes. Any biological differences that may exist between the races, such as in sodium metabolism (57,58), would be exacerbated by these environmental influences (see Chapter 6, this volume).

It is also important to note that moderate blood pressure concordance has been observed in couples living together even when risk factors such as age, obesity, dietary salt intake, and socioeconomic status are controlled (78,83,89). Suarez et al. (84), for example, suggested that blood pressure concordance is influenced by shared aspects of the marital relationship and noted that there are different degrees of shared behaviors for couples at different ages. This suggests that age, length of marriage, and extent of shared activities are among the mediators that must be considered when interpreting the meaning of familial aggregation of blood pressure in married or cohabiting couples.

The work by Baer and colleagues (9–11) and others also suggests that models of coping with conflict and anger provided by hypertensive parents may contribute additional risk in offspring above and beyond that which is attributable simply to biological inheritance. Personality characteristics such as denial and an unwillingness to admit to neurotic and aggressive feelings have been reported in a subgroup of young adults with a family history of hypertension (51). Gentry (31) also contends that anger-coping styles are learned and may be related to the psychological attributes of the dominant parent.

Although only a few studies have compared the family relationships and interaction patterns both within hypertensive families and between these families and the families of normotensives, the few that have made these comparisons suggest that negative behaviors (i.e., communication-disrupting behaviors) are associated with increases in blood pressure, and that communication skills training can reduce both hostile communication and the associated physiological reactivity in hypertensives during their interactions with their spouses (27,28).

In a series of studies with family triads, Baer and colleagues (10,11) reported greater gaze aversion in families with a hypertensive parent compared with families with normotensive parents. They suggested that this gaze aversion reflected conflict avoidance (i.e., by reducing information and confrontation), and suggested further that this style of coping with conflict may generate impaired anger management in the children and thereby increase their risk for developing the disorder. In one study, Baer et al. (11) measured blood pressures before and after a family conflict role-play task and found greater SBP reactivity in the offspring of hypertensives along with more parental conflict-avoidant nonverbal behavior. Similar results were noted by McClure and Myers (64) in a study with black hypertensive and normotensive mother–daughter pairs. These investigators found that the hypertensive mother–daughter dyads exhibited more avoidant behaviors than the normotensive dyads during discussions of conflictual family issues (e.g., dating). The hypertensive family dyads were more likely to avoid eye contact, introduce irrelevant topics, and maintain silence when a response was clearly warranted. They also exhibited higher DBP reactivity during the conflict discussion. This pattern of conflict coping is congruent with the evidence reported by Cumes-Rayner and Price (19,20) that hypertensives evidence a preference for self-concealment, especially in potentially nonsupportive social encounters (see Chapter 4, this volume). In contrast, the normotensive mother–daughter dyads exhibited both more negative verbal behavior (e.g., openly criticized and voiced disagreements) and more positive nonverbal behavior (e.g., more smiling and touching), engaged in more problem solving (e.g., accepted responsibility for their behavior and made compromises), and evidenced lower SBP and DBP reactivity to the conflict discussion task. It is still unclear from all of these studies, however, specifically how the conflict-management and general interpersonal styles of hypertensive parents affect their children, and whether these behaviors increase the risk of developing the disorder in these presumably biologically susceptible children. These questions can only be answered by more detailed longitudinal family process studies that could evaluate what proportion of risk for hypertension may be attributed to family context and family process variables versus what could be attributed to biological endowment.

Finally, the relative contribution of family factors to risk for hypertension has also been investigated using the stress-reactivity paradigm. Several researchers have proposed that exaggerated physiological responsivity to physically and psychologically challenging stimuli may be implicated in the development and clinical expression of hypertension or may accelerate the development of vascular and end-organ complications (55,59, and Chapter 11, this volume). For a more detailed discussion of the research on cardiovascular reactivity in hypertension in blacks see Chapter 6, this volume.

Although it is unclear if physiological hyperreactivity is an early marker of the disorder or part of the inherited predisposition to the disorder in the offspring of hypertensives, there is an impressive body of literature that suggests that children of hypertensives do in fact exhibit enhanced physiological responses to a variety of psychosocial stressors (61, and Chapter 3, this volume). In addition, profiles of cardiovascular reactivity to stresses have been shown to be more concordant in twin compared with nontwin siblings (13,14,23). McClure and Myers (64) also found moderate concordance of blood pressure reactivity in their black mother–daughter dyads. Thus, it may be concluded that the evidence on concordance in cardiovascular stress reactivity is clearly supportive of the genetic contribution hypothesis. However, we suggest that at least the results of the McClure and Myers (64) study could also be interpreted as indicating that cardiovascular responses to a conflict stressor may be mediated in part by shared or complementary coping strategies. If that is the case, then the results may be partly attributable to environmental influences that confer additional risk for this disease.

Since a variety of biological, psychological, and social factors are associated with resting and stress-induced blood pressures, focusing on families should be a useful strategy for determining the contribution these variables make, either separately or in interaction, to risk for essential hypertension.

THE CASE FOR AN INTERACTIONAL APPROACH

The evidence reviewed here indicates that several psychosocial stressors have been implicated in the excessive morbidity and mortality from essential hypertension suffered by blacks. Blacks from lower SES backgrounds who live in high socioecologically stressful and socially disorganized communities have higher resting blood pressures and are at substantially greater risk of developing this disease than both whites and other blacks from less oppressive backgrounds. Blacks who cope with life demands by compensating for limited instrumental resources by increasing effort and determination (i.e., high John Henryism) also run additional cardiovascular risks. The evidence is also accumulating that blacks, and especially black men, who characteristically respond to anger provocation with reflexive anger suppression or reflexive anger overreaction/expression are particularly at risk for hypertension. There is evidence that suggests that anger provoked by racially loaded experiences may be more cardiovascularly dysregulating for blacks than anger provoked by more racially neutral encounters. Finally, there is a growing body of evidence that suggests that family context and process variables also contribute to enhanced risk for developing essential hypertension.

Unfortunately, however, these bodies of research are developing in a haphazard and unintegrative fashion, and therefore, we are unable to appreciate fully the degree to which this evidence is potentially complementary. A good example of the complementary nature of the evidence is provided by Harburg, Gentry, and colleagues from the Detroit studies, which showed the highest resting BP and the greatest overall risk for hypertension to be in black males, living in low SES, high socioecologically stressful communities, who also characterized themselves as anger-suppressors. If we extend this line of evidence to include the data on John Henryism, we see the overlap of low SES, high socioecological stress, and high John Henryism as components of a high-risk profile. It would be very useful at this juncture for studies to begin incorporating all of these variables into their designs. For example, would black men with both high-risk socioecological backgrounds and high-risk psychological profiles (i.e., high John Henryism and anger-suppressing or anger-overreacting styles) evidence the highest resting blood pressures and the greatest cardiovascular reactivity to acute stresses compared with their black peers who only possess some of these risk factors? In other words, do these psychosocial risk factors confer risk in an additive fashion or do they interact synergistically to increase risk in some nonlinear fashion? How much additional risk is conferred by these factors above and beyond that attributable to other known lifestyle risks such as smoking, sedentary lifestyles, obesity, high sodium/low potassium, high sodium/low calcium, and high cholesterol diets? Also, does the source of stress and anger provocation (e.g., racially loaded versus racially neutral provocation) impact differently on the contribution that the other psychosocial and lifestyle risk factors make to elevated resting blood pressure, to cardiovascular stress reactivity to acute stresses, and to long-term risk for developing stable hypertension in blacks? Do these factors operate differently as a function of SES or gender?

These and similar questions beg to be answered and require that investigators approach their studies of the contribution of psychosocial stressors in hypertension in blacks from a multidimensional perspective. Such a perspective would include but not be limited to the following: (1) careful assessment and consideration of the major known lifestyle risk factors in their analyses; (2) assessment of personal/family socioeconomic status and of socioecological stress level of the neighborhoods in which the subjects reside; (3) assessment of coping styles, either in terms of constructs such as John Henryism or the coping styles suggested by Harrell for dealing with racism, and/or those suggested by Lazarus and colleagues for dealing with daily hassles; (4) more careful assessment of styles of coping specifically with anger provocation, with consideration of the psychological significance of the provocation (e.g., racial discrimination, ego insult, infringement on personal control, etc.) and the methodology used for measuring the variable (i.e., self-reports versus ratings of overt behavior). This research would make an even greater contribution to the field if both black men and women are studied, and if family context and family process factors are also incorporated into the study design (e.g., studies of cardiovascular reactivity to racially neutral versus racially loaded anger-provoking stressors as part of a family interaction task). Finally, the most significant lacunae in our knowledge of how psychosocial stressors contribute to the excess morbidity and mortality from hypertension suffered by blacks is the absence of longitudinal evidence similar to that provided by Framingham for whites. Such a study would provide the best test of the psychosocial stressors hypotheses discussed here.

REFERENCES

1. Adams, L. L., R. A. Washburn, G. T. Haile, and L. H. Kuller. Behavioral factors and blood pressure in black college students. *J. Chronic. Dis. 40:* 131–136, 1987.
2. Akinkugbe, O. O. *Cardiovascular disease in Africa.* Paper presented at the first All-Africa Cardiovascular Symposium, University of Ibadan, Nigeria, March 15–18, 1976.
3. Alexander, F. Emotional factors in essential hypertension: presentation of a tentative hypothesis. *Psychosom. Med. 1:* 175–179, 1939.
4. Anderson, N. B., H. F. Myers, T. Pickering, and J. S. Jackson. Hypertension in blacks: psychosocial and biological perspectives. *J. Hypertension 7:* 161–172, 1989.
5. Anderson, N., and J. S. Jackson. Race, ethnicity and health psychology. In: *Health Psychology; A Discipline and a Profession,* edited by G. D. Stone, S. M. Weiss, J. D. Matarazzo, N. E. Miller, J. Rodin, G. E. Schwartz, C. D. Belar, M. J. Follick, and J. E. Singer. University of Chicago Press, Chicago, 1987, pp. 265–283.
6. Armstead, C. A., K. A. Lawler, G. Gorden, J. Cross, and J. Gibbons. Relationship of racial stressors to blood pressure responses and anger expression in black college students. *Health Psychol. 8(5):* 541–556, 1989.
7. Ashcroft, M. T. Prevalence of hypertension and associated electrocardiographic abnormalities in Jamaica and West Africa. *W. Indian Med. J. 26:* 24–33, 1977.
8. Ashcroft, M. T., and P. Desai. Blood-pressure and mortality in a rural Jamaican community. *Lancet 1:* 1167–1170, 1978.
9. Baer, P. E. Conflict management in the family: the impact of paternal hypertension. *Adv. Fam. Int. Assessment Theory 3:* 161–184. 1: 1167–1170, 1983.
10. Baer, P. E., J. Vincent, B. Williams, G. G. Bourianoff, and P. Bartlett. Behavioral response to induced conflict in families with a hypertensive father. *Hypertension 2:* 70–77, 1980.
11. Baer, P. E., J. Reed, P. C. Bartlett, J. P. Vincent, B. J. Williams, and G. G. Bourianoff. Studies of gaze during induced conflict in families with a hypertensive father. *Psychosom. Med. 45:* 233–242, 1983.
12. Biron, P., and J. Mongeau. Familial aggregation of blood pressure and its components. *Pediatr. Clin. North Am. 25:* 1057–1063, 1978.
13. Carmelli, D., M. A. Chesney, M. M. Ward, and R. H. Rosenman. Twin similarity in cardiovascular stress response. *Health Psychol. 4:* 413–423, 1985.
14. Carroll, D., J. K. Hewitt, K. A. Last, J. R. Turner, and J. Sims. A twin study of cardiac reactivity and its relationship to parental blood pressure. *Physiol. Behav. 34:* 103–106, 1985.
15. Clark, V. R., and J. P. Harrell. The relationship among Type A behavior, styles used in coping with racism, and blood pressure. *J. Black Psychol. 8(2):* 89–99, 1982.
16. Connor, S. L., W. E. Connor, H. Henry, G. Sexton, and E. J. Keenan. The effects of familial relationships, age, body weight, and diet on blood pressure and the 24 hour urinary excretion of sodium, potassium, and creatinine in men, women, and children of randomly selected families. *Circulation 1:* 76–85, 1984.

17. Cooper, R. A note on the biologic concept of race and its application in epidemiologic research. *Am. Heart J. 108:* 715–723, 1984.
18. Cottington, E. M., B. M. Brock, J. S. House, and V. M. Hawthorne. Psychosocial factors and blood pressure in the Michigan Statewide Blood Pressure Survey. *Am. J. Epidemiol. 121:* 515–529, 1985.
19. Cumes-Rayner, D. P., and J. Price. Understanding hypertensives' behaviour. I. Preference not to disclose. *J. Psychosom. Res. 33:* 63–74, 1989.
20. Cumes-Rayner, D. P., and J. Price. Understanding hypertensives' behavior. II. Perceived social approval and blood pressure reactivity. *J. Psychosom. Res. 34(2):* 141–152, 1990.
21. Diamond, E. L. The role of anger and hostility in essential hypertension and coronary heart disease. *Psychol. Bull. 92:* 410–433, 1982.
22. Dimsdale, J. E., C. Pierce, D. Schoenfeld, A. Brown, R. Zusman, and R. Graham. Suppressed anger and blood pressure: the effects of race, sex, social class, obesity, and age. *Psychosom. Med. 48:* 430–436, 1986.
23. Ditto, B. Sibling similarities in cardiovascular reactivity to stress. *Psychophysiology 24:* 353–360, 1987.
24. Durel, L. A., C. S., Carver, S. B. Spitzer, M. M. Llabre, J. K. Weintraub, P. G. Saab, and N. Schneiderman. Associations of blood pressure with self-report measures of anger and hostility among black and white men and women. *Health Psychol. 8(5):* 557–575, 1989.
25. Dyer, A. R., J. Stamler, R. B. Shekelle, and J. Schoenberger. The relationship of education to blood pressure. Findings on 40,000 employed Chicagoans. *Circulation 54:* 987–992, 1976.
26. Epstein, F. H. How useful is a family history of hypertension as a predictor of future hypertension? *Ann. Clin. Res. 20:* 583–592, 1984.
27. Ewart, C. K., K. F. Burnett, and C. B. Taylor. Communication behaviors that affect blood pressure: an A-B-A-B analysis of marital interaction. *Behav. Modif. 7:* 331–344, 1983.
28. Ewart, C. K., C. B. Taylor, H. C. Kraemer, and W. S. Agras. Reducing blood pressure reactivity during interpersonal conflict: effects of marital communication training. *Behav. Ther. 15:* 473–484, 1984.
29. Frisancho, A. R., W. R. Leonard, and L. Bolletins. Blood pressure in blacks and whites and its relationship to dietary sodium and potassium intake. *J. Chronic Dis. 37:* 515–519, 1984.
30. Gentry, W. D., A. P. Chesney, H. E. Fary, R. P. Hall, and E. Harburg. Habitual anger-coping styles: effect of mean blood pressure and risk for essential hypertension. *Psychosom. Med. 44:* 195–202, 1982.
31. Gentry, W. D. Relationship of anger-coping styles and blood pressure among black Americans. In: *Anger and Hostility in Cardiovascular and Behavioral Disorders,* edited by M. A. Chesney and R. H. Rosenman. Hemisphere Publishing Corporation, Washington, 1985, pp. 139–147.
32. Grim, C. E., F. C. Luft, J. Z. Miller, P. L. Brown, M. A. Cannon, and M. H. Weinberger. Effects of sodium loading and depletion in normotensive first-degree relatives of essential hypertensives. *J. Lab. Clin. Med. 94:* 764–771, 1979.
33. Grolnick, L. A family perspective of psychosomatic factors in illness: a review of the literature. *Fam. Process. 11:* 457–486, 1972.
34. Harburg, E., E. H. Blakelock, and P. J. Roeper. Resentful and reflective coping with arbitrary authority and blood pressure: Detroit. *Psychosom. Med. 41:* 189–202, 1979.
35. Harburg, E., S. Julius, N. F. McGinn, J. McLoed, and S. W. Hoobler. Personality traits and behavioral patterns associated with systolic blood pressure levels in college males. *J. Chronic Dis. 17:* 405–414, 1964.
36. Harburg, E., J. C. Erfurt, L. Hauenstein, C. Chape, W. J. Schull, and M. A. Schork. Socioecological stress, suppressed hostility, skin color, and black-white male blood pressure: Detroit. *Psychosom. Med. 35:* 276–296, 1973.
37. Harburg, E., L. Geibermann, P. Roeper, M. A. Schork, and W. J. Schull. Skin color, ethnicity, and blood pressure. I: Detroit blacks. *Am. J. Public Health 68:* 1177–1188, 1978.
38. Harburg, E., L. Geibermann, P. Roeper, M. A. Schork, and W. J. Schull. Skin color, ethnicity, and blood pressure. II. Detroit whites. *Am. J. Public Health 68:* 1189–1198, 1978.
39. Harrell, J. P. Analyzing black coping styles: a supplemental diagnostic system. *J. Black Psychol. 5:* 99–108, 1979.
40. Harrell, J. P. Psychological factors in hypertension: a status report. *Psychol. Bull. 87:* 482–501, 1980.
41. Harris, R. E., M. Sokolow, L. G. Carpenter, M. Freedman, and S. P. Hunt. Response to psychologic stress in persons who are potentially hypertensive. *Circulation 7:* 572–578, 1953.

42. Higgins, M. W., J. B. Keller, H. L. Metzner, F. E. Moore, and L. D. Ostrander. Studies of blood pressure in Tecumseh, Michigan. II. Antecedents in childhood of high blood pressure in young adults. *Hypertension 2* (Suppl 1): 117–123, 1980.

43. Hypertension Detection and Follow-up Cooperative Group: Race, education, and prevalence of hypertension. *Am. J. Epidemiol. 106:* 351–361, 1977.

44. James, S. A. Psychosocial and environmental factors in black hypertension. In: *Hypertension in Blacks: Epidemiology, Pathophysiology and Treatment,* edited by W. D. Hall, E. Saunders, and N. B. Shulman. Year Book Medical Publishers, Chicago, 1985, pp. 132–143.

45. James, S. A., and D. G. Kleinbaum. Socioecologic stress and hypertension-related mortality rates in North Carolina. *Am. J. Public Health 66:* 354–358, 1976.

46. James, S. A., S. A. Hartnett, and W. D. Kalsbeek. John Henryism and blood pressure differences among black men. *J. Behav. Med. 6:* 259–278, 1983.

47. James, S. A., A. Z. LaCroix, D. G. Kleinbaum, et al. John Henryism and blood pressure differences among black men. II. The role of occupational stressors. *J. Behav. Med. 7:* 259–275, 1984.

48. James, S. A., D. S. Strogatz, S. B. Wing, and D. L. Ramsey. Socioeconomic status, John Henryism and hypertension in blacks and whites. *Am. J. Epidemiol. 126:* 664–673, 1987.

49. Johnson, E. H., N. J. Schork, and C. D. Spielberger. Emotional and familial determinants of elevated blood pressure in black and white adolescent females. *J. Psychosom. Res. 31:* 731–741, 1987.

50. Johnson, E. H., C. D. Spielberger, T. J. Worden, and G. A. Jacobs. Emotional and familial determinants of elevated blood pressure in black and white adolescent males. *J. Psychosom. Res. 31:* 287–300, 1987.

51. Jorgensen, R. S., and B. K. Houston. Family history of hypertension, personality patterns, and cardiovascular reactivity to stress. *Psychosom. Med. 48:* 102–117, 1986.

52. Julius, M., E. Harburg, E. M. Cottington, and E. Johnson. Anger-coping types, blood pressure, and all-cause mortality: a follow-up in Tecumesh, Michigan (1971–1983). *Am. J. Epidemiol. 124:* 220–233, 1986.

53. Kessler, R. C., and H. W. Neighbors. A new perspective on the relationships among race, social class and psychological distress. *J. Health Soc. Behav. 27:* 107–115, 1986.

54. Knight, R. G. G., J. M. Paulin, and H. J. Waal-Manning. Self-reported anger intensity and blood pressure. *Br. J. Clin. Psychol. 26:* 65–66, 1987.

55. Krantz, D. S., and S. B. Manuck. Acute psychophysiologic reactivity and risk of cardiovascular disease: a review and methodologic critique. *Psychol. Bull. 96:* 435–464, 1984.

56. Langford, H. G., F. P. J. Langford, and M. Tyler. Dietary profile of sodium, potassium, and calcium in U.S. blacks. In: *Hypertension in Blacks: Epidemiology Pathophysiology and Treatment,* edited by W. D. Hall, E. Saunders, and N. B. Shulman. Year Book Medical Publishers, Chicago, 1985, pp. 49–57.

57. Luft, F. C., C. E. Grim, N. Fineberg, and M. H. Weinberger. Effects of volume contraction in normotensive whites, blacks and subjects of different ages. *Circulation 59:* 643–650, 1979.

58. Luft, F. C., L. I. Rankin, R. Bloch, et al. Cardiovascular and humoral responses to extremes of sodium intake in normal white and black men. *Circulation 60:* 697–706, 1979.

59. Manuck, S. B., and D. S. Krantz. Psychophysiologic reactivity in coronary heart disease and essential hypertension. In: *Handbook of Stress, Reactivity, and Cardiovascular Disease,* edited by K. A. Matthews, S. M. Weiss, T. Detre, T. M. Dembroski, B. Falkner, S. B. Manuck, and R. B. Williams, Jr. John Wiley & Sons, New York, 1986, pp. 11–34.

60. Manuck, S. B., R. L. Morrison, A. S. Bellack, and J. M. Polefrone. Behavioral factors in hypertension: cardiovascular responsivity, anger, and social competence. In: *Anger and Hostility in Cardiovascular and Behavioral Disorders,* edited by M. A. Chesney and R. H. Rosenman. Hemisphere/McGraw-Hill, New York, 1985, pp. 149–172.

61. Matthews, K. A., and C. J. Rakaczky. Familial aspects of the Type A behavior pattern and physiologic reactivity to stress. Paper presented at the conference on "Biobehavioral Factors in Heart Disease." Winterscheid, Federal Republic of Germany, June 1984.

62. McCarron, D. A., D. A. Morris, and C. Cole. Dietary calcium in human hypertension. *Science 217:* 267–269, 1982.

63. McClure, F. H. Cardiovascular stress responses in black hypertensive and normotensive families. Paper presented at the meeting of the American Psychological Association, New Orleans, La., August 1989.

64. McClure, F. H., and H. F. Myers. Blood pressure responses in black hypertensive and normotensive families during conflict. Unpublished paper.

65. Miall, W. E., P. Heneage, T. Khosla, H. G. Lovell, and F. Moore. Factors influencing the degree of resemblance in arterial pressure of close relatives. *Clin. Sci. 33:* 271–283, 1967.

66. Mongeau, J. G., and P. Biron. The influence of genetics and of household environment in the transmission of normal blood pressure. *Clin. Exp. Hypertens. 3(4):* 593–596, 1982.

67. Myers, H. F. Stress, ethnicity and social class: a model for research on black populations. In: *Minority Mental Health,* edited by E. E. Jones and S. Korchin. Holt, Rinehart & Winston, New York, 1982, pp. 118–148.

68. Myers, H. F., (chair), et al. Summary of workshop. III. Working group on socioeconomic and sociocultural influences in coronary heart disease. *Am. Heart J. 108*(3 part 2): 706–710, 1984.

69. Myers, H. F. Family contributions in essential hypertension in blacks. Paper presented at the meeting of the American Psychological Association, Washington, D.C., August 22–26, 1986.

70. Myers, H. F., N. B. Anderson, and T. L. Strickland. A biobehavioral perspective on stress and hypertension in black adults. In: *Black Adult Development and Aging,* edited by R. L. Jones. Cobb & Henry, Berkeley, 1989, pp. 311–349.

71. Neser, W. B., H. A. Tyroler, and J. C. Cassel. Social disorganization and stroke mortality in the black population of North Carolina. *Am. J. Epidemiol. 93:* 166–175, 1971.

72. Perini, C., F. B. Muller, U. Rauchfleisch, R. Battegay, and F. R. Buhler. Hyperadrenergic borderline hypertension is characterized by suppressed aggression. *J. Cardiovasc. Pharmacol. 8*(Suppl. 5): S53–56, 1986.

73. Persky, V., W. H. Pan, J. Stamler, A. Dyer, and P. Levy. Time trends in the U.S. racial difference in hypertension. *Am. J. Epidemiol. 124:* 724–737, 1986.

74. Pilowski, I., D. Spalding, J. Shaw, and P. I. Korner. Hypertension and personality. *Psychosom. Med. 35:* 50–56, 1973.

75. Prineas, R. J., and R. F. Gillum. U.S. epidemiology of hypertension in blacks. In: *Hypertension in Blacks: Epidemiology, Pathophysiology and Treatment,* edited by W. D. Hall, E. Saunders, N. B. Schulman. Year Book Medical Publishers, Chicago, 1985, pp. 37–48.

76. Roberts, J., and M. Rowland. Hypertension in adults 25–74 years of age, United States, 1971–1975. Vital and Health Statistics, Series II, data from the National Survey No. 221 (DDHS publication No. (PHS) 81-1671). Hyattsville, Md., Dept. of Health and Human Services, 1981.

77. Rowland, M., and J. Roberts. National Center for Health Statistics. Blood pressure levels and hypertension in persons ages 6–74 years: United States, 1976–1980. Vital and Health Statistics, AdvanceData, No. 84, Public Health Service, Washington, U.S. Government Printing Office, 1982, 1–11.

78. Sackett, D. L., G. D. Anderson, R. Milner, et al. Concordance for coronary risk factors among spouses. *Circulation 52:* 589–595, 1975.

79. Schachter, J. Pain, fear, and anger in hypertensives and normotensives. *Psychosom. Med. 19:* 17–29, 1957.

80. Siegel, J. M. Anger and cardiovascular risk in adolescents. *Health Psychol. 3:* 293–313, 1984.

81. Simmons, D. Blood pressure, ethnic group, and salt intake in Belize. *J. Epidemiol. Community Health 37:* 38–42, 1983.

82. Smith, M. A., and B. K. Houston. Hostility, anger expression, cardiovascular responsivity, and social support, *Biol. Psychol. 24:* 39–48, 1987.

83. Speers, M. A., S. V. Kasl, D. H. Freeman, and A. M. Ostfield. Blood pressure concordance between spouses. *Am. J. Epidemiol. 123:* 818–829, 1986.

84. Suarez, L., M. H. Criqui, and E. Barrett-Connor. Spouse concordance for systolic and diastolic blood pressure. *Am. J. Epidemiol. 118:* 345–351, 1983.

85. Sutherland, M. E., and J. P. Harrell. Individual differences in physiological responses to fearful, racially noxious, and neutral imagery. *Imaging Cognitive Personality 6:* 133–150, 1986–1987.

86. Syme, S. L. Psychosocial determinants of hypertension. In: *Hypertension: Determinants, Complications and Interventions,* edited by E. Onesti and C. Klimt. Grune & Stratton, New York, 1979, pp. 95–99.

87. Tyroler, H. A. The Detroit project studies of blood pressure: a prologue and review of related studies and epidemiological issues. *J. Chronic Dis. 30:* 613–624, 1977.

88. Viega Jardim, P. C. B., O. Carniero, and S. B. Carniero. Blood pressure in an isolated community of predominant black population of Northern Goias, Brazil (abstract). *Cardiovasc. Dis. Epidemiol. Newsletter 40:* 162, 1986.

89. Winkelstein, W. Jr., S. Kantor, M. Ibrahim, and D. L. Sackett. Familial aggregation of blood pressure: a preliminary report. *J.A.M.A. 195:* 848, 1966.

90. Winkleby, M. A., D. R. Ragland, and S. L. Syme. Self-reported stressors and hypertension: evidence of an inverse association. *Am. J. Epidemiol. 127(1):* 124–134, 1988.

91. Zinner, S. H., P. S. Levy, and E. H. Kass. Familial aggregation of blood pressure in childhood. *N. Engl. J. Med. 284:* 401–404, 1971.

92. Zinner, S. H., B. Rosner, W. Oh, and E. H. Kass. Significance of blood pressure in infancy: familial aggregation and predictive effect on later blood pressure. *Hypertension 7:* 411–416, 1985.

6

Autonomic Reactivity and Hypertension in Blacks: Toward a Contextual Model

NORMAN B. ANDERSON AND MAYA MCNEILLY

The purpose of this chapter is threefold. For readers not familiar with the reactivity paradigm, we describe the underlying tenets and provide a summary of animal and human research examining the validity of the reactivity hypothesis. This is followed by a review of research on black–white differences in autonomic reactivity as a means of understanding the higher rates of hypertension among blacks. The chapter concludes with a description of a contextual model that provides a framework for understanding the research findings to date, and a stimulus for future research in this area.

THE REACTIVITY HYPOTHESIS: ANIMAL AND HUMAN EVIDENCE

Autonomic nervous system response to behavioral and environmental stimuli and its relation to the development of essential hypertension has become a widely investigated area of behavioral medicine. The study of acute autonomic responses, or "reactivity," as these acute changes have come to be known, emphasizes individual differences in the magnitude and patterns of physiological *changes* in response to specific stimuli, rather than resting or basal autonomic activity.

A number of animal and human experiments have examined the hypothesis that the magnitude of acute cardiovascular and hormonal changes in response to stress may be of pathophysiological significance to the development of hypertension. Although it is beyond the scope of the current chapter to provide an exhaustive review of the animal and human literature, there are several excellent summaries available (4,44,62,85,89,99,102).

Animal Studies

In the initial animal experiments, Henry and associates (62,63) demonstrated that factors such as territorial conflict, residential crowding, and disruptions in social status produced sustained high blood pressure in mice. This sustained high blood pressure was preceded by transient activation of the "defense" or "fight–flight" pattern of β-adrenergically-mediated sympathetic outflow, in-

volving increases in heart rate, blood pressure, muscle blood flow, catecholamine release, and activation of the renin–angiotensin–aldosterone system.
Another line of animal reactivity research was conducted using the spontaneously hypertensive rat (SHR). When exposed to chronic daily stress in their
prehypertensive state, these animals exhibit exaggerated autonomic responses
when compared with animals not genetically predisposed to hypertension
(56,98). Importantly, these exaggerated, stress-induced pressor responses occur prior to the development of sustained high blood pressure in the SHRs. In
fact, hypertension in the SHR could be delayed considerably by decreasing
behavioral and environmental stress via social isolation (55).

Taken together, the findings with the SHRs illustrate the interaction of a
genetic predisposition to hypertension with behavioral and environmental
stress. David Anderson has conducted a series of studies with dogs demonstrating that the combination of behavioral stress and dietary sodium act synergistically to augment blood pressure (5,6). In these experiments, dogs exposed to daily trials of shock avoidance tasks for 2 weeks exhibited a
significant increase in blood pressure, but only while on a high sodium diet (5).
Interestingly, neither the chronic daily stress nor the high sodium intake alone
was able to produce the sustained hypertension.

Human Studies

In a human reactivity experiment, measures of autonomic activity are obtained during baseline, stress, and recovery periods while subjects are either
seated or supine. Studies are typically conducted with the subject in a sound-
attenuated chamber and the physiological recording equipment in an adjacent
room. Extended baseline measurements are made, usually between 10 and 30
min, during which samples of autonomic functioning are obtained at regular
intervals (e.g., every minute). This extended baseline period allows for the sta-
bilization of cardiovascular and neuroendocrine activity while subjects receive
minimal environmental stimulation. Following this extended baseline period,
subjects participate in one or more "stressful" or challenging procedures. These
procedures may include any one or more of the following: mental arithmetic,
competitive and noncompetitive reaction time tasks, video games, anagrams,
speech stress, cold pressor test, handgrip, orthostasis, physical exercise, mirror
tracing, or the Stroop task. Following the stress period, there may be a recovery
period to measure physiological responses while the subject again rests quietly.

Of most interest in reactivity research is the magnitude of change in the
various autonomic indices (e.g., heart rate, cardiac output, blood pressure,
forearm blood flow, and catecholamines) from the resting baseline to the stress
period. Wide and consistent individual differences have been observed in response to these laboratory challenges, and it is hypothesized that the magnitude of autonomic reactivity may be positively associated with the development of essential hypertension (41,42,102,124).

In addition to the absolute magnitude of autonomic changes in response
to laboratory procedures, reactivity research is also concerned with the *patterns* of autonomic adjustment. In particular, two patterns of autonomic adjustments, the "β-adrenergic" and "α-adrenergic" patterns, have been investigated most thoroughly. The β-adrenergic reactivity pattern is characterized by

an increase in blood pressure associated with increases in cardiac output, stroke volume, heart rate, epinephrine and norepinephrine, and a decrease in total peripheral resistance. This pattern is most clearly observed in response to tasks such as mental arithmetic, competitive reaction time tasks, physical exercise, video games, and the preparation period of the speech stressor. In contrast to the β-adrenergic pattern, the α-adrenergic produces an increase in blood pressure via a large secretion of plasma norepinephrine accompanied by an increase in total peripheral resistance. Indeed, the increase in peripheral vascular resistance is the hallmark of the α-adrenergic pattern. Laboratory procedures that produce a predominantly α-pattern include the forehead, foot, and hand cold pressor tests, the speech stressor (speaking portion), mirror tracing, handgrip, and orthostasis. To date, most of the laboratory research has focused on the β-adrenergic pattern of reactivity, although the α-adrenergic pattern is beginning to receive increased attention. Interestingly, most of the longitudinal research on autonomic reactivity and the development of hypertension has utilized α-adrenergic stimuli (e.g., the cold pressor test). It is important to point out that the labeling of these patterns as β- or α-adrenergic is mainly for descriptive purposes, since the underlying receptor involvement in the cardiovascular patterns produced by most of the aforementioned laboratory stressors has not been confirmed using pharmacological blockade procedures.

Unlike the animal research, most experiments using the reactivity paradigm with humans have been cross-sectional rather than longitudinal. Studies have focused on comparisons between hypertensives and normotensives, or individuals at risk for hypertension due to a family history versus those with a negative family history (43,45,103). In general, these experiments have shown that in response to laboratory stressors: *(1)* whites with established or borderline hypertension exhibit cardiovascular hyperreactivity compared with subjects with normal blood pressure (46,66,135); and *(2)* whites with a parental history of hypertension exhibit greater cardiovascular responses than the offspring of normotensives (28,78,100).

Although there is considerable evidence that autonomic reactivity is correlated with hypertension status and risk for hypertension, there have been few prospective epidemiological studies that have evaluated whether heightened autonomic reactivity *predicts* the subsequent onset of hypertension. There is even less evidence that exaggerated autonomic reactivity *causes* hypertension in humans. Several studies, however, have uncovered significant and positive associations between exercise-induced reactivity and later hypertension development (68,146). Of the handful of prospective epidemiological studies conducted on non-exercise-induced reactivity and hypertension, the vast majority have used the cold pressor test to elicit reactivity (17,28,30,31,60,111,149). Of these studies, only two (111,149) have been able to demonstrate the predictive validity of the cold pressor test for subsequent hypertension development (125).

The majority of the negative studies, however, have suffered from methodological weaknesses including inadequate sample sizes, short duration follow-up, or inappropriate assessment of reactivity (99). In a study that was free of many of these methodological flaws (111), researchers studied 910 white male medical students whose blood pressure and pulse were measured before and during the cold pressor test. The students were tested between 1948 and 1964. In the follow-up period, ranging between 20 and 36 years, it was discovered that the maximal change in systolic blood pressure during the cold pressor test was significantly predictive of the incidence of hypertension by age 44. This association persisted after adjustments for age at study entry, Quetelet index, cigarette smoking, pretest systolic blood pressure, and paternal or maternal history of hypertension. Menkes et al. (149) note that the excess risk associated with systolic blood pressure reactivity was not apparent until the population aged some 20 years, and was most apparent among those in whom hypertension developed before age 45.

In a study using a behavioral rather than physical stressor, Borghi et al. (21) found that among borderline hypertensives with high intralymphocytic sodium levels, diastolic blood pressure reactivity and recovery from a mental arithmetic task were significant predictors of sustained hypertension after 5 years. Those persons who exhibited greater reactivity and who had recovery pressures at least 6% above baseline levels were at greatest risk for developing sustained hypertension.

Although recent epidemiological research has established an association between reactivity and hypertension, the exact nature of this association remains ambiguous. As Manuck et al. (99) note, autonomic reactivity may be linked to hypertension development in any of a number of ways. For example, reactivity may be a direct cause of hypertension, whereby increases in neurogenic input and cardiac output may, over time, lead to augmented peripheral resistance and structural changes in the arterial walls (40). Alternatively, reactivity may serve only as a risk marker, where it may predict subsequent hypertension yet be of no pathogenic significance. Third, autonomic reactivity may cause hypertension, but only if this response is frequently elicited over a protracted period of time. In this "diathesis-stress" model, some individuals may have a biological predisposition to exaggerated reactivity. Whether this predisposition leads to established hypertension is determined by the frequency with which the individual is exposed to environments that elicit the augmented cardiovascular response. The more frequently elicited, the greater the likelihood that the heightened reactivity would result in sustained high blood pressure. Finally, autonomic reactivity may act in synergy with other risk factors to enhance further the risk for hypertension. That is, reactivity may act to modulate the effects of other risk factors such as dietary sodium or family history of hypertension (99). For example, animal research reviewed earlier suggests that while neither sodium nor chronic stress alone produces sustained high blood pressure in dogs, their combined influence does (5). At this time, there are insufficient data to warrant advocating one model over another.

Although the relationship between autonomic reactivity and the development of essential hypertension remains to be specified, the reactivity laboratory paradigm has generated a considerable amount of research activity. In recent years, investigators have explored racial differences in reactivity in attempts to understand the higher rates of hypertension among blacks compared with whites. In this chapter, we provide a review of research on racial differences in reactivity in both children and adults. In order to highlight race differences in the patterns of reactivity (i.e., β- versus α-adrenergic) the review is organized into sections discussing cardiac responses (e.g., heart rate, cardiac output, etc.) and vascular responses (e.g., blood pressure, peripheral resistance, forearm blood flow). This review is based in part on an earlier review by Anderson (7), but has been updated to reflect more recent studies. Following this review, a conceptual model is presented that illustrates the possible biopsychosocial interactions that might underlie the racial differences in reactivity, and that might serve as a guide for future research.

BLACK–WHITE DIFFERENCES IN REACTIVITY

Table 6.1 provides a summary of studies on race differences in reactivity.

Cardiac Reactivity

Children
Investigations of cardiac reactivity in black children and white children have used both physical (e.g., exercise, forehead cold pressor, and postural tilt) and psychological (e.g., video game) challenges. Studies employing physical stimuli have produced inconsistent results, with some indicating higher levels of exercise-induced heart rate or cardiac index among whites relative to blacks (15,20,65,141), while others have yielded nonsignificant race differences in response to exercise, postural tilt, and forehead cold pressor (1,137,140). In contrast to these data from studies using physical challenges, psychological challenges such as video games have consistently elicited greater heart rate reactivity among black children than whites (114–116). In two of these studies, effects of experimenter race on heart rate responses were observed where children, particularly blacks, have shown greater heart rate reactivity when paired with a same-race experimenter (114,115). There was also a tendency for white children to have higher resting heart rates than black children when paired with a black experimenter. The authors speculated that same-race pairings possibly elicited an increased effort to perform well on the tasks, whereas the mixed-race pairings resulted in decreased challenge and involvement.

Adults
Similar to the data on cardiac reactivity among children, the data on heart rate reactivity in black adults and white adults are somewhat mixed. For example, studies have shown that younger blacks show diminished cardiac reactivity (indicated by lower heart rate or cardiac output responses) both at rest and in response to stressors such as mental arithmetic, video games, competitive and noncompetitive reaction time tasks, and mental arithmetic (9,32,44,92,118). Other studies have shown no race differences in heart rate or cardiac output reactivity among normotensives or hypertensives (10,11,30,90, 104,112,136,138). As will be elaborated in the next section, Light and Sherwood (90) reported a greater fall in cardiac output during a challenging reaction time task following β-adrenergic blockade in blacks with normal and elevated blood pressure compared with their white counterparts. In one study, higher heart rates among black hypertensives compared with white

TABLE 6.1. Black–White Difference in Reactivity[a]

Author	No./ Race	Age (yr)	Gender	Blood pressure status	Family history hypertension	Personality
1. Alpert, B. S. et al. (1)	184 B 221 W	6–15	M (NR) F (NR)	N	NR	NA
2. Alpert, B. S. et al. (1)	184 B 221 W	6–15	M (NR) F (NR)	N	NR	NA
3. Anderson, N. B. et al. (13)	41 B	26–63 X = 48.6	F	N	Type A: 4 +/3 − Type B: 9 +/9 − Type X: 10 +/7 −	7 Type A 18 Type B 17 Type X
4. Anderson N. B. et al. (14)	33 B	18–22	F	N	17 +/16 −	NA
5. Anderson, N. B. et al. (8,9)	10 B 10 W	18–21	M	N	NA	NA
6. Anderson, N. B. et al. (9)	17 B 20 W	18–22	M	N	NA	NA
7. Anderson, N. B. et al. (11)	42 B 32 W	18–22	F	N	B: 23 +/19 − W: 7 +/25 −	NA
8. Anderson, N. B. et al. (10)	27 B 29 W	18–22	M	N	B: 11 +/16 − W: 13 +/16 −	NA
9. Armstead, C. A. et al. (16)	24 B	College aged	12 M 12 F	NR	NR	NA
10. Arensman, F. W. et al. (15)	19 B 31 W	10	M	N	NR	NA
11. Berenson, G. S. et al. (20)	139 B 139 W	6–16	139 M 139 F	5 strata based on DBP	NR	NA
12. Dimsdale, J. E. et al. (27)	27 B 28 W	N: 32 ± 6 H: 35 ± 7	M	N H	+ FH − FH	NA

112

Procedures	Measures	Results
Continuous graded bicycle ergometer	SBP, HR	SBP: Bs > Ws (levels)
Continuous graded bicycle ergometer	HR, SBP, maximal workload physical working capacity. J point displacement, ST segment slope	SBP: Bs > Ws (levels) ST: Bs > Ws (levels) Workload: Bs > Ws for those with middle range body surface area
MA, SI	SBP, DBP, HR, speech components of SI	SBP, DBP: Type As > Type Bs and Type Xs in response to SI Potential for hostility and Type A speech components positively related to cardiovascular responses
MA	SBP, DBP, MAP, HR, FBF, FVR	SBP, DBP, FBF: $+$FH $<$ $-$FH (changes)
CP	SBP, DBP, MAP, HR, FBF, FVR	SBP, DBP, HR: Bs > Ws (changes)
MA	SBP, DBP, MAP, HR, FBF, FVR, mood state, aerobic fitness	SBP, DBP, HR: Bs < Ws (changes)
MA, CP	SBP, DBP, MAP, HR, FBF, FVR, mood state	SBP: Bs > Ws in response to CP (changes) DBP: Bs slower recovery vs Ws following MA (changes) Mood: Bs > Ws in anxiety, guilt, fear, restlessness and decreases in alertness, relaxation, and happiness in response to MA (changes)
MA, CP	SBP, DBP, MAP, HR, FBF, FVR	SBP, DBP: Bs > Ws in response to CP (levels)
Films viewed depicting (a) racist situations involving Bs, (b) anger-provoking nonracist situations, and (C) neutral scenes	BP, mood checklist, Trait and state anger	BP: greater for racist scenes vs other scenes (changes) State anger: increased to racist and anger-provoking scenes (changes) BP: positively correlated with trait anger
Graded bicycle ergometer	SBP, DBP, CI, CO, SVR	SVR: Bs > Ws at pre-exercise and maximal exercise, and early and late recovery (levels) CI: Ws > Bs at pre-exercise and maximal exercise, and early and late recovery (levels)
Children re-examined 1–2 yr after initial participation in the Bogalusa Heart Study. Tasks: orthostatic stress, handgrip, CP, and glucose tolerance test	SBP, HR, urinary NA^+ and K^+, PRA serum dopamine β-hydroxylase, plasma glucose	SBP: Bs with highest DBP showed highest stress-induced levels PRA: SBP negatively correlated in Bs with highest DBPs HR: Ws > Bs (levels) K^+: Ws > Bs (levels) Dopamine beta-hydroxylase: Ws > Bs Glucose: Ws > Bs
Dietary sodium loads: 200 mEq/day for 4 days and 10 mEq/day for 5 days, NE infusions	SBP, DBP, urinary NA^+	BP: linear dose-response curve with NE. Older subjects showed steeper slopes. High Na^+ diet produced steeper slopes, particularly among Bs, compared to low Na^+ diet. BHs > WHs for SS

(continued)

113

TABLE 6.1. Black–White Difference in Reactivity[a]—*Continued*

Author	No./ Race	Age (yr)	Gender	Blood pressure status	Family history hypertension	Personality
13. Durel, L. et al. (30)	72 B 63 W	25–44	81 M 54 F	N to H	No group differences	NA
14. Falkner, B. et al. (33)	40 B	18–23	NR	NR	B: 67% + W: 38% +	NA
15. Falkner, B. et al. (32)	83 B 38 W	18–23	NR	B: 48 N 35 H W: 30 N 8 H	NR	NA
16. Falkner, B. et al. (34)	83 B 38 W	18–23	NR	B: 48 N 35 H W: 30 N 8 H	NR	NA
17. Fredrickson, M. (44)	15 B 21 W	41–52	21 M 15 F	N, BdH, H	NR	NA
18. Hohn, A. R. et al. (65)	62 B 79 W	10–17	NR	N	B: 42 + /20 − W: 34 + /45 −	NA

Procedures	Measures	Results
SI, VG, CP, AMBP at home and work	SBP, DBP, Cook-Medley Hostility Scale, State-Trait Anger Scale, Cognitive-Somatic Anger Scale, Framingham & Harburg anger scales	SBP, DBP: Bs > Ws to CP; Ws > Bs to SI; Ms > Fs to VG Hostility: Bs > Ws; Trait anger: Bs < Ws; Somatic anger: Fs > Ms AMBP: Fs showed a positive correlation between all 4 anger scales and AMBPs at work Numerous correlations between personality, mood, and CV response
MA before and after 14-day dietary sodium load (10 g/day) added to subjects' usual diet	DBP, MAP, SS, Wt	DBP: after sodium loading, SS > Sin (levels) MAP: after sodium loading, SS Bs with +FH > Sin Bs with −FH (levels) WT: after sodium loading, +FH Bs > −FH Bs (changes)
MA before and after dietary sodium load (10 g/day) added to subjects' usual diet	SBP, DBP, HR, SS	SBP, DBP: Hs > Ns during MA before and after loading (levels) SBP: Ws > Bs after Na$^+$ loading during MA (levels and changes) HR: Ws > Bs before and after Na$^+$ loading (changes) SS (prevalence): Bs > Ws Wt.: Hs > Ns after Na$^+$ loading
MA before and after dietary sodium load (10 g/day) added to subjects' usual diet	MAP, HR, urinary Na$^+$, Wt	SS (prevalence): Bs > Ws NA$^+$ excretion: Sin > SS WT: SS > Sin MAP: −correlation between MAP change and Na$^+$ excretion; FH > −FH before and after Na$^+$ loading
Aversive RT	SBP, DBP, HR, RES, SKBF, SKVR, MBF, MVR, SCP, SCR	SBP, HR: BHs and BNs < WHs and WNs SCP, SCR: Bs < Ws SKVR, MVR: increased in Bs
Treadmill	SBP, DBP, urinary: Na$^+$, electrolytes, kallikrein, prostaglandin E-like material, PRA, NE	*Results for Hs* SBP, DBP: Bs with +FH > Bs with −FH; Bs > Ws at rest with exertion (levels) HR: Ws with +FH > Ws with −FH following exercise; Ws > Bs before and after exercise (levels) PRA: Bs with +FH > Bs with −FH; Ws > Bs before and after exercise NE: Ws with +FH < Ws with −FH following exercise NA$^+$ excretion: Bs > Ws before exercise K$^+$ excretion: Ws > Bs before exercise Prostaglandin E-like material: Ws with +FH > Ws with −FH before exercise *Results for Ns* Na$^+$, K$^+$ excretion: Bs > Ws (before exercise) PRA: Bs < Ws (before and after exercise) NE: Bs < Ws (after exercise)

(continued)

115

TABLE 6.1. Black–White Difference in Reactivity[a]—*Continued*

Author	No./ Race	Age (yr)	Gender	Blood pressure status	Family history hypertension	Personality
19. Johnson, E. H. et al. (75)	24 B	19–25	M	N	12 +/12 −	NA
20. Light, K. C. et al. (92)	109 B 119 W	18–22	M	BdH	NR	NA
21. Light, K. C. et al. (90)	20 B 20 W	18–22	M	N and Marginally elevated casual BP: 5 B/6 W	NR	NA
22. McAdoo, W. G. et al. (104)	47 B 70 W	18–30	66 M 51 F	N	NR	NA
23. McNeilly, M. et al. (110)	17 B 20 W	19–50	M	N, BdH, H	Groups matched	NA
24. Morrell, M. A. (112)	34 B 42 W	34–55 x = 43.01	M	N	B: 13 +/21 − W: 18 +/24 −	NA
25. Murphy, J. K. et al. (114)	109 B 104 W	6–18	125 M 88 F	N	NR	NA
26. Murphy, J. K. et al. (115)	68 B 411 W	9	237 M 242 F	NR	NR	NA

Procedures	Measures	Results
Anagrams, MA, home blood pressures	SBP, DBP, HR, State-Trait Personality Inventory, Anger Expression Scale, State Anger Reaction Scale, Jenkins Activity Scale, Submissive/Dominance subscales from the 16PF Scale	SBP, DBP: $+$FH $>$ $-$FH (resting, stress-induced and home levels) Trait anger, Anger-out, Submissiveness: $+$FH $>$ $-$FH
CP, competitive and noncompetitive RT with and without monetary incentives; 74 Bs and 84 Ws tested in same-race pairs with the remainder tested in different-race pairs	SBP, DBP, HR	SBP: BHs $>$ WHs (changes) DBP, Hr: BHs $>$ BNs to RT HR: Bs $<$ Ws at rest and during stress (levels) Bs and Ws with casually elevated blood pressure showed greater increases in BP and HR vs those without casually elevated BPs
Competitive RT task with propranolol (beta blocker)	SBP, DBP, HR, TPR, PEP, CO, SV	DBP: Bs with marginally elevated SBP $>$ Ws during stressor before and after beta blockade (changes) CO: Bs and Ws with marginally elevated SBP $>$ during task vs Ns preblockade (changes) TPR: Bs $>$ Ws in response to task (changes) SV, PEP, CO: Bs $<$ Ws to task with blockade (changes)
MA, Stroop, Mirror Draw Isometric handgrip, CP	SBP, DBP, HR	BP: Bs $>$ Ws in response to CP and DBP to handgrip; Ms $>$ Fs to all stressors HR: Ms $<$ Fs
Intravenous catherization	SBP, DBP, HR, plasma β-endorphin, urinary Na^+	SBP, DBP, HR: Hs $>$ Ns; BHs $>$ WHs (levels) β-endorphin: BHs $<$ BNs; WHs $>$ WNs (levels) Lower levels of β-endorphin and urinary Na^+ correlated with higher BP and HR (levels)
MA	SBP, DBP, HR, SCR SCP	DBP: Bs $>$ Ws at baseline and during task (levels) SCR: Bs $<$ Ws at baseline and during task (levels) No significant effects when baseline differences covaried.
VG and race of experimenter effects	SBP, DBP, HR	SBP, DBP: Bs $>$ Ws (changes) HR: same-race pairs $>$ mixed-race pairs (changes)
VG	SBP, DBP, HR	SBP, DBP, HR: Bs $>$ Ws (changes)

(continued)

117

TABLE 6.1. Black–White Difference in Reactivity[a]—*Continued*

Author	No./ Race	Age (yr)	Gender	Blood pressure status	Family history hypertension	Personality
27. Murphy, J. K. et al. (116)	135 B 175 W	6–18 x = 11.0	192 M 118 F	N	NR	NA
28. Musante, L. et al. (117)	16 B	11–14 x = 12.9±1.7	M	N	8 + FH 8 – FH	NA
29. Myers, H. F. et al. (118)	20 B 20 W	18–35 x = 22.78	M	N	B: 10+/10 – W: 10+/10 –	NA
30. Rowlands, D. B. et al. (131)	16 B 16 W	21–58	18 M 14 F	H	NR	NA
31. Strickland, T. L. et al. (136)	24 B 24 W	17–22	F	N	B: 12+/12 – W: 12+/12 –	NA
32. Tell, G. S. et al. (137)	302 B 614 W	14–16	500 M 416 F	N	NR	NA
33. Tischenkel, N. J. et al. (138)	44 B 39 W	25–44	47 M 36 F	N	NR	NA
34. Trieber, F. A. et al. (141)	24 B 51 W	4–6	37 M 38 F	N	NR	NA
35. Trieber, F. A. et al. (140)	20 W 20 B	10–14	M	N	NR	NA
36. Venter, C. P. et al.—study done in South Africa	16 B 16 W	NR	NR	N	NR	NA

118

Procedures	Measures	Results
VG and race of experimenter effects	SBP, DBP, HR	SBP: Ms > Fs (changes) DBP: main effect of experimenter—B > W; interaction between child's race and child's gender—BMs > WMs whereas BFs = WFs; same-race pairings (especially for Bs) > mixed-race pairings (changes) HR: same-race pairing for Bs > mixed-race pairings Repeated exposure to video game produced progressively higher levels of BP and HR
CP	SBP, DBP, HR, CO, SV, TPR	DBP, TPR: +FH > −FH (changes)
Caffeine (250 mg) vs placebo (3 mg caffeine) and MA	SBP, HR	SBP: caffeine > placebo; caffeine + stress > placebo; Bs with +FH showed slower recovery after stress vs Ws (changes) HR: Ws > Bs overall but not specific to caffeine or stress (levels)
Intraarterial AMBP, isometric exercise, dynamic exercise (bicycle ergometer) CP and phenylephrine challenge to test sinoaortic baroreflex activity	SBP, DBP, baroreflex activity, fasting cholesterol and triglycerides, resting PRA and NE, and urinary Na$^+$ and K$^+$	All NS
Caffeine (250 mg) vs placebo (3 mg caffeine) and MA	SBP, DBP, HR	SBP, DBP: increased with caffeine + stress HR: decreased with caffeine + stress
Orthostatic stress (supine to standing)	SBP, DBP, HR	SBP: decreased in response to stress; Bs > Ws (changes); decreases positively correlated with supine SBP DBP: increased in response to stress; Fs > Ms (changes); increases negatively correlated with resting DBP
SI, VG, CP, bicycle ergometer	SBP, DBP, HR; plasma E, NE, and PRA; urinary Na$^+$ and K$^+$	SBP: BFs > BMs or Ws to bicycle exercise (changes) DBP: Bs > Ws in response to CP (changes) SBP and DBP: Ms > Fs in response to VG (changes)
Treadmill	SBP, DBP, HR	SBP: Bs < Ws (changes and levels) HR: Bs < Ws (pre-exercise and peak levels); Fs > Ms (pre-exercise levels)
CP	SBP, DBP, HR, CO, and TPR	DBP: for both studies Bs > Ws (changes) TPR: for both studies Bs > Ws (changes)
Head-up tilt	SBP, DBP	SBP: increased only in Ws DBP: increased in both Bs and Ws

(continued)

TABLE 6.1. Black–White Difference in Reactivity[a]—*Continued*

Author	No./ Race	Age (yr)	Gender	Blood pressure status	Family history hypertension	Personality
37. Voors, A. W. et al. (142)	139 B 139 W	7–15	139 M 139 F	5 strata based on DBP	NR	NA

[a]Abbreviations: B = black; BF = black female; BH = borderline hypertensive; BM = black male; BP = blood pressure; CI = cardiac index; CO = cardiac output; CP = cold pressor; dB = decibels; DBP = diastolic blood pressure; F = female; FBF = forearm blood flow; +FH = positive family history; −FH = negative family history; FVR = forearm vascular resistance; g = gram; H = hypertensive; HR = heart rate; K⁺ = potassium; L = liter; M = male; MA = mental arithmetic; MAP = mean arterial blood pressure; MBF = muscle blood flow; mEq = millequivalents; mg = milligrams; MVR = muscle vascular resistance; N = normotensive; NA = not applicable; Na⁺ = sodium; NaCl = sodium chloride; NE = norepinephrine;

hypertensives were found in response to repeated exposure to the foot-immersion cold pressor task (110).

Vascular Reactivity

Children

In contrast to the cardiac reactivity data, results from studies on race differences in vascular reactivity have produced a more consistent pattern of findings. Studies conducted with children indicate that, compared with whites, black children show greater increases in blood pressure and total peripheral resistance in response to both physical (e.g., exercise, cold pressor, postural tilt) and behavioral (e.g., video games) stimuli (15,114–116,141). In a study investigating race differences in exercise-induced SBP, cardiac index (CI), and systemic vascular resistance, Arensman et al. (15) tested black and white 10-year-old boys in a supine, graded, maximal exercise test. Although there were no significant race effects on blood pressure responses, white males showed higher CI responses before, during, and after stress, whereas black males showed greater systemic vascular resistance throughout experimental periods. The authors concluded that although the blood pressure responses of black and white children were similar, the mechanisms sustaining blood pressure elevations in blacks were increased vascular resistance and diminished CI.

Adults

As with children, black adults generally show greater blood pressure, forearm vascular, and total peripheral resistance reactivity than whites (89,11,92,104, 110,138,139). Several studies, however, have yielded nonsignificant differences (139) or noted the lower blood pressure responses among blacks compared with whites (9,32,44). It should be noted, however, that in studies where blacks have been found to exhibit smaller blood pressure responses than whites, researchers have used stimuli that activate the β-adrenergic reactivity pattern. In these studies, therefore, there were also smaller heart rate responses among blacks.

Procedures	Measures	Results
Orthostatic stress, isometric exercise (handgrip), and CP	SBP, DBP, HR, PRA, serum and urine electrolytes	SBP, DBP: Bs > Ws; Bs with highest DBPs > other groups during stress (levels). Stress-induced pressures negatively correlated with PRA (levels) HR: Ws with highest DBPs > other groups during stress (levels)

NR = not reported; PEP = preejection period; PF = personality factor; PRA = plasma renin activity; RT = reaction time; SBP = systolic blood pressure; SC = skin conductance; SCP = skin conductance potential; SCR = skin conductance response; SI = structured interview; SkBF = skin blood flow; SkVR = skin vascular resistance; SS = sodium sensitivity; SV = stroke volume; SVR = systemic vascular resistance; TPR = total peripheral resistance; VG = videogames; W = white; WF = white female; WM = white male; x = mean.

In a study highlighting the complexities of race differences in patterns of cardiac and vascular reactivity to pharmacological and psychosocial challenges, Light and Sherwood (90) assessed race differences in patterns of cardiovascular responses to a competitive reaction time task with and without β-antagonist challenge (propranolol) among males with normal or marginally elevated SBP. Before blockade, subjects with elevated SBP, regardless of race, showed greater stress-induced increases in cardiac output than normotensives; blacks, however, showed greater diastolic reactivity responses than whites. After blockade, blacks with normal and elevated systolic pressure showed a greater attenuation of stressor-induced stroke volume, preejection period, and cardiac output than white subjects, and greater increases in total peripheral resistance. The increases in peripheral resistance suggest, as the authors point out, that blacks, especially those with elevated systolic pressure, may show greater α-adrenergic activity or sensitivity. The greater fall in cardiac factors following beta blockade suggest a *greater* β-adrenergic influence in blacks. At the time, however, the fact that blacks did not show a larger increase in cardiac factors prior to blockade makes this hypothesis less tenable. A more parsimonious explanation may be that the greater decline in cardiac factors among blacks following beta blockade was due partly to a larger vagal reflex in response to their higher peripheral resistance.

In another study investigating relationships between anger and cardiovascular responses across race and gender, Durel et al. (30) noted that vascular reactivity was influenced by the type of task. They observed that increases to the cold pressor task (a stimulus that elicits predominantly α-adrenergically-mediated vasoconstriction) were greater in blacks than whites, whereas whites showed greater blood pressure increases than blacks during the Type A structured interview (SI).

Neuroendocrine Responses

Catecholamines and certain neuropeptides such as renin and β-endorphin, regulate blood pressure, heart rate, and sodium balance through direct and indirect actions on the brain, heart, kidney, and vasculature.

Catecholamines

Studies indicate that along with showing exaggerated cardiovascular responses to stressors, hypertensives show augmented catecholamine responses to stressors (49). Few studies, however, have examined the relationship between catecholamines and race. For example, in reviewing the literature, Goldstein (49) reported only 8 of 78 comparative studies identified the racial makeup of the subject population. Of these, 5 involved only white patients.

More recent studies of catecholamine responses among blacks produced mixed results. For example, Hohn et al. (65) observed that black normotensives showed lower basal levels of norepinephrine than whites. Berenson et al. (20) observed that relative to whites, blacks showed smaller stress-induced increases in plasma levels of dopamine β-hydroxylase, a catecholamine metabolite less frequently studied in psychophysiological investigations. Other studies have produced nonsignificant results with respect to between- or within-race differences in catecholamine responses (131,138).

Neuropeptides

Research indicates that compared with whites, blacks generally show lower levels of plasma renin activity (PRA) and a greater preponderance of low-renin hypertension (52; see also Chapter 10, this volume). While a number of investigations have studied race differences in basal levels of PRA, fewer have studied PRA responses to stimulation. Most of these studies have found that black adults show lower levels than white adults, whether at rest or in response to stimulation (61,94,95). Hohn further observed that hypertensive blacks with a positive family history of hypertension showed higher PRA levels than blacks with a negative family history. In two studies in which PRA was measured in black children and white children (20,142), blood pressure reactivity was negatively correlated with PRA among black boys in the highest diastolic blood pressure strata. Nonsignificant effects of race on stress-induced PRA levels were obtained by Rowland et al. (131) and Tischenkel et al. (138), who exposed their subjects to a variety of both physical and psychosocial stressors.

Opioid inhibition of sympathetic activity is deficient in white individuals with or at risk for essential hypertension (106–108). Race differences in the opioid mediation of hypertension were investigated by McNeilly et al. (109,110), who observed that black hypertensives showed lower levels of β-endorphin, an opioid peptide, than black normotensives, whereas white hypertensives showed higher endorphin levels than their normotensive counterparts in response to repeated exposure to the foot immersion cold pressor task. In addition, lower levels of plasma β-endorphin were associated with higher blood pressure and heart rate, particularly among black hypertensives.

PREDICTORS OF REACTIVITY AMONG BLACKS

Most reactivity research that included blacks has consisted of racial comparisons of cardiovascular responses between blacks and whites. Since not all blacks are at higher risk for developing hypertension, researchers have begun to investigate predictors of reactivity and risk, such as family history of hypertension, blood pressure status, and personality *among* blacks. A review of this literature follows.

Family History of Hypertension

Although a number of studies have shown that family history of hypertension predicts cardiovascular reactivity among whites (103), this effect has been less consistent among blacks. Musante et al. (117) found that black children with a positive family history showed greater cardiovascular reactivity to the forehead cold pressor than those with a negative family history. Other studies, with adults, have found higher reactivity and stress-induced *levels,* rather than changes, in those individuals with a positive family history of hypertension (33,65,75). Most studies, however, have shown no significant effects of family history on reactivity (10,11,13,112,136), although Myers et al. (118) found slower recovery following stress in those subjects with a positive family history. Possible reasons for the lack of significant findings for family history are discussed later in this chapter.

Blood Pressure Status

The vast majority of studies comparing blacks at differing levels of blood pressure have shown that, among children and adults, individuals with higher blood pressure show greater reactivity to a variety of stressors than individuals with lower blood pressure (20,90,92,110,142). One study, studies, however, failed to obtain significant effects of blood pressure status on cardiovascular reactivity, although race differences in reactivity were observed (44).

Personality

Studies have shown that among blacks, elevated resting blood pressure and hypertension have been associated with suppressed anger and hostility (47,57,58,75,76). Similarly, investigations of cardiovascular reactivity and personality among blacks suggest that anger, hostility, and Type A behavior are associated with greater reactivity. The nature of this relationship, however, may depend on gender, family history of hypertension, personality constructs measured, and the experimental tasks and stimuli used. For example, Durel et al. (30) found that among black females, trait anger was associated with greater systolic and diastolic pressure at rest in the laboratory and at work, and with diastolic pressure during the cold pressor task. Among black males, however, positive correlations were observed only between cognitive anger and diastolic pressure at rest.

Relatedly, Anderson et al. (13) found that Type As showed greater blood pressure reactivity than Bs and Xs in response to the Type A structured interview but not to mental arithmetic. In addition, the potential for hostility and speech components of the interview responses were positively related to cardiovascular reactivity. Similarly, in another study, Clark and Harrell (23) found that Type A behavior was positively associated with diastolic blood pressure reactivity among blacks.

Johnson (75) observed interactive effects of personality and family history of hypertension on blood pressure. Black males with a positive family history showed higher levels of trait anger, anger-out, and submissiveness than those with a negative family history. These males also showed the greatest blood pressure levels at rest and during stress. Finally, Armstead et al. (16) tested the effects of exposure to racist stimuli on anger and cardiovascular reactivity among blacks. They observed that blood pressure increases were significantly greater after exposure to video clips depicting racist scenes than those showing nonracist, anger-provoking, and neutral scenes. Additionally, blood pressure responses were positively correlated with trait anger.

Summary of Research Findings

There have been a substantial number of studies on black–white differences in autonomic reactivity. These studies have been conducted with both children and adults, and have utilized a wide variety of laboratory stressors, experimental designs, physiological measures, and population subgroups. Yet, despite the diversity of approaches used, most studies have demonstrated that blacks show a greater blood pressure reactivity to laboratory stressors compared with their white counterparts. Perhaps more important is that the mechanisms responsible for producing the stress-induced elevation of blood pressure response may be different in blacks than in whites. Blacks have been found to exhibit greater blood pressure reactivity mediated by peripheral vasoconstriction (characteristic of the α-adrenergic pattern), while the blood pressure response of whites has shown a greater cardiac involvement (characteristic of the β-adrenergic pattern). These results, particularly the heightened peripheral vasoconstrictive responses in blacks, have been observed among children, adults, normotensives, and borderline hypertensives. It has been most clearly seen in studies using stressors, such as the forehead cold pressor test, that are specifically designed to produce a predominantly α-adrenergic pattern of reactivity. Fewer studies have been conducted on the variability of responses to laboratory stressors *among* blacks. The exception is the research on family history of hypertension and reactivity among blacks, where the studies have not consistently uncovered greater reactivity in black adults with a positive family history. The possible reasons for the lack of findings for family history will be discussed in a later section.

TOWARD UNDERSTANDING RACIAL DIFFERENCES IN VASCULAR REACTIVITY:
A CONTEXTUAL MODEL

The research reviewed in this chapter represents the first generation of studies investigating racial differences in reactivity. It is critical at this juncture to move beyond studies that simply describe racial group differences in autonomic responses, toward experiments aimed at understanding the basis of the observed differences. That is, designing studies that ask what factors are responsible for the greater vascular reactivity observed among blacks relative to whites, and, more importantly, what variables are predictive of heightened vascular reactivity *within* the black population? It is these questions that the proposed contextual model is designed to address.

Anderson and McNeilly (8), in their discussion of a contextual perspective of psychophysiological research, noted that physiological or psychophysiological measurements taken in an experimental laboratory are partly a function of the ecological niche that the subject occupies at that time. This ecological niche may comprise several interdependent and overlapping systems or levels of analyses, including sociocultural, interpersonal, situational, temporal, and biological. According to Revenson (129), a contextual approach emphasizes the "reciprocal, bidirectional nature of relationships between persons and their contexts" or environments. This bidirectional causality implies that each of the contextual levels may potentially influence, and may be influenced by other contextual levels. With regard to racial differences in reactivity, it may be argued that the degree of black–white differences in vascular reactivity and essential hypertension may in large be partly due to racial differences in the ecological niches that the two groups occupy in the United States.

Figure 6.1 illustrates a proposed working contextual model for investigations of stress-induced vascular reactivity in blacks. The principal tenet of the

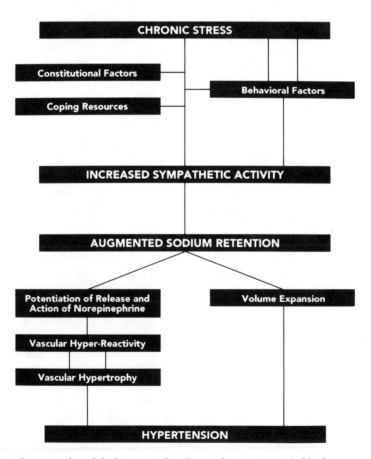

FIGURE 6.1. Contextual model of stress-induced vascular reactivity in blacks.

proposed contextual model is that exaggerated peripheral vascular reactivity observed in many blacks relative to whites is a function of a number of biological, psychological, and behavioral, environmental, and sociocultural factors. The model begins with the premise that in reactivity research, *race should be viewed as a proxy for effects of differential exposure to chronic social and environmental stressors, rather than as a proxy for the effects of genetic differences.* Blacks, on average, are exposed to a greater array of chronic stressors than their white counterparts. These chronic stressors interact with biological, behavioral, and psychological risk factors to increase sympathetic nervous system activity that, in turn, leads to enhanced sodium retention at the kidney. The resulting higher sodium levels in the body not only increase blood volume but also potentiate the effects of norepinephrine on the vasculature. Thus, when norepinephrine is released in response to laboratory stressors, the higher prevailing levels of plasma sodium augment the effects of norepinephrine, thereby resulting in increased vascular reactivity. Over time, and with repeated stressor-induced autonomic arousal, this increased vascular reactivity may lead to structural changes on the vascular wall (e.g., increased wall to lumen ratio), which further augments reactivity. If repeated frequently over a number of years, this process leads to sustained hypertension. Chapter 11, this volume, shows the cellular biophysical and molecular mechanisms accounting for the above sequence. The remainder of this chapter is devoted to providing the rationale and justification for each component of this model and the relevance of each to research on race differences in reactivity.

CHRONIC STRESSORS

Based on the writings on Cooper (24,25) and others (143), race is viewed as a sociological designation that indicates exposure to common life experiences. According to the current model, one of the features that distinguishes the life experiences of blacks and white Americans is the greater exposure to chronic life stressors in black than in whites. As Cooper and David (25) note, "blacks in the United States have a historically determined structural relationship to the social system" (p. 113). This structural relationship has involved several hundred years of institutional discrimination and government-sanctioned racism (80,148), which has only recently been remediated through legislation (for example, the Civil Rights legislation of the 1960s). As a consequence of this history, and the continued race-consciousness of our society, blacks currently experience a greater array of chronic stressors relative to whites. These include higher poverty rates and low income levels, residential crowding, substandard housing, socioecological stress, higher unemployment, lower status occupations, and lower social status (35,36,74,86,147).

Many of these chronic social and environmental stressors have been related to hypertension among blacks. For example, socioeconomic status (SES) shows a strong inverse relationship with hypertension among blacks (67). Additionally, Harburg et al. (58) have found that blacks residing in neighborhoods high in socioecological stress, characterized by low SES and high social instability (SIS) (defined as high crime rate, high divorce rate), exhibited significantly higher systolic and diastolic blood pressures than blacks living in low SES but more stable neighborhoods. Among whites, socioecological stress did not influence blood pressure. Similarly, James and Kleinbaum (70) have found that for black males aged 45–54, high stress (low SES, high SIS) counties of North Carolina were associated with significantly higher hypertension-related mortality (e.g., hypertensive heart disease, stroke) than low stress counties. As in Harburg's Detroit studies, no stress–mortality relationship was found for white males. Thus, not only are blacks exposed more frequently to chronic stressors, but these social and environmental factors may have a greater impact.

CHRONIC STRESS AND VASCULAR REACTIVITY: PHYSIOLOGICAL MEDIATORS

If the differential exposure to chronic stressors is related to acute cardiovascular reactivity, as we have proposed, it should be possible to identify specific physiological mechanisms linking these phenomena in blacks. It is proposed that exposure to chronic stressors enhances sympathetic nervous system activity that results in augmented sodium retention. Augmented sodium retention may, in addition to increasing blood volume, contribute to the greater vascular reactivity responses in blacks.

Sympathetic Nervous System Effects

Of critical importance is whether exposure to chronic stress is associated with this hypothesized physiological scenario. Research from animal and human studies has demonstrated that exposure to acute and chronic stress may be linked to increased resting sympathetic nervous system activity, increased sodium retention, and increased sympathetic reactivity. In a series of studies, in which the effects of stress and sodium retention were measured in dogs (89), saline-infused dogs, who were exposed to a daily shock avoidance task, exhibited significant reductions in sodium and fluid excretion with an associated rise in blood pressure (54). In additional studies, it was discovered that the inhibited sodium excretion during stress was directly mediated by renal sympathetic nerves, given that the increased renal tubular reabsorption could be prevented by surgical denervation of the kidneys (84). In a study of spontaneously hypertensive rats (SHRs) and normotensive Wistar-Kyoto rats (WKYs), Koepke and DiBona (83) found that stress significantly increased renal sympathetic nerve activity and antinatriuresis in SRHs, but had no effect on renal sympathetic nerve activity or sodium excretion in the WKYs. Similar effects of stress on renal functioning and sympathetic activity in the SHRs have been reported by Lundin and Thoren (98). In perhaps the first study of stress and sodium retention in humans, Light et al. (91) discovered that a stressful laboratory task (competitive reaction time) decreased urinary sodium excretion in individuals at risk for hypertension, including both borderline hypertensives and persons with a parental history of hypertension.

Research with animals and humans has demonstrated that chronic stress may augment resting sympathetic tone and enhance sympathetic reactivity to acute stress. Animals exposed to daily chronic stress have shown increases in resting levels of catecholamine compared with nonstressed animals. Additionally, chronically stressed animals have exhibited augmented catecholamine responses following exposure to *novel* stressors. That is, when exposed to a unique stressor, chronically stressed animals showed more pronounced autonomic responses than animals not previously exposed to chronic stress (79,105). Among humans, chronic stress results in higher resting sympathetic activity, and greater acute sympathetic reactivity to novel laboratory stressors. For example, for as many as 3 years following the nuclear power accident, residents of Three Mile Island had higher resting levels of urinary epinephrine and norepinephrine than control groups (19,26,39,132). In a study of residential crowding, Fleming et al. (38) found that individuals living in more crowded neighborhoods had greater blood pressure and heart rate reactivity during a challenging behavioral task than those who lived in less crowded neighborhoods.

Sodium Effects

There are at least three reasons why sodium is proposed as a principal physiological mediator of heightened vascular reactivity in blacks. First, there is now considerable evidence that the heightened sympathetic nervous system (SNS) may induce sodium retention (144). Second, although the dietary sodium intake of blacks may not be significantly higher than that of whites (52), blacks tend to excrete less sodium in urine, and exhibit greater pressor responses to sodium loading (93,97). Thus, blacks may be more susceptible to the blood pressure effects of sodium, despite a similar dietary intake relative to whites. It is possible, then, that the greater sodium retention in blacks is related to increased sympathetic activity. Third, research suggests that sodium may augment cardiovascular reactivity in subjects at risk for hypertension (2,3,34). For example, Ambrosioni et al. (3) studied the effects of a moderate dietary salt restriction on intralymphocytic sodium content and pressor responses to behavioral stress in 25 young borderline hypertensives. It was discovered that sodium reduction significantly attenuated both intralymphocytic sodium content and diastolic blood pressure responses to behavioral stressors (mental arithmetic, handgrip, and bicycle exercise). Finally, there is some indication that sodium may exert its effects on blood pressure via heightened vasoconstriction rather than by increasing cardiac output. For instance, sodium has been found to increase resting forearm vascular resistance in borderline hypertensives (101). High sodium intake has also been shown to augment adrenergically mediated vasoconstrictor responses in SHRs but not in the WKYs (120). Thus, given the influence of the SNS on sodium retention, the greater sodium sensitivity among blacks, and the effects of sodium on both reactivity and vascular resistance, sodium may be the pivotal physiological mechanism responsible for the observed race differences in vascular reactivity.

How might sodium contribute to increased vascular resistance? As shown in Figure 6.1, sodium may lead to heightened vascular resistance through its effects on plasma norepinephrine release and action. Sodium loading increases plasma and urinary norepinephrine levels, and sodium deprivation has the inverse effect (18,22,37,96,119,130). Furthermore, high sodium intake has been shown to potentiate the effects of norepinephrine on the vasculature (127). High dietary sodium intake has also been associated with increased pressor responses to infused norepinephrine in black hypertensives relative to white hypertensives (27). Thus, if blacks exhibit an exaggerated antinatriuresis, this may lead to an increased release or vasoconstrictive action of plasma norepinephrine. This chain of events would increase peripheral vascular resistance in blacks. Moreover, chronic stressors, which in themselves stimulate the release of plasma norepinephrine, would interact with higher prevailing sodium levels to further stimulate vascular reactivity. It is hypothesized that the heightened vascular reactivity observed in blacks may ultimately result in structural changes (i.e., hypertrophy) in the peripheral vasculature, which, in turn, may further augment vascular hyperreactivity (41,42). A long-term consequence of this process could be sustained hypertension (41,42), the biophysical basis of which is reviewed in Chapter 11, this volume.

In summary, there is compelling evidence that blacks are systematically exposed to a wider array of chronic psychosocial stressors than their white counterparts. These stressors involve lower SES, higher rates of poverty, higher unemployment, lower status occupations, exposure to racism, and more crowded and ecologically stressful residential environments. Many of these stressors have been related to elevated blood pressure and increased hypertension prevalence. Research with humans and animals suggests that exposure to chronic stress may increase tonic SNS activity, acute autonomic reactivity, and urinary sodium retention. Future studies may determine whether the types of stressors that many blacks confront on a daily basis are related to the pathogenesis of hypertension.

BEHAVIORAL AND PSYCHOLOGICAL FACTORS

It is possible that chronic social stressors may operate through specific behavioral or psychological factors to increase sodium retention (see Chapters 4 and 5, this volume). Behavioral and psychological factors have been linked to elevated blood pressure and hypertension among blacks (12,69). For example, suppressed anger and hostility have been associated with elevated blood pressure and hypertension in both adolescents and adults (47,57,59,76,77). In general, this literature has indicated that blacks who suppress their anger when provoked, or who express their anger without reflection, have higher resting blood pressure levels than those who routinely express their anger, or who express it only after some reflection. Among black women at work, the experience of frequent anger is related to higher ambulatory blood pressures (30).

Another behavioral factor associated with high blood pressure among blacks is the "John Henryism" behavioral pattern (70–73; see Chapter 5, this volume). At this time, research has not examined whether inhibited anger expression or John Henryism are related to inhibited sodium excretion among blacks. It is clear, however, that anger-suppression and John Henryism may be elicited by the social environment. For example, for anger-expression to increase risk for elevated blood pressure, there must be frequent exposure to provocational environmental circumstances. The anger blacks experience concerning their historical treatment is well documented (51). Yet, historically, there have also been sanctions against the overt expression of this anger (i.e., reprisals of various sorts from the dominant culture). In essence then, the social milieu in which many blacks exist not only contributes to the experience of angry feelings but simultaneously punishes their expression. On the other hand, the behavior of individuals high in John Henryism may actually increase their exposure to stressful social and environmental circumstances. Because of their determination and work ethic, these individuals strive to improve their life opportunities. However, among those with a low educational level, there may be numerous barriers that block the achievement of their goals, or make accomplishing them more difficult (see Chapters 4 and 5, this volume). Furthermore, their efforts to gain control over a difficult-to-control, high-stress environment may inadvertently increase stress exposure. Thus, compared with people low in John Henryism, those high in John Henryism may actually expose themselves more frequently to frustrating and stressful situations. That is, they will continue to strive to gain control in spite of the barriers. Whether this exposure to behaviorally mediated chronic stress results in enhanced SNS and altered sodium regulation remains to be empirically determined. It has been reported, however, that active behavioral coping with acute laboratory stressors enhances sodium retention (91). It is this active coping with real-life stressors that is the sine qua non of the John Henryism pattern.

Chronic social stressors may also have other psychological and emotional effects that could potentially influence sodium retention. For example, low income blacks have been found to report more psychological distress than lower and higher income whites and higher income blacks, perhaps due to the combined burden of poverty and racism (81). Additionally, the stressful residential environments to which many blacks are exposed (e.g., crowding, crime) are related to stress symptoms such as anxiety, depression, and somatic complaints, and lower levels of perceived control (19,26,39,132).

BIOLOGICAL/GENETIC FACTORS

Genetic variables have been identified as important factors determining sodium excretion in both blacks and whites. By means of family history and twin models, a strong heritability component to sodium retention has been observed (53). In discussing the role of genetic factors in black–white differences in sodium excretion, however, several issues should be considered. First, although blacks with a parental history of hypertension are at increased risk for developing the disorder compared with the offspring of normotensives, epidemiological evidence indicates that the association of parental history and risk for hypertension is not as strong among blacks as it is among whites (134). Consequently, there would be a weaker association between parental history and any suspected pathogenic process, such as sodium retention or cardiovascular reactivity. Indeed, no published studies have observed the expected relationship between parental history of hypertension and cardiovascular reactivity (i.e., changes rather than levels) among black adults (10,11,13,112), although this relationship has been found fairly consistently among whites (45). It is at present unclear why the parental history of hypertension and cardiovascular reactivity relationship has not been found among black adults. An explicit assumption in the parental history literature is that offspring of hypertensives inherit the genetic risk for the disorder and its pathophysiological concomitants. Yet, given the strong influence of psychosocial stressors in the pathogenesis of hypertension among blacks (12), it is unclear whether offspring of hypertensives whose disorder has a psychosocial origin would be at greater risk for developing the disorder or exhibiting its pathophysiological consequence. Psychosocial stressors may serve to overshadow the influence of parental history such that risk for hypertension and reactivity are augmented even in persons with a negative parental history. This would result in a diminished ability to detect differences between parental history groups among blacks. It is interesting to note, however, that one study with black children has uncovered the effects of parental history on reactivity (117). This may suggest that if the effects of chronic stress overshadow those of parental history, they may not do so until the adult years (i.e., after an accumulation of exposures). Second, although sodium retention may have a genetic component (53), it may also be stimulated by psychosocial stressors. To the degree that blacks, particularly low income blacks, experience more psychological stress than do whites or upper income blacks (81), they may consequently be more susceptible to inhibited sodium excretion.

Finally, the fact that there is a genetic contribution to sodium excretion does not necessarily imply that genetic factors are responsible for the *race* differences in sodium retention. Indeed, the genetic distinction between blacks and whites is, at best, ambiguous. It has been noted that the gene pool of American blacks comprises a heterogeneous mixture of genes from genetically diverse populations of Africa (64,113), and those from the U.S. white population (48,126). Reed (128) and Lewontin (87) have argued that blacks and whites in the United States are not separate genetic populations. To the contrary, Reed estimates that up to 50% of the genes of black Americans are derived from Caucasian ancestors, while Lewontin and associates (87,88) report that genetic differences between *individuals* within a race have a substantially greater impact on the total species genetic variation than genetic differences between *races*. Although sodium retention may have a genetic component that contributes to *within*-race variability in sodium regulation, it may be overly simplistic to assume that the *between*-race differences in sodium excretion are due to heritable factors. Psychosocial explanations may be equally viable for both between-race and within-race differences in sodium excretion. This is not to imply that biological (i.e., constitutional) factors do not play a role in reactivity in blacks, but that they probably influence *within-race* variability more than between-race variability in autonomic responses. For example, blacks with borderline hypertension may be those who are genetically predisposed to hypertension. These are individuals who also exhibit greater reactivity (92).

COPING RESOURCES

Although there may be social and behavioral factors that increase sodium retention among blacks, there may also be sociocultural factors that buffer the effects of chronic stress in this group. Specifically, cultural traditions of black Americans may serve to counteract the sympathetic and hypertensinogenic effects of chronic stress. A number of authors have advocated the view that black Americans share many characteristics, both social and behavioral, that have their origin in African traditions (29,121–123,145). As summarized in Anderson (7), these African traditions include, among other things, a strong spiritual orientation; a deep sense of kinship and identification with the "tribe" and larger group, rather than a strictly individualistic orientation; a reverence for the oral tradition and the spoken word; a flexible concept of time, which is marked by events rather than the clock or calendar, that is, an emphasis on the past and present rather than the future; and an unashamed use of emotional expressiveness.

The presence of these African traditions in the black culture is apparent, for example, in the expression of both verbal and nonverbal behaviors (84,136); the importance of extended family, which may include in addition to blood relatives, individuals who are given the same status and responsibilities as blood relatives (121); the central role of religion and spirituality and the unique style and emotional expressiveness of the black church service, even though the content of the hymns and readings may be Euro-American (145); and the strong sense of group solidarity, racial identity, or "we-ness" in the black community (122,123).

According to the contextual model, these cultural traditions should decrease the effects of stress and, consequently, the effects of stress on SNS activity, sodium retention, and blood pressure level. It has been found, for example, that among whites, regular church attendance is associated with lower resting blood pressure levels than less frequent attendance (50). It would be of interest to determine whether blacks exposed to chronic psychosocial stressors (e.g., low income blacks), but who also have a high cultural "buffer" (e.g., strong religious orientation, social support, or extended family network), exhibit lower tonic SNS activity, lower sodium retention, and lower cardiovascular reactivity than those individuals less connected with cultural resources.

TESTING THE CONTEXTUAL MODEL: DIRECTIONS FOR RESEARCH

The contextual model presented in this chapter was designed to provide a stimulus both for examining the basis for racial differences in vascular reactivity as well as for exploring within-race variability in vascular responses among blacks. Toward these ends, the model suggests a number of testable hypotheses and research questions. Various components of the model could be tested using either field or laboratory methodologies. For example, the model predicts that blacks who are exposed to higher levels of chronic stress should have higher resting stress hormone levels (e.g., catecholamines, cortisol) and exaggerated responses to novel stimuli, suggesting increased sympathetic nervous system activity compared with blacks experiencing lower levels of chronic stress. Second, chronic stress should also be positively associated with increased sodium retention (i.e., lower sodium excretion rates) and greater vascular reactivity in blacks. Third, the combination of chronic stress exposure and behavioral and psychological factors such as anger-suppression and John Henryism should be positively associated with both increased SNS activity and greater sodium retention. Furthermore, dietary sodium loading (or saline infusions) should potentiate vascular reactivity in blacks experiencing chronic stress; these effects should be diminished by α-adrenergic blockade. Finally, if the adverse physiological effects of chronic stress can be demonstrated, the contextual model would predict that blacks with more coping resources (e.g., high social support, strong religious orientation, and racial identity) will show lower SNS activity and decreased sodium retention relative to those with fewer coping resources.

SUMMARY AND CONCLUSIONS

In summary, according to the proposed model, race is viewed as a sociocultural designation that denotes differential exposure to chronic psychosocial stressors. It is proposed that blacks are exposed to significantly more chronic psychological and social stressors than whites. Many of these chronic psychosocial stressors have been associated with hypertension prevalence in epidemiological studies. Furthermore, chronic stress has been shown to augment cardiovascular reactivity to acute stress in both animals and humans, and to increase sodium retention in SHRs. Acute stress has also been demonstrated to increase sodium retention in humans. The essential element to our model is that chronic psychosocial stressors that are more represented within the black American population due to historical factors are related to an increase in sodium sensitivity and retention. This altered sodium metabolism secondary to chronic psychosocial stressors may be augmented by both biological, behavioral, and psychological risk factors for hypertension, and modulated by stress coping resources. It is hoped that this model will serve as a stimulus for further research on the biopsychosocial aspects of autonomic reactivity and hypertension in blacks.

REFERENCES

1. Alpert, B. S., E. V. Dover, D. L. Booker, A. M. Martin and W. B. Strong. Blood pressure response to dynamic exercise in healthy children—black versus white. *J. Pediatr.* 99: 556–560, 1981.
2. Ambrosioni, E., F. V. Costa, L. Montebugnoli, C. Borghi, and B. Magnani. Intralymphocytic sodium concentration as an index of response to stress and exercise in young subjects with borderline hypertension. *Clin. Sci.* 61(Suppl. 7): 25, 1981.
3. Ambrosioni, E., F. V. Costa, C. Borghi, L. Montebugnoli, M. F. Giordani and B. Magnani. Effects of moderate salt restriction on intralymphocytic sodium and pressor response to stress in borderline hypertension. *Hypertension* 4: 789–794, 1982.
4. Anderson, D. E. Interactions of stress, salt, and blood pressure. *Annu. Rev. Physiol.* 46: 143–153, 1984.
5. Anderson, D. E., W. D. Kearns, and W. E. Better. Progressive hypertension in dogs by avoidance conditioning and saline infusion. *Hypertension* 5: 286, 1983.
6. Anderson, D. E., W. D. Kearns, and T. J. Worden. Potassium infusion attenuates avoidance-saline hypertension in dogs. *Hypertension: 5,* 415, 1983.
7. Anderson, N. B. Racial differences in stress-induced cardiovascular reactivity and hypertension: current status and substantive issues. *Psychol. Bull.* 105(11): 89–105, 1989.
8. Anderson, N. B., and M. McNeilly. Age, gender, and race variables in psychophysiological

assessment: sociodemographics in context. *Psychological Assessment: A Journal of Consulting and Clinical Psychology 3:* 376–384, 1991.

8a. Anderson, N. B., Lane, J. D., Muranaka, M., Williams, R. B., & Houseworth, S. Racial differences in blood pressure and forearm vascular responses to the cold face stimulus. *Psychosomatic Med. 50,* 57–63, 1988.

9. Anderson, N. B., J. D. Lane, H. Monou, R. B. Williams, Jr., and S. J. Houseworth. Racial differences in cardiovascular reactivity to mental arithmetic. *Int. J. Psychophysiol. 6:* 161–164, 1988.

10. Anderson, N. B., J. D. Lane, F. Taguchi, and R. B. Williams, Jr. Patterns of cardiovascular responses to stress as a function of race and parental hypertension in men. *Health Psychol. 8*(5): 525–540, 1989.

11. Anderson, N. B., J. D. Lane, F. Taguchi, R. B. Williams, Jr., and S. J. Houseworth. Race, parental history of hypertension, and patterns of cardiovascular reactivity in women. *Psychophysiology 26*(1): 39–47, 1989.

12. Anderson, N. B., H. F. Myers, T. Pickering, and J. S. Jackson. Hypertension in blacks: psychosocial and biological perspectives. *J. Hypertens. 7:* 161–172, 1989.

13. Anderson, N. B., R. B. Williams, Jr., J. D. Lane, T. Haney, S. Simpson, and S. J. Houseworth. Type A behavioral, family history of hypertension, and cardiovascular responses among black women. *Health Psychol. 5:* 393–406, 1986.

14. Anderson, N. B., R. B. Williams, Jr., J. D. Lane, S. Houseworth, and M. Muranaka. Parental history of hypertension and cardiovascular responses to behavioral stress in young black women. *J. Psychosomatic Res., 31,* 723–729, 1987.

15. Arensman, F. W., F. A. Trieber, M. P. Gruber, and W. B. Strong. Exercise induced differences in cardiac output, blood pressure and systemic vascular resistance in a healthy biracial population of ten year old boys. *Am. J. Dis. Child. 143:* 212–216, 1989.

16. Armstead, C. A., K. A. Lawler, G. Gorden, J. Cross, and J. Gibbons. Relationship of racial stressors to blood pressure responses and anger expression in black college students. *Health Psychol. 8*(5), 541–556, 1989.

17. Barnett, P. H., K. A. Hines, A. Schirger, and R. P. Gage. Blood pressure and vascular reactivity to the cold pressor test. *J.A.M.A. 183:* 845–848, 1963.

18. Battarbee, H. D., D. P. Funch, and J. W. Dailey. The effect of dietary sodium and potassium upon blood pressure and catecholamine excretion in rat. *Proc. Soc. Exp. Biol. Med. 161:* 32, 1979.

19. Baum, A., R. J. Gatchel, and M. A. Schaeffer. Emotional behavioral, and physiological effects of chronic stress at Three Mile Island. *J. Consult. Clin. Psychol. 51:* 565–572, 1983.

20. Berenson, G. S., A. W. Voors, L. S. Webber, E. R. Dalferes, Jr., and D. W. Harsha. Racial differences of parameters associated with blood pressure levels in children—The Bogalusa Heart Study. *Metabolism 28*(12): 1218–1228, 1979.

21. Borghi, C., F. V. Costa, S. Boschi, A. Mussi, and E. Ambrosioni. Predictors of stable hypertension in young borderline subjects: a five-year follow-up study. *J. Cardiovasc. Pharmacol. 8:* S138–S141, 1986.

22. Carriere, S., G. Lalumiere, A. Daigneault, and J. Champlain. Sequential changes in catecholamine plasma levels during isotonic volume expansion in dogs. *Am. J. Physiol. 235:* F119, 1978.

23. Clark, V., and J. Harrell. The relationship among Type A behavior, styles used in coping with racism, and blood pressure. *J. Black Psychol. 8:* 89–99, 1982.

24. Cooper, R. A note on the biologic concept of race and its application in epidemiologic research. *Am. Heart J. 108:* 715–723, 1984.

25. Cooper, R., and R. David. The biological concept of race and its application to public health and epidemiology. *J. Health Polit. Policy Law 11*(1): 97–116, 1986.

26. Davidson, L. M., R. Fleming, and A. Baum. Chronic stress, catecholamines, and sleep disturbance at Three Mile Island. *J. Hum. Stress 13:* 75–83, 1987.

27. Dimsdale, J. E., R. Graham, M. G. Ziegler, R. Zusman, and C. C. Berry. Age, race, diagnosis and sodium effects on the pressor response to infused norepinephrine. *Hypertension 10:* 564–569, 1987.

28. Ditto, B. Parental history of essential hypertension, active coping, and cardiovascular reactivity. *Psychophysiology 23:* 62–70, 1986.

29. Dixon, V. J. World views and research methodology. In: *African Philosophy: Assumptions and Paradigms for Research on Black Persons,* edited by L. King, F. Dixon, and W. Nobles. Fanon Center, Los Angeles, 1976.

30. Durel, L. A., C. S. Carver, S. B. Spitzer, M. M. Llabre, J. K. Weintraub, P. Saab, and N. Schneiderman. Associations of blood pressure with self-report measures of anger and hostility among black and white men and women. *Health Psychol. 8*(5): 557–575, 1989.

31. Eich, R. H., and E. C. Jacobensen. Vascular reactivity in medical students followed for 10 years. *J. Chronic Dis. 20:* 583–592, 1967.

32. Falkner, B., and H. Kushner. Race differences in stress-induced reactivity in young adults. *Health Psychol. 8*(5): 613–627, 1989.

33. Falkner, B., H. Kushner, D. K. Khalsa, M. Canessa, and S. Katz. Sodium sensitivity, growth and family history of hypertension in young blacks. *J. Hypertens. 4:* S381–S383, 1986.

34. Falkner, B., G. Onesti, and E. T. Angelakos. Effect of salt loading on the cardiovascular response to stress in adolescents. *Hypertension 3*(Suppl. II): 195–199, 1981.

35. Farley, R. *Blacks and Whites: Narrowing the Gap?* Harvard University Press, Cambridge, Mass., 1984.

36. Farley, R., and W. R. Allen. *The Color Line and the Quality of Life in America.* Oxford University Press, New York, 1989.

37. Faucheux, B., N. T. Buu, and O. Kuchel. Effects of saline and albumin on plasma and urinary catecholamines in dogs. *Am. J. Physiol. 232:* F123, 1977.

38. Fleming, I., A. Baum, L. M. Davidson, E. Rectanus and S. McArdle. Chronic stress as a factor in psychologic reactivity to challenge. *Health Psychol. 6:* 221–238, 1987.

39. Fleming, I., A. Baum, and L. Wess. Social density and perceived control as mediators of crowding stress in high-density residential neighborhoods. *J. Pers. Soc. Psychol. 52:* 899–906, 1987.

40. Folkow, B. Cardiovascular structural adaptation: its role in the initiation and maintenance of primary hypertension. The Fourth Volume Lecture. *Clin. Sci. Mol. Med. 55:* 35, 1978.

41. Folkow, B. Physiological aspects of primary hypertension. *Psychol. Rev. 62:* 347, 1982.

42. Folkow, B. Psychosocial and central nervous influences in primary hypertension. *Circulation 76*(Suppl. I.): I-10-I-19, 1987.

43. Fredrickson, M. Behavioral aspects of cardiovascular reactivity in essential hypertension. In: *Biological and Psychological Factors in Cardiovascular Disease,* edited by T. H. Schmidt, T. M. Dembroski, and G. Blumchen. Springer-Verlag, Berlin, 1986, pp. 418–446.

44. Fredrikson, M. Racial differences in reactivity to behavioral challenge in essential hypertension *J. Hypertens. 4:* 325–331, 1986.

45. Fredrikson, M., and K. A. Matthews. Cardiovascular responses to behavioral stress and hypertension: a meta-analytic review. *Soc. Behav. Med. 12:* 30–39, 1990.

46. Fredrikson, M., U. Dimberg, M. Frisk-Hamber, and G. Strom. Hemodynamic and electrodermal correlates of psychogenic stimuli in normotensive and hypertensive subjects. *Biol. Psychol. 15:* 63–73, 1982.

47. Gentry, W. D., A. P. Chesney, H. E. Gary, P. P. Hall, and E. Harburg. Habitual anger-coping styles: effects on mean blood pressure and risk for essential hypertension. *Psychosom. Med. 44k:* 195–202, 1982.

48. Glass, B., and C. C. Li. The dynamics of racial intermixture: an analysis based on the American Negro. *Am. J. Hum. Genet. 5:* 1–20, 1953.

49. Goldstein, D. S. Plasma catecholamines and essential hypertension: an analytical review. *Hypertension 5:* 86–99, 1983.

50. Graham, T. W., B. H. Kaplan, J. C. Cornoni-Huntley, S. A. James, C. Becker, C. G. Hames, and S. Heyden. Frequency of church attendance and blood pressure elevation. *J. Behav. Med. 1*(1): 37–43, 1978.

51. Grier, W. H., and P. M. Cobbs. *Black Rage.* Basic Books, New York, 1968.

52. Grim, C., F. Luft, J. Miller, G. Meneely, H. Batarbee, C. Hames, and K. Dahl. Racial differences in blood pressure in Evans County, Georgia: relationship to sodium and potassium intake and plasma renin activity. *J. Chronic Dis. 33:* 87–94, 1980.

53. Grim, C., F. Luft, M. Weinberger, J. Miller, R. Rose, and J. Christia. Genetic, familial, and racial influences on blood pressure control systems in man. *Aust. N.Z. J. Med. 14:* 453–457, 1984.

54. Gringnolo, A., J. P. Koepke, and P. A. Obrist. Renal function, heart rate and blood pressure during exercise and shock avoidance in dogs. *Am. J. Physiol. 242,* R482, 1982.

55. Hallback, M. Consequence of social isolation on blood pressure, cardiovascular reactivity and design in spontaneously hypertensive rats. *Acta Physiol. Scand. 93:* 455, 1975.

56. Hallback, M., and B. Folkow. Cardiovascular response to acute mental "stress" in spontaneously hypertension rats. *Acta Physiol. Scand. 90:* 684–693, 1974.

57. Harburg, E., E. H. Blakelock, and P. J. Roper. Resentful and reflective coping with arbitrary authority and blood pressure: Detroit. *Psychosom. Med. 41:* 189–202, 1979.

58. Harburg, E., J. Erfurt, L. Hauenstein, C. Chape, W. Schull, and M. Schork. Socioecological stress, suppressed hostility, skin color, and black-white blood pressure: Detroit. *J. Chronic Dis. 26:* 595–611, 1973.

59. Harburg, E., J. C. Erfurt, L. S. Hauenstein, C. Chape, W. J. Schull, and M. A. Schork. Socioecological stress, suppressed hostility, skin color and black-white male blood pressure: Detroit. *Psychosom. Med. 35:* 276–296, 1973.

60. Harlan, W. R., R. K. Osborne, and A. Graybiel. Prognostic value of the cold pressor test and the basal blood pressure: based on an 18-year follow-up study. *Am. J. Cardiol. 13:* 683–687, 1964.

61. Helmer, O. M., and W. E. Judson. (1968). Metabolic studies on hypertensive patients with suppressed plasma renin activity not due to hyperaldosteronism. *Circulation 38:* 965–976, 1968.

62. Henry, J. P., and J. Cassel. Psychosocial factors in essential hypertension: recent epidemiologic and animal experimental evidence. *Am. J. Epidemiol. 90:* 171–200, 1969.

63. Henry, J. P., P. M. Stephens, and G. A. Santisteban. A model of psychosocial hypertension showing reversibility and progression of complications. *Circ. Res. 36:* 156, 1975.

64. Hiernaux, J. *The People of Africa.* Scribner's Press, New York, 1975.

65. Hohn, A. R., D. A. Riopel, J. E. Keol, C. B. Loadholt, H. S. Margolius, P. V. Halushka, P. J. Privitera, J. G. Webb, E. S. Medley, S. H. Schuman, M. I. Rubin, R. H. Pantell, and M. L. Braustein. Childhood familial and racial differences in physiologic and biochemical factors related to hypertension. *Hypertension 5:* 56–70, 1983.

66. Hollenberg, N. K., G. H. Williams, and D. F. Adams. Essential hypertension: abnormal renal vascular and endocrine responses to a mild psychological stimulus. *Hypertension 3:* 11–17, 1981.

67. Hypertension Detection and Follow-up Program Cooperative Group. Race, education and prevalence of hypertension. *Am. J. Epidemiol. 106:* 351–361, 1977.

68. Jackson, A. S., W. G. Squires, Grimes, et al. *J. Cardiac Rehab. 3: 263–268, 1983.*

69. James, S. A. Psychosocial and environments factors in black hypertension. In: *Hypertension in Blacks: Epidemiology, Pathophysiology and Treatment,* edited by W. Hall, E. Saunders, and N. Schulman. 132–143. Year Book Publishers, Chicago, 1985.

70. James, S. A., and D. G. Kleinbaum. Socioecologic stress and hypertension-related mortality rats in North Carolina. *J. Public Health 66:* 354–358, 1976.

71. James, S. A., S. A. Hartnett, W. D. Kalsbeek. John Henryism and blood pressure differences among black men. *J. Behav. Med. 6:* 259–278, 1983.

72. James, S. A., A. Z. LaCroix, D. G. Kleinbaum, and D. S. Strogatz. John Henryism and blood pressure differences among black men. II. The role of occupational stressors. *J. Behav. Med. 7:* 259–275, 1984.

73. James, S. A., D. S. Strogatz, S. B. Wing, and D. L. Ramesy. Socioeconomic status, John Henryism, and hypertension in blacks and whites. *Am. J. Epidemiol. 126:* 664–673, 1987.

74. Jaynes, G. D., and R. M. Williams. Jr. *A Common Destiny: Blacks and American Society.* National Academy Press, Washington, D.C., 1989.

75. Johnson, E. H. Cardiovascular reactivity, emotional factors, and home blood pressures in black males with and without a parental history of hypertension. *Psychosom. Med. 51:* 390–403, 1989.

76. Johnson, E. H., N. J. Schork, and C. D. Spielberger. Emotion and familial determinants of elevated blood pressure in black and white adolescent females. *J. Psychosom. Res. 31:* 731–741, 1978.

77. Johnson, E. H., C. D. Spielberger, T. J. Worden, and G. A. Jacobs. Emotional and familial determinants of elevated blood pressure in black and white adolescent males. *J. Psychosom. Res. 31:* 287–300, 1987.

78. Jorgensen, R. S., and B. K. Houston. Family history of hypertension, gender, and cardiovascular reactivity and stereotype during stress. *J. Behav. Med. 4:* 175–189, 1981.

79. Kant, G. J., T. Eggleston, L. Landman-Roberts, C. C. Kenion, G. C. Driver, and J. L. Meyerhoff. Habituation to repeated stress in stressor specific. *Pharmacol. Biochem. Behav. 22:* 631–634, 1985.

80. Katz, P., and D. Taylor. eds. *Eliminating Racism.* Plenum, New York, 1988.

81. Kessler, R. C., and H. W. Neighbors. A new perspective on the relationships among race, social class, and psychological distress. *J. Health Soc. Behav. 27:* 107–115, 1986.

82. Kochman, T. *Black and White Styles in Conflict.* University of Chicago Press, Chicago, 1981.

83. Koepke, J. P., and G. F. DiBona. High sodium intake enhances renal nerve and antinatriuretic responses to stress in SHR. *Hypertension 7:* 357, 1985.

84. Koepke, J. P., K. C. Light, and P. A. Obrist. Neural control of renal excretory function during behavioral stress in conscious dogs. *Am. J. Physiol. 245:* R251, 1983.

85. Krantz, D. S., and S. B. Manuck. (1984). Acute psychophysiologic reactivity and risk of cardiovascular disease: a review and methodologic critique. *Psychol. Bull. 96:* 435–464, 1984.

86. Lawrence, G. *The Black Male*. Beverly Hills, Sage, 1981.
87. Lewontin, R. C. The appointment of human diversity. *Evolutionary Biol. 6:* 381–398, 1973.
88. Lewontin, R. C., S. Rose, and L. J. Kamin. *Not in Our Genes: Biology, Ideology, and Human Nature*. Pantheon Books, New York, 1984.
89. Light, K. C. Psychosocial precursors of hypertension: experimental evidence. *Circulation 76*(Suppl. I): I67–I76, 1987.
90. Light, K. C., and A. Sherwood. Race, borderline hypertension, and hemodynamic responses to behavioral stress before and after beta-adrenergic blockade. *Health Psychology 8:* 577–595, 1989.
91. Light, K. C., J. P. Koepke, P. A. Obrist, and P. W. Willis. Psychological stress induces sodium and fluid retention in men at high risk for hypertension. *Science 220:* 429, 1983.
92. Light, K. C., P. A. Obrist, A. Sherwood, S. James, and D. Strogatz. Effects of race and marginally elevated blood pressure on cardiovascular responses to stress in young men. *Hypertension 10:* 555–563, 1987.
93. Luft, F., C. Grim, N. Fineberg, and M. Weinberger. Effects of volume expansion and contraction in normotensive whites, blacks, and subjects of different ages. *Circulation 59:* 643–650, 1979.
94. Luft, F., C. Grim, J. Higgins, Jr., and M. Weinberger. Differences in response to sodium administration in normotensive white and black subjects. *J. Lab. Clin. Med. 90:* 555–562, 1977.
95. Luft, R., L. Rankin, R. Block, A. Weyman, L. Willis, R. Murray, C. Grim, and M. Weinberger. Cardiovascular and humoral responses to extremes of sodium intake in normal black and white men. *Circulation 60:* 697–706, 1979.
96. Luft, F. C., L. I. Rankin, D. P. Henry, R. Bloch, C. E. Grim, A. E. Weyman, R. H. Murry, and M. H. Weinberger. Plasma and urinary norepinephrine values at extremes of sodium intake in normal man. *Hypertension 1:* 261, 1979.
97. Luft, F., C. Grim, and M. Weinberger. Electrolyte and volume homeostasis in blacks. In: *Hypertension in Blacks: Epidemiology, Pathophysiology, and Treatment,* edited by W. Hall, E. Saunders, and N. Shulman. Year Book Medical Publishers, Chicago, 1985, pp. 115–131.
98. Lundin, S., and P. Thoren. Renal function and sympathetic activity during mental stress in normotensive and spontaneously hypertensive rats. *Acta Physiol. Scand. 115:* 115, 1982.
99. Manuck, S. B., A. L. Kasprowicz, and M. F. Muldoon. Behaviorally-evoked cardiovascular reactivity potential associations. *Ann. Behav. Med. 12*(1): 17–29, 1990.
100. Manuck, S. B., and J. M. Proietti. Parental hypertension and cardiovascular response to cognitive and isometric challenge. *Psychophysiology 19:* 481–489, 1982.
101. Mark, A. L., W. J. Lawton, F. M. Abbound, A. E. Fitz, W. E. Cannor, and D. D. Heistad. Effects of high and low sodium intake on arterial pressure and forearm vascular resistance in borderline hypertension. *Circ. Res. 36*(Suppl. I): I194–I198, 1975.
102. Matthews, K., S. Weiss, T. Detre, T. Dembroski, B. Falkner, S. Manuck, and R. Williams, eds. *Handbook of Stress Reactivity and Cardiovascular Disease*. Wiley, New York, 1986.
103. Matthews, K. A., and C. J. Rakacsky. Familial aspects of the Type A behavioral pattern and physiologic reactivity to stress. In: *Biological and Psychological Factors in Cardiovascular Disease.,* edited by T. H. Schmidt, T. M. Dembroski, and G. Blumchen. Springer-Verlag, Berlin, 1986, pp. 228–245.
104. McAdoo, W. G., M. H. Weinberger, J. Z. Miller, N. S. Fineberg, and C. E. Grim. Race and gender influence hemodynamic responses to psychological and physical stimuli. *J. Hypertens. 8:* 961–967, 1990.
105. McCarthy, R., K. Horwatt, and M. Konarska. Chronic stress and sympathetic-adrenal medullary responsiveness. *Soc. Sci. Med. 26:* 333–341, 1988.
106. McCubbin, J. A., R. S. Surwit, and R. B. Williams. (1985). Endogenous opiates, stress reactivity and risk for hypertension. *Hypertension 7:* 808–811, 1985.
107. McCubbin, J. A., R. S. Surwit, R. B. Williams, C. B. Nemeroff, and M. McNeilly. Altered pituitary hormone response to naloxone in hypertension development. *Hypertension 14:* 636–644, 1989.
108. McCubbin, J. A., R. S. Surwit, and R. B. Williams. Opioid dysfunction and risk for hypertension: naloxone and blood pressure responses during different types of stress. *Psychosom. Med. 50:* 8–14, 1988.
109. McNeilly-Singh, M. Neuropeptide mediation of hypertension and cardiovascular reactivity in blacks and whites. Ph. D. dissertation, University of Georgia, Athens, 1987.
110. McNeilly, M., A. Zeichner. Neuropeptide and cardiovascular responses to intravenous

catheterization in normotensive and hypertensive blacks and whites. *Health Psychol.* 8(5): 487–501, 1989.

111. Menkes,, M. S., K. A. Matthews, D. S. Krantz, et al. Cardiovascular reactivity to the cold pressor test as a predictor of hypertension. *Hypertension 14:* 524–530, 1989.

112. Morrell, M. A., H. Myers, D. Shapiro, I. Goldstein, and M. Armstrong. Cardiovascular reactivity to psychological stressors in black and white normotensive males. *Health Psychol. 7:* 479–501, 1988.

113. Mourant, A. E. *Blood Relations: Blood Groups and Anthropology.* Oxford University Press, New York, 1983.

114. Murphy, J., B. Alpert, D. Moses, and G. Somes. Race and cardiovascular reactivity: a neglected relationship. *Hypertension 8:* 1075–1083, 1986.

115. Murphy, J. K., B. S. Alpert, S. S. Walker, and E. S. Willey. Race and cardiovascular reactivity: a replication. *Hypertension 11:* 308–311, 1988.

116. Murphy, J. K., B. S. Alpert, E. S. Willey, and G. W. Somes. Cardiovascular reactivity to psychological stress in healthy children. *Psychophysiology 25:* 144–152, 1988.

117. Musante, L., F. A. Trieber, W. B. Strong, and M. Levy. Family history of hypertension and cardiovascular reactivity to forehead cold stimulation in black male children. *J. Psychosom. Res. 34*(1): 111–116, 1990.

118. Myers, H. F., D. Shapiro, F. McClure, and R. Daims. Impact of caffeine and psychological stress on blood pressure in black and white men. *Health Psychol. 8*(5): 597–612, 1989.

119. Nicholls, M. G., W. Kiowski, A. J. Zweifler, S. Julius, M. A. Schork, and J. Greenhouse. Plasma norepinephrine variations with dietary sodium intake. *Hypertension 2:* 29, 1980.

120. Nilsson, H., D. Fly, P. Friberg, G. E. Kalstrom, and B. Folkow. Effects of high and low sodium diets on the resistance vessels and their adrenergic vasoconstrictor fibre control in normotensive (WKY) and hypertensive (SHR) rats. *Acta Physiol. Scand. 125:* 323–334, 1985.

121. Nobles, W. Africanity: its role in black families. *The Black Scholar:* 10–16, June, 1974.

122. Nobles, W. African philosophy: foundations for black psychology. In: *Black Psychology,* 2nd ed., edited by R. L. Jones. Harper & Row, New York, 1980.

123. Nobles, W. Extended self: rethinking the so-called Negro self concept. In *Black Psychology,* 2nd ed., edited by R. L. Jones. Harper & Row, New York, 1980.

124. Obrist, P. A. *Cardiovascular Psychophysiology: A Perspective.* Plenum Press, New York, 1981.

125. Pickering, G., and W. Gerin. Area review: blood pressure reactivity. Cardiovascular reactivity in the laboratory and the role of behavioral factors in hypertension: a critical review. *Ann. Behav. Med. 12*(1): 3–16, 1990.

126. Pollitzer, W. S. The Negroes of Charleston, SC: a study of hemoglobin types, serology, and morphology. *Am. J. Phys. Anthropol. 16:* 241–263, 1958.

127. Rankin, L. I., F. C. Luft, D. P. Henry, P. S. Gibbs, and M. H. Weinberger. Sodium intake alters the effects of norepinephrine on blood pressure. *Hypertension 3:* 650–656, 1981.

128. Reed, T. Caucasian genes in American Negroes. *Science 165:* 762–768, 1969.

129. Revenson, T. A. All other things are not equal: an ecological approach to personality and disease. In: *The Disease Prone Personality,* edited by H. Friedman. New York: Wiley, 65–94.

130. Romoff, M. S., G. Keush, V. M. Campese, M-S. Wang, R. M. Friedler, P. Weidman, and S. G. Massry. Effect of sodium intake on plasma catecholamines in normal subjects. *J. Clin. Endocrinol. Metab. 48:* 26–31, 1979.

131. Rowlands, D., J. De Givanni, R. McLeay, R. Watson, T. Stallard, and W. Littler. Cardiovascular response in black and white hypertensives. *Hypertension 4:* 817–820, 1982.

132. Schaeffer, M. A., and A. Baum. Adrenal cortical response to stress at Three Mile Island. *Psychosom. Med. 46:* 227–237, 1984.

133. Smith, E. J. Cultural and historical perspectives in counseling blacks. In: *Counseling the Culturally Different: Theory and Practice,* edited by D. W. Sue. 141–185. Wiley, New York, 1981.

134. Stamler, R., J. Stamler, W. Riedlinger, G. Algera, and R. Roberts. Family (parental) history and prevalence of hypertension: results of a nationwide screening program. *J.A.M.A. 241:* 43–47, 1979.

135. Steptoe, A., D. Melville, and A. Ross. Behavioral response demands, cardiovascular reactivity and essential hypertension. *Psychosom. Med. 46:* 33–48, 1984.

136. Strickland, T. L., H. F. Myers, and B. B. Lahey. Cardiovascular reactivity with caffeine and stress in black and white normotensive females. *Psychosom. Med. 51:* 381–389, 1989.

137. Tell, G. S., R. J. Prineas, and D. Gomez-Marin. Postural changes in blood pressure and

pulse rate among black adolescents and white adolescents: the Minneapolis children's blood pressure study. *Am. J. Epidemiol. 128*(2): 360–369, 1988.

138. Tischenkel, N. J., P. G. Saab, N. Schneiderman, R. A. Nelesen, R. D. Pasin, D. A. Goldstein, S. B. Spitzer, R. Woo-Ming, and D. J. Weidler. Cardiovascular and neurohumoral responses to behavioral challenge as a function of race and sex. *Health Psychol. 8*(5): 503–524, 1989.

139. Trieber, F. A., L. Musante, D. Braden, F. Arensman, W. B. Strong, M. Levy, and S. Leverett. Racial differences in hemodynamic responses to the cold face stimulus in children and adults. *Psychosom. Med. 52:* 286–296, 1990.

140. Trieber, F. A., L. Musante, W. B. Strong, and M. Levy. Racial differences in young children's blood pressure. *Am. J. Dis. Child. 143:* 720–723, 1989.

141. Venter, C., Joubert, P., Strydon, W. The relevance of ethnic differences in hemodynamic responses to the head-up tilt maneuver to clinical pharmacologic investigations. *J. Cardiovasc. Pharmacol. 7,* 1009–1010,

142. Voors, A., L. Webber, and G. Berenson. Racial contrasts in cardiovascular response tests for children from a total community. *Hypertension 2:* 686–694, 1980.

143. Washington, E., and V. McLloyd. The external validity of research involving American minorities. *Hum. Dev. 25:* 324–339, 1982.

144. Weinberger, M., F. Luft, and D. Henry. The role of the SNS in the modulation of sodium excretion. *Clin. Exp. Hypertens. A4:* 719–735, 1982.

145. White, J. L. Toward a black psychology. In: *Black Psychology,* 2nd ed. edited by R. L. Jones. Harper & Row, New York, 1980.

146. Wilson, N. V., and B. M. Meyer. *Prev. Med. 10:* 62–68, 1981.

147. Wilson, W. J., ed. The ghetto underclass: social science perspectives. *The Annals of the American Academy of Political and Social Science 501,* 1989.

148. Wilson, W. *The Declining Significance of Race.* University of Chicago Press, Chicago, 1980.

149. Wood, D. L., S. G. Sheps, L. R. Eleback, and A. Schirger. Cold pressor test as a predictor of hypertension. *Hypertension 6:* 301–306, 1984.

IV

SALT SENSITIVITY, NUTRITION, INTRACELLULAR IONS, RENIN: PHYSIOLOGICAL CONSIDERATIONS

7

Salt Sensitivity and Hypertension in African Blacks

JACOB MUFUNDA AND HARVEY V. SPARKS, JR.

Hypertension is a relatively new disease in Africa, and it appears that its increasing prevalence is related to the adoption of living patterns similar to those found in Europe and North America. Since in the developing countries of Africa, large numbers of people are migrating to urban areas where they tend to adopt a more Western lifestyle, hypertension is of increasing concern to Africans. Among the many changes associated with Westernization that could be responsible for increased hypertension are an increase in psychosocial stress, higher intake of alcohol, more obesity, reduction in dietary fiber, increased dietary fat and simple carbohydrates, and altered dietary electrolytes.

American blacks have a higher prevalence of hypertension than American whites (55, 70, 73, 81), and hypertension-related mortality is higher among American blacks than whites (70). The reasons for these unfortunate statistics are not fully understood. It is tempting to believe that if we understood the cause of the rising prevalence of hypertension in Africa it would provide clues about hypertension in blacks in America. However, it is inappropriate to lump all blacks into one racial group without noting the wide variation in physical and cultural characteristics of populations indigenous to the African continent and the degree of miscegenation in America and elsewhere (2,15). In fact, "black" in this context refers to one or more ethnic groups with some commonality of social, economic, dietary, and other habits, as well as physical characteristics (14). Despite these reservations, learning more about the blood pressure of groups of Africans may be useful in understanding hypertension in the African diaspora, including American blacks.

We will begin by summarizing the epidemiological evidence that hypertension among Africans is largely a disease of Westernization. Then we will discuss the effect of dietary salt on the blood pressure of American and African blacks and the mechanisms by which a high salt diet may raise blood pressure.

EPIDEMIOLOGY

Absence of Hypertension in Traditional Cultures

Before 1965, hypertension was virtually absent and blood pressure did not increase with age in un-Westernized populations native to Africa. This contrasts

143

with the case in Europe and the United States, where the prevalence of hypertension among blacks and whites was greater than 10% and blood pressure was known to increase with age (see 62 for references). In 1929, Donnison (19) reported blood pressure measurements on 1,000 healthy indigenous residents of South Kenya, ranging in age from 15 to 60 years old. Blood pressure significantly decreased from 123/82 mm Hg at 15 years to 105/67 mm Hg in individuals over 60 years of age. Williams failed to detect hypertension in his 1941 study of 394 pastoral and agricultural Ugandan residents (88). In both men and women blood pressure did not increase after 30 years of age.

Kaminer and Lutz (34) confirmed Donnison's original observations by demonstrating the absence of hypertension and failure of blood pressure to increase with age in individuals whose lifestyles had not been changed by Western influence. They studied the blood pressure on the !San, a traditionally nomadic tribe of the Kalahari Desert. There were 78 nomadic adults and 21 adult farm workers and prisoners in the study. Average blood pressure of the nomads was 108/66 mm Hg for men and 112/70 mm Hg for women. The blood pressure was significantly higher for the male farm laborers and prisoners than for the male nomads. The researchers proposed that increased stress resulting from more contact with Western living conditions may have been responsible for the higher pressures observed in the farm laborers and prisoners.

Un-Westernized Africans are not the only ones who do not develop high blood pressure with age; similar findings were observed in the traditional indigenous populations of Australia, China, Alaska, South America, and the Pacific Islands (see 62 for references).

Maddocks (51) proposed that there can be two blood pressure distribution curves in any population. The first curve is a normal physiological curve that is present in every population. The second is an abnormal curve to the right side of the physiological curve. These two curves overlap each other, giving a bimodal distribution for blood pressure in Westernized communities. He proposed that the right shifted abnormal curve is acquired, usually as a result of stress, and represents hypertensives. Regardless of the cause of the shift, it appears that the abnormal curve was not yet present at the time of the aforementioned studies of traditional communities of Africa.

Emergence of Hypertension

After 1965, numerous investigators reported a significant incidence and prevalence of hypertension in African populations. In addition, both systolic and diastolic pressure began to increase with age in some African populations. The new pattern of high blood pressure was quite similar to what was reported in both American blacks and whites. The following studies illustrate this new blood pressure pattern.

East Africa

In 1969, Forsyth (21) described a 1.1% prevalence of hypertension in a rural, mainland Tanzanian population. At the same time, the prevalence of hypertension in Zanzibar, an island off the coast of Tanzania, was 4.9%. This represented different hypertension prevalences in two subpopulations from the that when blood pressures of rural and urban populations in Zaire were compared by age group, rural people had slightly higher pressures and that blood pressure increased with age in both groups. This finding differs from all other studies done in Africa.

Southern Africa

Seedat (74) used a randomized house-to-house survey to study 1,000 members of the South African Zulu tribe who had migrated to an urban environment. Blood pressure increased with age in this population. They reported a prevalence of hypertension (WHO definition) of 25% in men and 27% in women. These investigators also surveyed 987 rural Zulu people. The prevalence of hypertension was lower for the rural group than for the urban group, 8.7% for men and 10% for women.

Hypertension prevalence was more recently reported to be 25% in urban Zimbabwe (32). A survey in a rural area of Zimbabwe, which is 200 miles from the capital city, involved 1,000 adults. The population was contacted through the medical personnel in the area, the local chief, and political leaders, and rendezvous places were announced. People gathered at these sites to have their blood pressure measured. All people older than 15 years were included in the study. The prevalence of hypertension was 7%. This survey is biased for those who wanted to have their blood pressures measured, but indicates that as in South Africa and Nigeria, blood pressure is lower in rural populations than in urban populations.

Urbanization and Blood Pressure of Blacks outside of Africa

Urbanization is usually associated with increased average pressures and a higher prevalence of hypertension in Africa, but studies of blacks living in the United States and the Caribbean Islands have not demonstrated this effect. Miall et al. (53) studied 1,550 females and 1,130 males in urban and rural Jamaica. The urban population was from Kingston, the capital of Jamaica, and the rural population was from an area 20 miles from Kingston. Members of the rural population were engaged in vegetable gardening and commuted between their rural home and the city to sell their produce. At all ages, from 15 to 75 years, the females from the rural area had significantly higher average pressures than those from the urban area.

Kotchen and Kotchen (40) investigated the geographical effect on racial blood pressure differences in American black and white adolescents. Blood pressure of high school students from an urban area, Washington D.C., and a rural area, Bourbon County, Kentucky, were compared. Briefly, blood pressure was not different between races in the rural area, but systolic pressure was significantly higher in urban blacks than in urban whites. Furthermore, systolic pressures of rural students were higher than those of urban students of both races.

The conclusion from these and other studies is that urbanization in the Western Hemisphere does not have the same effect on the blood pressure of blacks as does urbanization in Africa. A possible difference is that in the Western Hemisphere, both rural and urban people have a Western lifestyle. This

same genetic pool but in different environments. This study was
earliest to document an increase in hypertension prevalence with a
It is interesting that the subpopulation with the higher prevalen
tension lived on the island, which was more urbanized and Weste
the mainland.

A similar finding of increased blood pressure with age was
Parry (66), who studied 1,500 men and 700 women living traditior
Ethiopian highlands. Although the prevalence of hypertension v
corded, average blood pressure increased with age.

It was not until Shaper et al. (75) emphasized the probable
environment in the development of hypertension in Africans that ex
were sought through longitudinal studies. Members of a traditionall
Kenyan tribe, Samburu, were drafted into the Kenyan army. The
markedly changed with adoption of Western culture. For example,
recruits were supplied with daily food rations that provided 15 g of
pared with less than 4 g/day in the traditional environment. Blood p
the army recruits significantly increased compared with their cou
still living traditionally. There was a positive correlation between th
of years spent in the army and the increase in both systolic and dias
sure. When grouped according to age, blood pressure in these sub
much higher than that of their counterparts still leading a traditiona
life. It is unknown if the higher salt intake caused the enhanced blood
increase with age or if some other factor associated with joining th
responsible. However, these data, in addition to those of Page et al.
Oliver et al. (58), suggest that increased intake of sodium may be re
for the observed increase in blood pressure with Westernization.

Poulter et al. (68,69) studied the Kenyan Luo subsistence farmer
rural environment and after they had migrated to Nairobi. The prev
hypertension was not reported, but average blood pressures were high
urban than the rural traditional subjects. Spot urine collections fro
subjects showed higher sodium to potassium ratio in the urban tha
rural population. This and other studies raise the possibility that it
be absolute sodium intake that is most closely related to blood pres
crease with urbanization. It may be that dietary sodium to potassium
a better predictor of the increase in blood pressure. This ratio has bee
to be positively correlated to blood pressure in both animal and human
(see, for example, 17 and 32). We will return to this point later.

West Africa
The study of West Africans has been considered especially relevant to
derstanding of hypertension in American blacks because West Africa
primary locus of the American slave trade (2). Akinkugbe and Ojo (3) pu
the blood pressures of 2,000 rural and 2,000 urban Nigerian men and
Approximately 200 subjects in each decade of life from 15 to 55 years
were studied. This study suggests that average blood pressure increas
nificantly with age in both environments and in both sexes; however,
creases were much greater in the urban than in the rural population.
lence of hypertension was not reported. M'Bayamba-Kabangu et al. (47)

leads to the idea that it is the Westernization of lifestyle that causes blood pressure to increase when Africans migrate to the city.

Cause of Effect of Westernization on Blood Pressure

Wilson (89) proposes on the basis of historical evidence that in tropical areas of West Africa dietary salt was in short supply until the last few decades. Given a hot environment that promoted sodium loss and in which sodium supply was scanty, it would make sense that a population with an unusual capacity to conserve sodium would evolve. Wilson proposes that individuals descended from Africans of this area might be sensitive to sodium because they are unusually capable of retaining salt. Those descended from Africans in areas where salt was always plentiful would be expected to be more resistant to salt. Because the American slave trade concentrated on West Africa, it would follow from this hypothesis that many present-day black Americans would have a genetic predisposition toward enhanced sodium retention. The combination of the high sodium intake typical of Western life and a tendency for sodium retention would then lead to increased body sodium and hypertension. More would have to be known about the availability of salt in other areas of Africa where hypertension is as common as in Western Africa before the validity of this hypothesis can be judged.

Several other mechanisms may contribute to the higher average pressures in blacks who have experienced Westernization. These mechanisms could include decreased dietary potassium (83), calcium (50,71), or fiber (11), and increased intake of carbohydrate (1), alcohol (4), polyunsaturated fatty acids (67), as well as psychosocial stress (76) and obesity (8). As indicated previously, we will confine our attention to the possible role of sodium and its relationship to potassium.

SODIUM AND HYPERTENSION

Epidemiological Evidence

The hypothesis that high dietary sodium is a major cause of hypertension continues to generate controversy. Older (see 62 for references) and more recent (32) cross-cultural epidemiological studies demonstrate a positive correlation between blood pressure and dietary sodium intake. When population groups in more than 20 independent surveys were classified on the basis of sodium intake, three groups of populations were recognized: low, medium, and high sodium populations. The low sodium populations consumed less than 100 mEq, the medium sodium populations between 100 and 200 mEq sodium per day, and the high sodium groups in excess of 200 mEq of sodium per day. The low sodium populations have lower blood pressure than either medium or high sodium populations (62). The low sodium–low blood pressure populations are best typified by the Yanomamo Indians of northern Brazil and southern Venezuela (58). Their sodium intake is less than 2 mEq per day. In this population, blood pressure does not increase with age, and hypertension is rare. The high sodium–high blood pressure groups are best exemplified by the native inhabitants of northern Japan, where sodium intake is in excess of 400 mEq per day and hypertension is very common (39).

The majority of population groups are classified as medium sodium–medium blood pressure with sodium intake ranging between 100 and 200 mEq sodium per day. It is this medium sodium group that has been most extensively studied. In general, studies of individual ethnic groups in this medium population have failed to show a positive correlation between blood pressure and either sodium intake or sodium to potassium ratio. The narrow range of sodium intake within a culture has been given as a possible explanation for the absence of correlation between pressure and sodium intake.

There have been a few exceptions to the absence of positive correlation between blood pressure and sodium intake within cultures. Kesteloot et al. (36) reported a positive correlation between urinary sodium excretion and blood pressure in China. A negative correlation between blood pressure and potassium was also present in this study. The researchers suggested that success in obtaining a positive correlation between blood pressure and sodium may have related to other dietary factors of the Chinese that resulted in concomitant high sodium and low urinary potassium excretion. Another exception are the Bantus of urban Zaire in which M'Buyamba-Kabangu et al. (47) found a correlation between sodium excretion and urinary sodium to potassium ratio and blood pressure.

In summary, epidemiological studies suggest a relationship of sodium chloride intake to high blood pressure and hypertension but usually the relationships are found with extremes of sodium intake across population groups. These studies suggest that if sodium intake is between 100 and 200 mEq, other causative factors become significant. One of these could be the concomitant intake of potassium.

Experimental Studies

Experimental Studies on Animals

The aforementioned epidemiological studies have provided partial evidence for a role for dietary sodium chloride in the development of essential hypertension. An animal model of hypertension that is dependent on a genetic sensitivity to sodium was developed by Dahl et al. (16) Dahl sensitive (S) rats exhibited increased blood pressure when subjected to 8% sodium chloride diet, whereas the Dahl resistant (R) rats did not. It was not simply the absolute amounts of sodium chloride that influenced blood pressure. When the Dahl S rats were fed a fixed sodium chloride intake but with increasing amounts of potassium, the increase in blood pressure was inversely dependent on the amount of potassium chloride.

The Dahl S hypertension model has been well characterized. The animal has been shown to be unable to excrete a sodium load as quickly as Dahl R rats. This inability to excrete sodium appears to be localized to the kidney. Bilateral nephrectomy in these Dahl S rats and transplantation of normal Sprague-Dawley rat donor kidneys prevent the development of hypertension on 8% sodium diet. Transplantation of donor Dahl S rats kidneys to recipient

Dahl R rats increases blood pressure in the Dahl R rats on 8% sodium diet. The pathogenesis appears to involve a humoral step, because parabiosis of Dahl S with Dahl R rats on high sodium diet increases blood pressure in both animals. However, the precise cellular mechanism or nature of this humoral factor has not been worked out. In many ways, the Dahl S rat may be a good model for humans who exhibit salt sensitivity (27).

Experimental Studies on Humans

Investigations that pursue individual variations in response to changes in sodium balance have led to the development of the concept of sodium sensitivity and sodium resistance of blood pressure changes to sodium ingestion (87). At present there is no uniform definition of sodium sensitivity or resistance and the criteria for sodium sensitivity or sodium resistance vary according to the design of the study. A decrease of mean arterial pressure of at least 10 mm Hg when intravenous salt loading was followed by furosemide-induced diuresis was used as sodium sensitivity by Weinberger et al. (87). Skrabal et al. (77) used the reduction of mean arterial pressure of 5 mm Hg or more following reduced sodium intake. Other studies have used an increase in mean arterial pressure following an oral or intravenous sodium load as evidence for sodium sensitivity. In addition to different methods of sodium challenge, these investigations vary in the conditions of the study (for example, home, hospital, or research unit), the prestudy sodium balance, and the control of other dietary factors.

A number of studies have been done on normotensive subjects to explore the mechanism of sodium-related increases in blood pressure without the potentially confounding effects of hypertension on target organs. Luft et al. (46) studied seven black and seven white normotensive men on different levels of sodium intake. All subjects received 10 mEq sodium per day for 7 days. Daily urinary excretion of sodium was measured. The subjects approached sodium balance after 3 days. Next, the dietary sodium was sequentially increased to 300, 600, 800, 1,200, and 1,500 mEq per day for 4 days on each diet. All the subjects were studied on the 10 and 300 mEq per day diets. Three whites and three blacks were studied on the 600 and 1,200 mEq diet. Four blacks and four whites were studied on 800 and 1,500 mEq sodium diets. To enable intakes of 1,200 and 1,500 mEq, intravenous saline solution was administered in addition to dietary salt. Blood pressure, sodium and potassium excretion, plasma renin activity, and plasma aldosterone were measured at the end of each diet. In blacks but not whites systolic blood pressure rose in response to the graded increase in dietary sodium from 10 to 600 and 800 mEq per day. Systolic blood pressure of whites did not increase until an intake of 1,200 mEq sodium per day was reached. Diastolic pressure significantly increased from the 10 mEq sodium to the 800 mEq sodium diet in blacks but not in whites. Plasma renin activity and plasma aldosterone concentration decreased to a similar extent regardless of race. These researchers concluded that blacks are more sensitive to the pressor effects of sodium than whites.

Three blacks and three whites were restudied while maintaining a zero potassium balance as sodium intake was increased. Zero potassium balance was effected by replacing the previous day 24 h potassium excretion by means of potassium tablets. Maintenance of zero potassium balance attenuated the pressure increase due to sodium loading. The authors suggested that the greater sensitivity to salt may contribute to the higher prevalence of hypertension in American blacks than in whites. However, the small number of subjects and the unknown degree of genetic heterogeneity of the blacks in this study made generalization of this finding to all blacks questionable.

Sowers et al. (79) studied 14 normotensive American blacks who were maintained on diets containing 40 mmol of sodium per day for 2 weeks and then 180 mmol/day for the next 2 weeks. Mean arterial pressure rose by 7%. Atrial natriuretic peptide (ANP) did not increase with increased sodium intake in this group. Weinberger et al. (87) used a more acute intervention to study salt sensitivity in large numbers of subjects. They infused 2 liters of 0.9% sodium chloride and then the next day induced sodium depletion with a 10 mmol/day diet and furosemide. With this protocol, 26% of normotensives exhibited a mean arterial blood pressure change of at least 10 mm Hg. There was no difference between blacks and whites.

Rikimaru et al. (72) examined the pressor response to sodium in natives of the highlands of Papua New Guinea to see whether salt sensitivity was present in individuals whose traditional lifestyle includes low dietary sodium. Normotensive men received a low sodium diet for 3 days. This was followed by a high sodium diet for another 10 days. Blood pressure, 24 h sodium and potassium excretion, plasma renin activity, and aldosterone concentration were measured at the end of each diet. Blood pressure significantly increased from the low sodium to the high sodium diet. Plasma aldosterone and renin activity both decreased as expected with increase in dietary sodium. The decrease in aldosterone and renin activity argues against a possible role for these two hormones in causing the blood pressure rise that was observed on the high salt diet.

Other studies support the contention by Luft et al. that whites are characteristically resistant to sodium. Kirkendall et al. (37) studied normotensive American whites on a diet that provided 410 mEq sodium per day for 4 weeks. Blood pressure and total peripheral resistance did not change for the entire period of study. Burstzyn et al. (12) trebled the sodium intake of British whites for 2 weeks and found no increase in blood pressure.

A recent study by Dustan and Kirk (20) reminds us of the danger of generalizing about a large ethnic group from small numbers. They studied 69 normotensive black subjects at the University of Alabama. Three days of a control diet containing 150 mmol of sodium were followed by 4 days of salt depletion achieved by a 9 mmol/day diet and furosemide. The subjects then continued the low salt diet for 3 more days while receiving 3.88 mmol/kg/day of sodium chloride intravenously. Twenty-nine other subjects underwent the same protocol except that salt loading preceded salt depletion. The most important finding was that the blood pressure response to salt loading was heterogeneous. There was a wide range in blood pressure responses, which were not correlated with the amount of sodium retained during loading. Furthermore, more pressor responses occurred when the salt loading occurred before the salt depletion.

We have recently studied the pressor response to dietary sodium in normotensive Zimbabwean medical students, urban hospital workers, and subsistence farmers (56,57). We followed a protocol that was similar to that used by Luft et al. (46). We measured blood pressure and a number of other variables after 4 days on diets containing 10 mEq and 800 mEq per day of sodium. The 19 medical students, who averaged 19 years of age, were drawn from a class in which there was one hypertensive out of 59 black students. All of the subjects included in the study were normotensive. They exhibited no increase in mean arterial pressure, but had a significant increase in systolic and decrease in diastolic pressure on high salt (Fig. 7.1). This is unlike whites, who exhibited no change in either systolic or diastolic pressure when subjected to this increase in dietary sodium (44). On the high salt diet, pulse pressure and the body weight increased substantially, indicating physiologically significant volume expansion. Any hypertensive effect of the volume expansion was apparently buffered by control mechanisms that maintained mean arterial pressure constant. We found a significant decrease in heart rate, which could be taken as evidence of a compensatory baroreceptor response to the elevation of systolic and pulse pressure. Angiotensin II and aldosterone fell on the high salt diet as expected, but ANP did not change. The lack of increase in ANP was surprising, but not unique. Hollister et al. (30) showed that upright posture was able to counteract the positive effect of a sodium load on ANP, which suggests that in the sitting position there may not always be adequate stretch of the atria to cause ANP release (82). As mentioned previously, normotensive American blacks did not exhibit an increase in ANP when dietary sodium was increased (79).

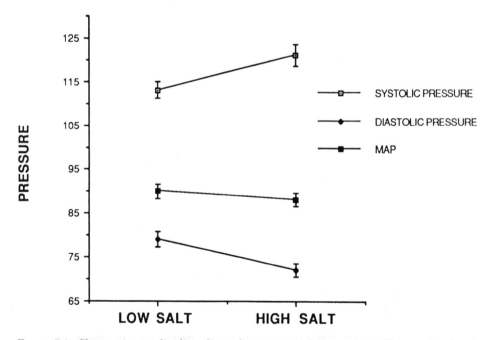

FIGURE 7.1. Changes in systolic, diastolic, and mean arterial pressure (mm Hg) associated with increase in salt intake from 10 to 800 mEq/day for 4 days in 19 Zimbabwean medical students.

Jin et al. (33) showed that an increase in the salt intake of WKY rats caused an increase in ANP, but that the same increase in salt intake by SHRs had no effect on ANP. SHRs are more sensitive to the pressor effects of sodium than are WKY rats. This raises the possibility that some individuals, perhaps those susceptible to the pressor effects of sodium, do not increase ANP in response to a sodium load. As will be discussed later, this could be of adaptive advantage when the environmental availability of salt is low, but also could cause more retention of a sodium load.

The Zimbabwean medical students were able to compensate for the increased salt intake so as to prevent an increase in mean arterial pressure, but the same was not true of the hospital workers and farmers. The average age of the urban workers and rural farmers was 37 and 39, respectively. The urban workers were drawn from the group used in Zimbabwe's portion of the Intersalt study, in which the local prevalence of hypertension was 25%. In a survey of 1,000 people living in the general area from which the farmers were drawn, the prevalence of hypertension was found to be 7%. However, when the blood pressures of 200 subsistence farmers were measured in the same area, the prevalence of hypertension was less than 2%. The higher prevalence in the larger group probably reflects the admixture of teachers, health care workers, merchants, and others living in a Western style in contrast to the local farmers with a traditional rural lifestyle. Thus our rural and urban subjects are drawn from populations with very different prevalences of hypertension, although they are all normotensive.

When given the high salt diet, both of these groups exhibited significant increases in systolic, mean, and pulse pressures (Figs. 7.2, 7.3). There was no decrease in heart rate or diastolic pressure. The weight gain was the same as

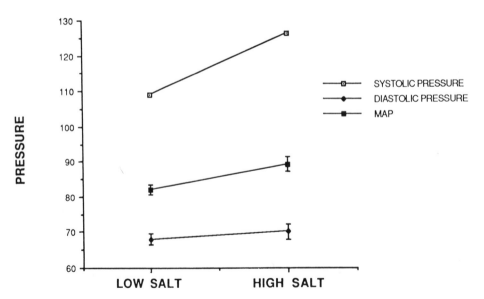

FIGURE 7.2. Changes in systolic, diastolic, and mean arterial pressure (mm Hg) associated with increase in salt intake from 10 to 800 mEq/day for 4 days in 21 Zimbabwean hospital workers.

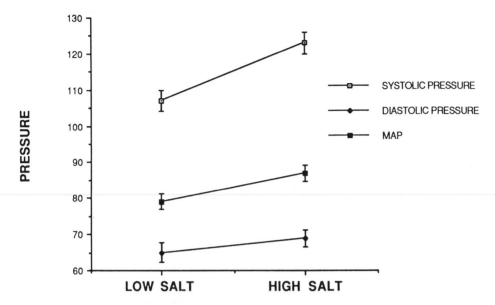

FIGURE 7.3. Changes in systolic, diastolic, and mean arterial pressure (mm Hg) associated with increase in salt intake from 10 to 800 mEq/day for 4 days in 20 Zimbabwean subsistence farmers.

the medical students, suggesting similar volume expansion. Taken together, these data suggest that, like the medical students, these older individuals retained a large amount of the ingested sodium, but did not avoid a rise in mean arterial pressure because diastolic pressure and heart rate did not fall. This is more like the pattern observed in American blacks by Luft et al. (45), although they exhibited an increase in diastolic pressure as well. The response of the urban and rural adults was more homogeneous than that observed by Dustan and Kirk in American blacks. Figure 7.4 shows that of the 41 subjects, 33 exhibited an increase in mean arterial pressure and 40 an increase in systolic pressure.

These observations lead us to think that salt sensitivity among blacks is not limited to the North American continent. We have already mentioned the idea that there could be adaptive advantage to an unusual ability to retain salt for populations living in regions where dietary salt is scarce and loss through sweat tends to be high because of high ambient temperatures. These conditions pertain in the West African forests, which were the source of slaves transported to North America and also at a much earlier time the starting point of the migration of Bantus to southern Africa, including Zambabwe.

Our studies of rural farmers, among whom hypertension is uncommon, suggest that increased salt sensitivity is not the result of urban living. Instead, it appears that the sensitivity to salt is present, but does not in itself result in hypertension. We do not have enough data to know if intake of salt differs between these rural and urban populations. It is possible that alterations in the ratio of sodium to potassium in the diet, as observed by Poulter (68,69), could be at least partially responsible for the higher prevalence of hypertension in the city.

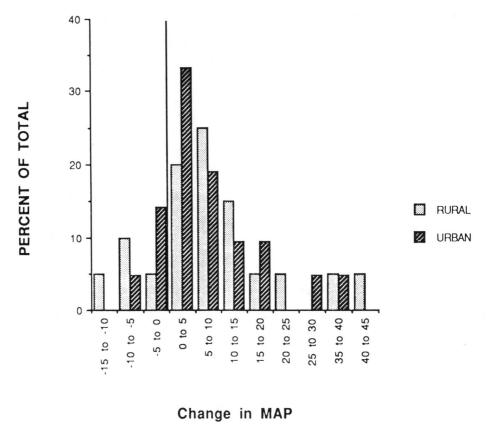

Change in MAP

FIGURE 7.4. Distribution of change in mean arterial pressure (MAP) for rural and urban Zimbabweans in response to increase in dietary salt.

The phenomenon of sodium sensitivity is clearly present in some normotensive humans, but it is necessary to identify the same phenomenon in essential hypertensives if the salt-sensitivity concept bears relevance to human essential hypertension. If salt sensitivity is a causal factor in hypertension, it should be possible to find evidence for high salt sensitivity in at least some hypertensives. Kawasaki et al. (35) studied 19 essential hypertensives. Antihypertensive medication was stopped for a month prior to the study. The patients received a sequence of three diets providing 10 mEq, 100 mEq, and 250 mEq sodium per day each for 7 days. Potassium intake was kept constant at 70 mEq per day. Subjects who exhibited an increase in blood pressure of more than 10% when sodium intake increased from 10 mEq to 250 mEq were called sodium sensitive. The sodium-sensitive subjects retained more sodium and gained more weight than resistant controls. These results were replicated by Fujita (22), who used the same protocol on 18 essential hypertensives. With a high sodium diet, sodium-sensitive subjects gained more weight and retained more sodium, as found by Kawasaki et al. In addition, sodium-sensitive subjects exhibited a greater increase in cardiac output and higher plasma norepinephrine. The sodium-sensitive subjects also displayed lesser decrements in plasma renin activity, and plasma aldosterone concentration on the high sodium diet when compared with sodium-resistant subjects. The concentration of prostaglandin E_2, a vasodilator and natriuretic agent, did not change in the sodium-sensitive subjects, whereas it increased in the sodium-resistant subjects on the 250 mEq sodium diet. These results together suggest that the greater increase in blood pressure in sodium-sensitive patients on the 250 mEq sodium diet can be attributed to greater sodium retention and in turn to an increased cardiac output. The persistence of autonomic drive in sodium-sensitive subjects may contribute to the relative sodium retention with sodium loads and the observed increase in blood pressure.

Sowers et al. (79) studied 11 hypertensive blacks given 40 mmol/day sodium for 2 weeks followed by 180 mmol/day for 2 weeks. Mean arterial pressure increased 6%. A major finding was much lower urinary dopamine in hypertensive than in normotensive subjects, both on low and high salt. In both groups, dopamine did not increase as much as has been reported for whites.

Dustan and Kirk (20) also studied hypertensives, using their protocol described earlier. They found that although on average, sodium loading increased blood pressure, there was marked heterogeneity in the responses and that the order of salt loading and depletion influenced the results.

Weinberger et al. (86) have shown that measurement of phenotypes of haptoglobin can help identify salt-sensitive and resistant subjects. Both normotensive and hypertensive subjects were tested for sodium sensitivity. Subjects with haptoglobin 1-1 phenotype are more likely to be sodium sensitive than phenotypes 1-2 or 2-2. Subjects with phenotype 2-2 are more likely to be salt resistant. This finding was supported by a study in another population, in which adults with haptoglobin phenotype 1-1 had higher pressure than those with phenotype 2-2.

In summary, the available data indicate that African and American blacks are more sensitive to sodium loading than whites and that hypertensives may be more sensitive than normotensives. Aging may also be associated with increased salt sensitivity (44). However, it should be remembered that there is considerable heterogeneity among the responses of any group. The mechanism of salt sensitivity is not completely understood, but a number of possibilities are under investigation and will be discussed later. Before that we will deal with the interaction of sodium and potassium.

Interaction between Sodium and Potassium

Epidemiological Evidence

One of the strongest pieces of evidence supporting a role of dietary sodium as a cause of hypertension is the blood pressure in low sodium–low blood pressure populations. However, these populations also have a high potassium intake. Furthermore, the ratio of sodium to potassium excretion is better correlated to blood pressure than sodium excretion alone (32).

All surveys comparing American blacks and whites have shown a higher excretion of potassium by whites than blacks (see 40 for references). Grim and colleagues (24) in Evans County, Georgia, used dietary recall and 24 h urinary excretion to estimate sodium and potassium intake. As expected, blacks had higher blood pressures than whites. Whites ate and excreted more sodium than blacks. However, potassium intake and excretion were also higher in whites than in blacks so that the dietary and urinary sodium to potassium ratio was higher in blacks than in whites. The higher sodium to potassium ratio in blacks may explain the paradox presented by the whites having had higher sodium intake but lower blood pressure. Barlow et al. (6) found the same differences between the races with respect to sodium and potassium excretion in South Africa.

We have already mentioned Poulter's study (68,69), which shows that when rural Kenyans move to Nairobi, blood pressure goes up as does the ratio of sodium to potassium in urine.

Potassium Intervention Studies

Luft et al. (46) found that when potassium balance was maintained during sodium loading, the pressor effects of sodium ingestion was inhibited. Parfrey and coworkers (64) showed in a random crossover study that mild hypertensives had lower blood pressures on a high potassium diet than on a high sodium diet. In a subsequent study the same group (65) showed that the blood pressures of normotensive students with a family history of hypertension, but not students with a normotensive family are sensitive to the depressor effects of dietary potassium.

We were unable to prevent the pressor effects of sodium with a supplement of 100 mEq of potassium per day in our studies of rural and urban Zimbabweans. Other studies on whites have also failed to demonstrate a depressor effect of potassium (12,54). Perhaps the negative studies are the result of administering too little potassium or perhaps, as is suggested by the studies by Parfrey et al. (64,65), the response to potassium depends on the genetic substratum.

Mechanism of the Pressor Effect of Sodium

If we accept that, on average, blacks are more sensitive to dietary sodium than are whites, it follows that an understanding of the precise mechanism(s) responsible for the pressor effect of sodium could lead us to a better understanding of the reason for the higher prevalence of hypertension in blacks. Unfortunately, a precise answer to this question is not available. Instead, we know of a number of possible explanations, more than one of which is probably partially true.

Cellular Transport of Sodium

Before considering the specific cause of sodium sensitivity, it would be useful to discuss differences in cation transport phenomena between blacks and whites. Several investigators have been able to establish differences among different types of hypertension and racial groups. Losse et al. (43) demonstrated that intraerythrocyte sodium was increased in essential hypertensives compared with normotensives or secondary hypertensives. Others have made similar observations, although there are some exceptions (see 91 for a complete listing of these studies). Again, with some exceptions, most studies show that intraerythrocyte sodium concentration is higher in blacks than in whites for both normotensives and hypertensives (23, 48, 78, 84, but see 85). This is true of African blacks as well (49).

Increased intraerythrocyte sodium concentration could result from reduced sodium-potassium pump activity, reduced outward sodium-potassium cotransport, or increased passive permeability to sodium. At present there is no consensus concerning racial differences in these transport systems. Different investigators have found depressed sodium-potassium pump activity or pump sites (48, 78), reduced sodium-potassium cotransport (23, 85), or both. Some investigators have also found evidence for lower sodium-sodium countertransport in blacks (84), but it is unclear how this relates to intracellular sodium concentration.

Whatever the primary mechanism for the increased intracellular sodium concentration in hypertension, this characteristic may contribute to the observed increase in total peripheral resistance in hypertension and to sodium sensitivity. Blaustein (9) hypothetically linked sodium-calcium exchange to hypertension. According to this hypothesis, increased intracellular sodium would cause increased intracellular calcium concentration by inhibiting calcium exit by way of a sodium-calcium countertransport system that depends on the influx of sodium down its electrochemical gradient to extrude calcium. If vascular smooth muscle experienced this increase in calcium ion concentration, increased total peripheral resistance could occur (28).

In support of a relationship between calcium, salt sensitivity, and hypertension is the observation by Oshima et al. (60) of increased intracellular calcium in salt-sensitive hypertensives on high sodium diet. These researchers studied 12 moderately hypertensive subjects after stabilizing blood pressure and sodium balance on 10 g salt per day. Subjects received 3 g of salt per day for 7 days followed by 20 g of salt per day for another 7 days. Mean arterial pressure increased on the high salt diet. Calcium excretion increased and total serum calcium decreased as compared with the low salt diet. Quin 2–monitored intracellular calcium concentration of lymphocytes significantly increased on the high salt diet. The elevation of mean arterial pressure was closely and positively correlated with the increase in intracellular free calcium and the increase in the hypotensive effect of nifedepine after sodium loading. These investigators concluded that salt sensitivity is mediated by increased intracellular free calcium. The assumption is that this increased intracellular calcium occurs in the relevant cell type, vascular smooth muscle.

Perhaps the most direct explanation for sensitivity is that in sodium-sensitive individuals increased dietary sodium causes an increase in vascular smooth muscle sodium, which in turn results in vasoconstriction. However, there are other possibilities, some of which may also rely on increased intracellular sodium as the triggering event. One way to put together the available information is to start with the observation that American blacks exhibit slower natriuresis in response to intravenous saline infusion than whites (44). This was shown in studies of the response of 94 black and 94 white normotensives to volume expansion resulting from intravenous administration of 2 liters of normal saline over a 4 h period. The volume expansion was followed the next day by a period of volume contraction caused by a low sodium diet and furosemide. Blacks excreted less salt than whites, especially during the daylight hours immediately following the administration of sodium. During the subsequent administration of furosemide the blacks excreted more sodium than the whites. During volume contraction, the blacks exhibited lower renin levels than did the whites. It is reasonable to assume that the tendency for blacks to excrete a load of sodium slowly is related to special characteristics of renal function that are an adaptive advantage in low salt environments. This characteristic could be explained by a difference in the responsiveness of the kidney to neural and hormonal control or to a difference in the intrinsic transport properties of renal tubular cells. Aviv (5) has proposed a role for sodium-hydrogen ion antiport in hypertension and this could be an explanation for reduced sodium excretion in sodium-sensitive individuals. There are also possible explanations involving hormonal and neural control mechanisms and the following discussion deals with these.

Sympathetic Nervous System

We commented earlier on Fujita's hypothesis that salt sensitivity involves inappropriate sympathetic nervous system activity. The firing rate of sympathetic neurons increases during the developmental phase in SHRs fed a high salt diet compared with age-matched rats fed low or basal salt diets. Dietz and Schomig (18) observed increased plasma and urinary norepinephrine and an exaggerated depressor response to ganglionic blockade in SHRs fed high salt. In addition, the increase in plasma norepinephrine in salt loaded rats is exaggerated during cold stress test. These findings suggest that in the developmental phase of hypertension in SHRs, increased sympathetic nervous system activity sets off a chain of events that leads to systemic hypertension.

Chen et al. (13) confirmed that increased salt intake increases blood pressure in SHRs but not in WKYs, and secondly that the sodium-induced hypertension in SHRs was associated with decreased norepinephrine stores and turnover in the anterior hypothalamus, a region that suppresses central sympathetic outflow when chemically or electrically stimulated. In addition, norepinephrine stores in the medulla and spinal cord of salt-fed SHRs were greater than in control WKY rats. These findings are consistent with the hypothesis that salt loading exacerbates the severity of hypertension in SHRs by decreasing the synthesis or release of norepinephrine from noradrenergic terminals in the anterior hypothalamus and increasing the release of norepinephrine from terminals in cardiovascular control centers in the brain stem.

Koepke et al. (38) determined the responsiveness of central α_2-adrenergic receptors by comparing the dose response curves for the effects of cumulative intracerebroventricular injections of guanabenz, an α_2-agonist, on changes in mean arterial pressure, renal sympathetic activity, and urinary sodium excretion in SHR and WKY rats. In the presence of high sodium chloride intake, renal sympathetic activity urinary and sodium excretion were more sensitive to guanabenz in SHRs and less sensitive in WKY rats. The responses to guanabenz were similar for SHR and WKY rats on control salt. They concluded that the responsiveness of central nervous system α_2-adrenergic receptors projecting to the kidney is increased by intake in conscious SHR but not in WKY rats.

The other mechanisms that have been proposed to link sodium to the sympathetic nervous system and the pathogenesis of systemic hypertension include alterations in baroreceptor sensitivity, vascular reactivity to α-adrenergic agonists, sensitivity of presynaptic and postsynaptic mechanisms that govern the release of and reuptake of biogenic amines as well as the synthesis, storage, and turnover of biogenic amines in central and peripheral neurons (59). Clearly more studies need to be done to ascertain the cellular and molecular level of sodium involvement in sympathetic system activity.

Atrial Natriuretic Peptide

As mentioned earlier, Jin et al. (33) demonstrated abnormal ANP regulation in SHRs. They fed 7-week-old SHR and WKY rats 1% and 8% sodium chloride diets for 2 weeks. The 8% salt diet increased blood pressure in SHR but not in WKY rats. Plasma ANP levels were significantly higher in WKYs fed 8% salt than WKYs fed 1% salt. Plasma ANP did not differ between the SHRs and WKY rats on the 1% salt diet, and an 8% salt diet did not increase ANP in SHRs. The observation that dietary sodium chloride stimulated ANP release in WKY rats and not in SHRs suggests that the exacerbation in hypertension seen in salt loaded SHRs may be related to an impairment in ANP release. In addition, ANP stores were elevated in the anterior hypothalamus of SHRs fed either diet compared with WKYs. The role of this alteration in central nervous system ANP in the pathogenesis of sodium chloride–sensitive hypertension remains to be determined. While the relevance of these observations in SHRs to studies in normotensive humans is unclear, the failure of ANP to increase in our subjects on high sodium chloride diet may be due to a similar mechanism.

Renal Circulation

Lawton et al. (42) studied normotensive and borderline hypertensive white males on 10 mEq and 400 mEq sodium diets. After 6 days of a low salt diet, orthostasis lowered diastolic pressure in normotensives but did not have an effect in borderline hypertensives, despite similarly reduced renal plasma flow and increased renal vascular flow in both groups. After 6 days of the high salt diet, orthostasis decreased renal plasma flow and increased renal vascular resistance index by 14% and 48% in the normotensive and borderline hypertensives, respectively. Upright posture also reduced the free water clearance to a greater extent in the borderline hypertensives than in the normotensives. Thus, a high sodium diet appears to unmask an abnormality in the neurohormonal control of the renal circulation in borderline hypertensives that may contribute to the development of hypertension in these subjects.

Digitalislike Substance

A humoral factor that appears to be important in the regulation of sodium excretion is the digitalislike activity of plasma (27). This substance, which has been purified and is ouabain or a closely related isomer (29), is elevated during volume expansion caused by sodium loading and in low-renin hypertension. This substance inhibits the sodium-potassium pump of plasma membranes leading to vasoconstriction, natriuresis, and increased vascular responsiveness to a variety of vasoconstrictors. Perhaps in salt-sensitive individuals, including many blacks, some of these control mechanisms do not cause a sufficiently rapid excretion of a sodium load. As volume expansion occurs, the digitalislike activity of plasma comes into play. This activity increases sodium excretion by (1) inhibiting Na^+/K^+-ATPase activity of the basolateral membrane of renal tubular cells, and (2) raising blood pressure causing a pressure diuresis. Thus pressure diuresis becomes a significant mechanism for regulating sodium excretion in sodium-sensitive individuals, because they rely more heavily than sodium-resistant individuals on the digitalislike substance.

Interaction of Sodium and Potassium

We described the fact that Westernization of Africans is associated with an increase in the ratio of sodium to potassium in the diet. Furthermore, in the United States, blacks have a higher ratio of dietary sodium to potassium. Both of the populations with higher sodium to potassium ratios have higher blood pressures. This could be another element of the explanation of the role of sodium in hypertension in blacks. The mechanism of the antagonistic effect of potassium on sodium's hypertensive effect is not completely understood but probably contains the following elements.

Potassium as a Natriuretic Agent

Potassium infusion into a dog renal artery causes prompt diuresis and natriuresis that is thought to be due to inhibition of sodium reabsorption in the proximal tubule. The diuretic effect of potassium has been shown in normotensive and hypertensive humans (7,10). By acting directly, the adrenal cortex high potassium intake increases plasma aldosterone, which should have antinatriuretic and hypertensive effects (83). Although potassium induces a rise in aldosterone levels, various studies have shown that a high potassium intake is natriuretic (90), although aldosterone may limit the loss of sodium. The natriuresis induced by high potassium could play a significant role in its hypotensive effects. Indeed, both salt loaded rats and spontaneously hypertensive rats whose blood pressure is reduced by a high potassium diet have a diminished exchangeable sodium space (53). Iimura et al. (31) reported a decrease in body weight, total exchangeable sodium, extracellular fluid space, and plasma volume in hypertensive patients treated with a high potassium diet.

Potassium's Effect on the Nervous System

Dietary potassium supplementation lowered the threshold for baroreceptor activity and increased the sensitivity of aortic arch receptors in normotensive humans (77). This increased baroreceptor sensitivity would buffer acute changes in blood pressure and could counteract the tendency for high blood pressure to develop.

Direct Dilator Effect of Potassium

Potassium exerts a direct vasodilator effect on resistance vessels at plasma concentrations that might be found with a high potassium intake (25). Intraarterial infusion of potassium causes prompt vasodilation, and this vasodilator response is abolished by ouabain, which suggests that it works by stimulating the sodium-potassium pump (26, 80). Overbeck and Clark were the first to suggest that the presence of a digitalislike substance in plasma of some individuals with hypertension may be responsible for an observed impairment of the vasodilatory response to potassium (61).

SUMMARY

It is evident that salt is an important factor in understanding hypertension in African and other blacks. The ability of some blacks to retain ingested salt is almost certainly of great adaptive advantage in situations when the availability of salt is low and the potential for the loss of salt is high. These conditions would have pertained in earlier times in many areas of Africa. We now know that blacks in both hemispheres are more likely than whites to exhibit a pressor sensitivity to dietary salt. However, we also know that sensitivity to salt in itself is not sufficient to cause hypertension, because hypertension is relatively rare among African blacks who have not adopted Western living habits. Furthermore, not all blacks with hypertension exhibit equal sensitivity to salt. An important element of Westernization may be an increase in the ratio of sodium to potassium in the diet. Other factors such as psychosocial stress, increased intake of alcohol, increased prevalence of obesity, reduction in dietary fiber and calcium, as well as increase in dietary fat and simple carbohydrates have not been discussed here, but must be given full consideration.

REFERENCES

1. Ahrens, R. A. Sucrose, hypertension and heart disease. An historical perspective. *Am. J. Clin. Nutr. 27:* 403–22, 1974.
2. Akinkugbe, O. O. World Epidemiology of hypertension in blacks. In: *Hypertension in Blacks,* edited by W. D. Hall, E. Saunders, and N. B. Shulman. Year Book Medical Publishers, Chicago, 1985, pp. 3–17.
3. Akinkugbe, O. O., and O. A. Ojo. Arterial pressures in rural and urban populations in Nigeria. *Br. Med. J. 2:* 222–224, 1969.
4. Arkwright, P. D. Effects of alcohol use and other aspects of lifestyle on blood pressure levels and prevalence of hypertension in a working population. *Circulation 66:* 60–66, 1982.
5. Aviv, A. The link between cytosolic calcium ion and the sodium-hydrogen ion antiport: a unifying factor for essential hypertension. *J. Hypertens. 6:* 685–691, 1988.
6. Barlow, R. J., M. A. Connell, B. J. Levendig, J. S. S. Gear, and J. Milne. A comparative study of urinary sodium and potassium excretion in normotensive urban black and white South African males. *S. Afr. Med. J. 62:* 939–941, 1982.
7. Bauer, J., and W. Gaunter. Effect of potassium on plasma renin activity and aldosterone during sodium restriction in normal man. *Kidney Int. 15:* 286–293, 1979.
8. Bjorntorp, P. Obesity and the risk of cardiovascular disease. *Ann. Clin. Res. 17:* 3–9, 1985.
9. Blaustein, M. P. Sodium ions, blood pressure regulation and hypertension. A reassessment and a hypothesis. *Am. J. Physiol. 232: (Cell Physiol. 2):* C165–C173, 1977.
10. Brunner, H. R., L. Baer, and J. E. Sealey. The influence of potassium administration and of potassium deprivation on plasma renin activity in normotensives and hypertensives. *J. Clin. Invest. 49:* 2128–2138, 1970.
11. Bursztyn, P. G., and D. R. Husbands. Fat induced hypertension in rabbits. *Cardiovasc. Res. 14:* 185–191, 1978.
12. Bursztyn, P., D. Hornall, and C. Watchdon. Sodium and potassium intake and blood pressure. *Br. Med. J. 281:* 537–539, 1980.
13. Chen, Y. F., Q. Meng, M. Wyss, H. Jin, and S. Oparil. High sodium chloride diet reduces hypothalamic norepinephrine turnover in hypertensive rats. *Hypertension 11:* 55–62, 1988.
14. Cooper, R. A note on the biologic concept of race and its application in epidemiologic research. *Am. Heart J. 108:* 715–723, 1984.

15. Cruickshank, J. K., and D. G. Beevers. Preface. In: *Ethnic Factors in Health and Disease,* edited by J. K. Cruickshank and D. G. Beevers. Wright, London, 1989, pp. vii–ix.

16. Dahl, L., M. Heine, and L. Tassinari. Effects of chronic excess salt ingestion. Evidence that genetic factors play an important role in susceptibility to experimental hypertension. *J. Exp. Med. 115:* 173, 1962.

17. Dahl, L., G. Leitt, and M. Heine. Influence of dietary potassium and sodium potassium ratio on development of salt hypertension. *J. Exp. Med. 138:* 318–330, 1972.

18. Dietz, R., and A. Schomig. Enhanced sympathetic activity caused by salt loading in SHR. *Clin. Sci. 59:* 171S–173S, 1980.

19. Donnison, C. P. Blood pressure in the African native: the bearing upon the aetiology of hyperpiesia and arteriosclerosis. *Lancet 1:* 6–7, 1929.

20. Dustan H. P., and K. A. Kirk. Relationship of sodium balance to arterial pressure in black hypertensive patients. *Am. J. Med. Sci. 31:* 378–383, 1988.

21. Forsyth, F. Hypertension in Tanzania; preliminary communication. *East Afr. Med. J. 46:* 309–312, 1969.

22. Fujita, R. Factors influencing blood pressure in salt sensitivity patients with hypertension. *Am. J. Med. 69:* 334–344, 1980.

23. Garay, P. R., C. Nazaret, G. Dagher, E. Bertrand, and P. Meyer. A genetic approach to the geography of hypertension. Examinations of sodium/potassium cotransport in Ivory Coast Africans. *Clin. Exp. Hypertens. 3:* 861–870, 1981.

24. Grim CE, FC Luft, JZ Miller et al. Racial differences in blood pressure in Evans County, Georgia: Relationship to sodium and potassium intake and plasma renin activity. *J. Chronic Dis., 33:* 87–94, 1980.

25. Haddy, F. Sodium potassium pump in low renin hypertension. *Ann. Intern. Med. 98:* 781–784, 1983.

26. Haddy, F. Potassium effect on contraction of arterial smooth muscle mediated by Na^+/K^+ ATPase. *Fed. Proc. 42:* 239–245, 1983.

27. Haddy, F. Endogenous digitalis like factor or factors. *N. Engl. J. Med. 316:* 621–623, 1987.

28. Haddy, F. J., M. B. Pamnani, and D. L. Clough. Alterations of sodium transport in vascular smooth muscle in hypertension. In: *Membrane Abnormalities in Hypertension,* vol. I, edited by C-K. Kwan. C.R.C. Press, Boca Raton, Fl., 1989, pp. 15–30.

29. Mathews, W. R., D. W. DuCharme, J. M. Hamlyn, D. W. Harris, F. Mandel, M. A. Clark, and J. H. Ludens. Mass spectral characterization of an endogenous digitalislike factor from human plasma. *Hypertension 17:* 930–935, 1991.

30. Hollister, S. A., I. Tanaka, T. Imada, J. Onrot, I. Biaggioni, D. Robertson, and T. Inagami. Sodium loading and posture modulate human ANP plasma levels. *Hypertension* (Supp II) *8:* 106–111, 1986.

31. Iimura, F., T. Kijima, and K. Kikuchi. Studies on the blood pressure lowering effect of potassium in essential hypertension. *Clin. Sci. 61:* 775–805, 1981.

32. Intersalt 1986. Cooperative research group: an international cooperative study on the relation of blood pressure to sodium and potassium excretion. *Br. Med. J. 297:* 319–328, 1988.

33. Jin, H., J. Chen, R. Yang, and S. Oparil. Impaired release of ANP in sodium chloride loaded SHR. *Hypertension 11:* 739–744, 1988.

34. Kaminer, B., and W. P. Lutz. Blood pressure in the Bushmen of the Kalahari. *Circulation 22:* 287–295, 1960.

35. Kawasaki, T., C. Delea, F. Bartter, and H. Smith. The effect of increasing sodium and decreasing sodium intakes on blood pressure and other related variables in human subjects with idiopathic hypertension. *Am. J. Med. 64:* 193–198, 1977.

36. Kesteloot, H., D. X. Huang, Y. Li, J. Geboers, and J. Joosens. The relationship between cations and blood pressure in the Peoples Republic of China. *Hypertension 9:* 654–659, 1987.

37. Kirkendall, M. W., W. E. Connor, F. Abboud, S. Rastog, T. Anderson, and M. Fry. The effect of dietary sodium chloride on blood pressure, body fluids and electrolytes, renal function and serum lipids of normotensive men. *J. Lab. Clin. Med. 87:* 418–434, 1976.

38. Koepke, J., S. Jones, and G. DiBona. Sodium responsiveness of central alpha-2 adrenergic receptor in SHR. *Hypertension 11:* 326–333, 1988.

39. Komachi, Y., and T. Shimamoto. Salt intake and its relationship to blood pressure in Japan past and present. In: *Epidemiology of Arterial Blood Pressure,* edited by H. Kesteloot and J. V. Joossens. Martinus Nijhof, The Hague, 1980, pp. 395–400.

40. Kotchen, J. M., and T. A. Kotchen. Geographic effect on racial blood pressure differences in adolescents. *J. Chronic Dis. 31:* 581–586, 1978.

41. Langford, H. G., F. P. J. Langford, and M. Tyler. Dietary profile of sodium, potassium, and

calcium in U. S. blacks. In: *Hypertension in Blacks,* edited by W. D. Hall, E. Saunders, and N. B. Shulman. Year Book Medical Publishers, Chicago, 1985, pp. 49–58.

42. Lawton, W. C., Sinkey, and A. Fitz. Dietary salt produces abnormal renal vasoconstrictor responses to upright posture in borderline hypertensive subjects. *Hypertension 11:* 529–536, 1988.

43. Losse, H., W. Zideck, H. Zumkley, F. Weel, and H. Vetter. Intracellular Na^+ as a genetic marker for essential hypertension. *Clin. Exp. Hypertens. 3:* 627–640, 1981.

44. Luft, F. C., C. E. Grim, N. Fineberg, and M. H. Weinberger. Effects of volume expansion and contraction in normotensive whites, blacks, and subjects of different ages. *Circulation 59:* 643–650, 1979.

45. Luft, F. C., C. E. Grim, and M. H. Weinberger. Electrolyte and volume homeostasis in blacks. In: *Hypertension in Blacks,* edited by W. D. Hall, E. Saunders, and N. B. Shulman Year Book Medical Publishers, Chicago 1985, pp. 115–131.

46. Luft, F. C., L. I. Rankin, R. Bloch, A. E. Weyman, L. R. Willis, R. H. Murray, C. E. Grim, and M. H. Weinberger. Cardiovascular and humoral responses to extremes of sodium intake in normotensive black and white men. *Circulation 60:* 697–705, 1979.

47. M'Bayamba-Kabangu J. R., R. Fagard, P. Lijnen, R. Mbuy wa Mbuy, J. Staessen, and A. Amery. Blood pressure and urinary cations in urban Bantu of Zaire. *Am. J. Epidemiol. 124:* 957–968, 1986.

48. M'Bayamba-Kabangu, J., P. Lijen, D. Groeegennoke, J. Staessen, W. Lissens, W. Goossens, R. Fagard, and A. Amery. Racial differences in intracellular and transmembrane fluxes of sodium and K^+ in erythrocytes of normal male subjects. *J. Hypertens. 2:* 647–651, 1984.

49. M'Bayamba-Kabangu J.R., P. Lijnen, R. Fagard, and A. Amery. Intraerythrocyte sodium concentration in black families with and without hypertension. *Methods Find. Exp. Clin. Pharmacol. 8:* 437–442. 1986.

50. McCarron, D. A., C. Morris, and C. Cole. Dietary calcium in human hypertension. *Science 217:* 267–270, 1982.

51. Maddocks I. Possible absence of essential hypertension in two complete Pacific Islands populations. The Lancet 2: 396–399, 1961.

52. Meneeley, G. R., and C. T. Ball. Experimental evidence of chronic sodium chloride toxicity and protective effect of potassium chloride. *Am. J. Med. 25:* 713–725, 1958.

53. Miall W. E., E. H. Kass, J. Ling, and K. L. Stuart. Factors influencing arterial pressure in the general population in Jamaica. *Br. Med. J. 2:* 492–497, 1961.

54. Miller, J., M. Weinberger, and J. Christian. Blood pressure response to potassium supplementation in normotensive adults and children. *Hypertension 10:* 437–442, 1987.

55. Moser, M., R. Morgan, H. Hale, S. Hoobler, R. Remington, J. Dodge, and A. Macaulay. Epidemiology of hypertension with particular reference to the Bahamas. *Am. J. Cardiol. 7:* 727–733, 1959.

56. Mufunda, J., J. E. Chimoskey, J. Matenga, C. Musabayane, and H. V. Sparks. Blood pressure response to acute changes in dietary sodium intake in young Zimbabwean men. *J. Hypertens. 10:* 279–285, 1992.

57. Mufunda, J., J. Chimoskey, C. Musabayane, J. Matenga, and H. Sparks. Effect of dietary potassium on the blood pressure response to extremes of sodium intake in black men. *FASEB J. 2:* A1525, 1988.

58. Oliver, W. J., E. L. Cohen, and J. V. Neel. Blood pressure, sodium intake and sodium related hormones in the Yanomamo Indians, a "no salt" culture. *Circulation 52:* 146–151, 1975.

59. Oparil, S. Increased sympathetic nervous system activity in salt dependent hypertension. In: National Institutes of Health, USA-Poland symposium, cardiovascular disease, Washington, D.C. U.S. Dept. of Health and Human Services, 1986, pp. 41–47.

60. Oshima, T., H. Matsuura, K. Matsumoto, K. Kido, and G. Kaijiyama. Role of cellular calcium in salt sensitivity of patients with essential hypertension. *Hypertension 11:* 703–707, 1988.

61. Overbeck, N. W., and D. W. J. Clark. Vasodilator response to potassium in genetic hypertension and renal hypertension. *J. Lab. Clin. Med. 86:* 973–983, 1975.

62. Page, L. Epidemiology of hypertension. In: *Hypertension,* edited by J. Genest, O. Kuchel, P. Hamet, and M. Cantin. McGraw-Hill, New York, 1983.

63. Page, L., A. Dammon, and R. Mollering. Antecedents of cardiovascular disease in 6 Solomon Island societies. *Circulation 49:* 1132–1146, 1974.

64. Parfrey, P. S., P. Wright, F. J. Goodwin, M. J. Vandenburg, J. M. P. Holly, S. J. W. Evans, and J. M. Ledingham. Blood pressure and hormonal changes following alteration in dietary sodium and potassium in mild essential hypertension. *Lancet 1:* 59, 1981.

65. Parfrey, P. S., P. Wright, J. M. P. Holly, S. J. W. Evans, K. Condon, M. J. Vandenburg, F. J.

Goodwin, and J. M. Ledingham. Blood pressure and hormonal changes following alteration in dietary sodium and potassium in young men with and without a familial predisposition to hypertension. *Lancet 1:* 113, 1981.

66. Parry, H. Ethiopian cardiovascular studies. III. The casual blood pressure in the Ethiopian highlands of Addis Ababa. *East Afr. Med. J. 46:* 246–256, 1969.

67. Pekka, P., A. Nissinen, E. Vartiainen, R. Dougherty, M. Multanen, J. Iacono, H. Korhonen, P. Pietinen, U. Lieno, S. Moisio, and J. Hultunen. Controlled randomized trial of effect of dietary fat on blood pressure. *Lancet 1:* 1–5, 1983.

68. Poulter, N. Blood pressure in urban and rural East Africa: the Kenyan Luo migrant study. In: *Ethnic Factors in Health and Disease,* edited by J. K. Cruickshank and D. G. Beevers. Wright, London, 1989, pp. 61–68.

69. Poulter, N., K. T. Khaw, B. Hopwood, M. Mugambi, S. Peart, G. Rose, and P. Sever. Blood pressure and its correlates in an African tribe in urban and rural environments. *J. Epidemiol. Community Health 38:* 181–186, 1984.

70. Prineas, R. J., and R. Gillum. United States epidemiology of hypertension in blacks. In: *Hypertension in Blacks* edited by W. D. Hall, E. Saunders, and N. B. Shulman. Year Book Medical Publishers, Chicago, 1985, pp. 17–36.

71. Resnick, L., J. Nicholson, and J. Laragh. Calcium metabolism in essential hypertension. Relationship to altered renin system activity. *Fed. Proc. 45:* 2739–2745, 1986.

72. Rikimaru, T., Y. Fujita, T. Okuda, N. Kajiwara, S. Miyatani, M. Alpers, and H. Koishi. Response of sodium balance, BP and other variables to sodium loading in Papua New Guinea Highlanders. *Am. J. Clin. Nutr. 47:* 502–508, 1988.

73. Saunders, G. M., and H. Bancroft. Blood pressure studies on negro and white men and women living in the Virgin Islands of the United States of America. *Am. Heart J. 23:* 410–423, 1942.

74. Seedat, Y. K. Race, environment and blood pressure: the South African experience. *J. Hypertens. 1:* 7–12, 1983.

75. Shaper, A. G., P. J. Leonard, K. W. Jones, and M. Jones. Environmental effects on the body build, blood pressure, and blood chemistry of nomadic warriors serving in the army in Kenya. *East Afr. Med. J. 46:* 282–289, 1969.

76. Simmons, D., G. Barbour, J. Congleton, J. Levy, P. Meacher, H. Saul, and T. Sowerby. Blood pressure and salt intake in Malawi: an urban and rural study. *J. Epidemiol. Community Health 40:* 188–192, 1986.

77. Skrabal, F., J. Aubock, H. Hortnagl, and H. Braunsteiner. Effect of moderate sodium restriction and increase in potassium on the pressor hormones response to noradrenaline and baroreceptor function in man. *Clin. Sci. 59:* 1575–1605, 1980.

78. Smith, J. B., M. B. Wade, N. S. Fineberg, and M. H. Weinberger. Influence of race, sex, and blood pressure on erythrocyte sodium transport in humans. *Hypertension 12:* 251–258, 1988.

79. Sowers, J., M. Zemel, P. Zemel, F. Lock, M. Walsh and E. Zawada. Salt Sensitivity in Blacks, Salt intake and natriuretic substances. *Hypertension 12:* 485–490, 1988.

80. Sparks, H. V. Effect of local metabolic factors on vascular smooth muscle: vessel wall pO_2 K^+ and osmolarity. In: *Handbook of Physiology. Circulation: Vascular Smooth Muscle,* edited by D. F. Bohr, A. P. Somlyo, and H. V. Sparks. Am. Physiol. Soc., Washington D.C., 1980.

81. Stamler, J., R. Stamler, W. F. Riedlinger, G. Algera, and R. H. Roberts. Hypertension of one million Americans: community hypertension evaluation clinic program 1973–75. *J.A.M.A. 235:* 2299–2306, 1976.

82. Tang, J., D. Song, M. Suen, and C. Wixie. Alpha-human ANP in normal volunteers and patients with heart failure or hypertension. *Peptides 7:* 33–37, 1986.

83. Tannen, J. Effects of potassium on blood pressure control. *Ann. Intern. Med. 98:* 773–780, 1983.

84. Trevisan, M., R. Cooper, D. Ostrow, C. Sempos, S. Sparks, S. Nanas, W. Miller, and J. Stamler. Red cell cation transport: differences between black and white school children. *J. Hypertens. 1:* 245–249, 1983.

85. Weder, A. B., B. A. Torretti, and S. Julius. Racial differences in erythrocyte cation transport. *Hypertension 6:* 115–123, 1984.

86. Weinberger, M., J. Miller, N. Fineberg, F. Luft, C. Grim, and J. Christian. Association of haptoglobin with sodium sensitivity and resistance of blood pressure. *Hypertension 10:* 443–446, 1987.

87. Weinberger, M. H., J. Z. Miller, F. C. Luft, C. G. Grim, and N. S. Fineberg. Definitions and characteristics of sodium sensitivity and blood pressure resistance. *Hypertension* 8(Suppl II): 127–134, 1986.

88. Williams, A. W. Blood pressure of Africans. *East Afr. Med. J. 18:* 109–117, 1941.

89. Wilson, T. W. History of salt supplies in West Africa and blood pressures today. *Lancet 1:* 784–786, 1986.

90. Young, D. B., R. E. McCaa, Y. Pan, and A. C. Guyton. The natriuretic and hypotensive effects of potassium. *Circ. Res. 38*(Suppl II): 84, 1976.

91. Zhu, D. L., G. S. Zhao, and H. Wang. Cation transport in blood cells from Chinese patients with essential hypertension. In: *Membrane Abnormalities in Hypertension,* vol. II, edited by C-K. Kwan. C.R.C. Press, Boca Raton, Fl., 1989, pp. 150–180.

8

Role of Nutrition in Black Hypertension: Calcium and Other Dietary Factors

JAMES R. SOWERS, PAULA C. ZEMEL, AND MICHAEL B. ZEMEL

A number of studies have shown that, on average, blacks in the Western Hemisphere have higher blood pressure than blacks from sub-Sahara Africa (2,77,92,123). Considerable regional variations in blood pressure also exist among blacks in the Western Hemisphere (6,42,49,90). This geographical heterogeneity in the prevalence of hypertension in various black populations around the world suggests that environmental factors play a critical role in determining the prevalence of hypertension in blacks (90). The importance of environment in contributing to the prevalence of hypertension in blacks is reinforced by the observation that when rural Africans undergo changes to more urban, Western lifestyles and diets, blood pressure increases (2,23,90,93, see Chapter 7, this volume). The information in this chapter examines one important environmental factor, nutrition, and its role in contributing to high blood pressure in urbanized, Westernized blacks (Table 8.1).

OBESITY AND HYPERTENSION IN BLACKS

An association between hypertension and obesity has been well documented in numerous clinical and epidemiological studies (44,80,82,119,121). Data from the Framingham study showed that subjects who were overweight at the start of the study later developed hypertension more often than subjects who were not overweight (47). In the Evans County, Georgia, study (121), a weight gain over a 6-year period was clearly associated with twice the likelihood that hypertension would develop. Further, obesity at the start of the study with no further weight gain was also associated with a fivefold greater chance of reaching hypertensive levels of blood pressure, and the relative risk of hypertension was eight times greater in those who were both overweight at the outset and who also gained weight during the 6-year study. The Evans County study also showed that the rate of remission of "hypertensive" blood pressure into the normal range was twice as great for subjects who lost 4.5 kg (10 lb) or more over 6 years as for those who gained 4.5 kg (10 lb) or more during the same interval. Data from a study done on former students of the University of Pennsylvania showed that obesity during the college years was one of the characteristics predictive of hypertension in middle life (74). This association be-

TABLE 8.1. Nutritional Factors Likely to Play a Role in the Pathogenesis of Hypertension in the African American Population

---

Obesity (particularly central obesity)
Effects of hyperinsulinemia to enhance sympathetic nervous system activity and to increase salt retention

Effects of insulin resistance contributing to increased peripheral vascular resistance

Low dietary calcium intake
Decreased natriuresis and associated volume expansion

Increased vasoconstriction

Compensatory increases in parathyroid hormone, parathyroid hypertensive factor, and 1,25 $(OH)_2$ D levels, all of which may increase intracellular calcium

Decreased cellular calcium pump activity

Low dietary magnesium intake
Increased peripheral vascular resistance

Decreased activity of the sodium-potassium membrane pump and the calcium extrusion pump

Low potassium intake
Increased vascular resistance

Decreased natriuresis and volume expansion

Loss of functional integrity of the vascular endothelium

---

tween overweight and blood pressure is present in children and adolescents, as was shown in the Bogalusa Heart Study (5). In children aged 5–15, body weight was correlated with blood pressure levels (see Chapter 3, this volume). Data from the hypertension detection and follow-up program found that 60% of the participants were more than 20% above ideal body weight (43) in contrast to 24% and 14% of all American women and men, respectively (99). The Meharry Cohort Study (71) evaluated the relationship between body weight and blood pressure of 433 physicians measured at the initial evaluation and the follow-up after 23 years. The results demonstrated that weight gain was more closely related to the development of hypertension than initial body weight or the weight at the end of the study period. These observations suggest that the relationship between obesity and blood pressure is a dynamic one.

Obesity as a risk factor for the development of hypertension is likely to be important in the African American population in whom 30% of males and 49% of females have been estimated to be obese [Table 8.1; (68,87)]. Indeed, there is a significant inverse association between relative weight, hypertension, and duration of formal education (43,69,83). In the United States a disproportionate number of blacks have limited education and financial resources (83). Among black women, the presence of obesity clearly varies inversely with socioeconomic status (30,69,72,83,87). Nevertheless, controlling for socioeconomic status does not eliminate the obesity prevalence differences between black and white women (2:1 prevalence of overweight in blacks compared with white women) (45).

Upper body fat (central obesity) is much more strongly linked to hypertension, diabetes, and cardiovascular disease than is peripheral fat distribution in several populations, including African American men and women (11,22,36). The relative excess of central obesity is greater than the excess of extremity obesity in black women (11). Further, there is evidence that increased central obesity can be detected in black children of both sexes (11,65). In the NHANES I data, blood pressures in black women were positively associated with subscapular skinfold thickness (measurement of central obesity). There is also a strong association between type II diabetes mellitus and central obesity in black women (39). Furthermore, central obesity in blacks may explain the loss of elevated high density lipoprotein cholesterol levels seen among some black adults and children of both sexes compared with whites (8,37). Indeed, a significant inverse correlation of body mass index and high density lipoprotein cholesterol was noted in a random sample of low socioeconomic status black women in Baltimore (37). Finally, it should be noted that obesity-related risks in blacks may be enhanced by an excess of multiple risk factors (107).

A higher prevalence of central obesity may explain, in part, the increased prevalence of type II diabetes (70,89) as well as essential hypertension in the black population (Table 8.2). Insulin resistance appears to be strongly linked to body fat distribution (109). That insulin resistance and accompanying hyperinsulinemia associated with central obesity is important in the genesis of hypertension in Westernized, industrialized blacks is further evidenced by recent studies demonstrating the role of insulin resistance/hyperinsulinemia in hypertension (24,28,81,95,97). Hyperinsulinemia may contribute to hypertension via activation of the sympathetic nervous system and renal salt retention (105). Insulin resistance appears to contribute to hypertension through increasing peripheral vascular resistance in association with altered cellular cation transport [Table 8.1; (106)]. Central obesity may also be an important factor explaining the high prevalence of hypertension in those individuals with type II diabetes (109). Recent studies conducted by Falkner et al. (21) demonstrated that insulin resistance exists in young black men with borderline hypertension. This observation further emphasizes the importance of insulin resistance in the pathogenesis of hypertension in black individuals (see Chapter 3, this volume).

TABLE 8.2. Pathophysiological Characteristics of Hypertension in African Americans

Expanded intravascular volume

Increased peripheral vascular resistance

Altered cellular cation transport leading to increased intracellular free calcium concentration

Increased renal vascular resistance and reduced renal blood flow

Reduced renal generation of natriuretic substances such as dopamine and kallikreins

Salt sensitivity related to the two preceding characteristics and likely accentuated by a suboptimal dietary calcium intake and perhaps by suboptimal dietary potassium intake

Increased hyperinsulinemia/insulin resistance

Low-renin state of hypertension

Increased urinary calcium excretion contributing to a relative "calcium deficiency" state

Increased frequency of type II diabetes in association with hypertension

DIETARY CATIONS AND HYPERTENSION IN BLACKS

High blood pressure in African Americans is generally characterized by a low-renin, hypervolemic salt-sensitive state of hypertension [Table 8.2; (27,55,60, 61,103)]. Hemodynamically, hypertension in this population is characterized by increased peripheral vascular resistance and a tendency toward reduced cardiac output (27). Pratt et al. (78) showed that black school children also have lower aldosterone secretion rates than white children, even when corrected for dietary potassium intake. This may reflect, in part, salt retention due to increased salt sensitivity at an early age in the black population. Blood pressures among these black children were significantly higher. A higher incidence of salt sensitivity occurs in blacks in spite of the apparent lack of differences in sodium and salt intakes between the two racial groups (34,53, 131). Volume expansion, in part, may theoretically explain the low-renin state that is often observed in the black hypertensive (27,61). Recent evidence has been presented to show that the underlying mechanism of renin hyporesponsivity may be more complex than previously believed (see Chapter 10, this volume). Mechanisms involved in the relatively high incidence of salt sensitivity in blacks, both normotensive and hypertensive, are poorly understood. However, an impaired natriuretic response to a salt load in these individuals could result from decreased renal blood flow (increased vascular resistance) (27) or reduced ability to generate renal natriuretic substances such as dopamine (17,103) and kallikreins [Table 8.2; (55)].

A promising mechanism involved in this differential salt sensitivity between blacks and whites is differences in dopamine responses to salt loading. In response to a salt load, individuals normally increase dopamine excretion in parallel with sodium excretion. Several investigators have pointed out that in salt-sensitive hypertensives there is both an impaired natriuretic response and a diminished response in renal dopamine generation (31,33). Chritchley et al. (17) observed that West Africans, even when normotensive, failed to increase dopamine secretion after a salt load. Sowers et al. (103) confirmed the decreased dopamine response to salt loading in hypertensive black subjects, and have also pointed out that hypertensive white subjects show heightened natriuretic and hypotensive responses to exogenous dopamine (101,102). Thus, decreased renal dopamine production may be one mechanism that helps explain increased salt sensitivity in blacks (Table 8.2).

Racial differences in cell cation metabolism have been observed by a number of investigators (see Chapter 9, this volume). Erythrocyte sodium levels are considerably higher in blacks (16,54,59,66,119). A higher level of platelet intracellular calcium ($[Ca^{2+}]_i$) has been noted in black hypertensives (16). Assuming that platelet $[Ca^{2+}]_i$ reflects vascular smooth muscle $[Ca^{2+}]_i$, this could, in turn, explain the increased vascular contractility and elevated peripheral vascular resistance observed in blacks with essential hypertension (4,19,26,58). Both a reduction in erythrocyte Na^+/K^+-ATPase (54,120) and Ca^{2+}-ATPase (134) have been observed in blacks, particularly those with hypertension. Canessa et al. (12) have described low sodium-potassium-chloride cotransport in blacks compared with whites. They have also shown that abnormalities of the cotransport system are predictors of sodium sensitivity in young blacks, both normotensive and hypertensive (13). A higher sodium-hydrogen antiport activity has been observed in cultured skin fibroblasts from blacks than in fibroblasts from whites (40). This increased sodium-hydrogen antiport activity in skin fibroblasts from blacks is also associated with a greater mobilization of calcium and increased cellular turnover of this cation (67). These cation transport abnormalities likely contribute to the altered cellular calcium and sodium metabolism and an increased prevalence of salt sensitivity observed in blacks with essential hypertension (Table 8.2).

CALCIUM METABOLISM, DIETARY CALCIUM, AND SALT SENSITIVITY

There are no consistent and significant differences between dietary salt ingestion in African Americans and whites (34,53,137). The observation that the increased prevalence of salt sensitivity in blacks compared with whites cannot be attributed to differences in sodium intake suggests that other dietary differences may be involved (Table 8.1). Dietary calcium is lower in blacks than in whites (53,137), possibly due to the high incidence of lactose intolerance (96) in blacks. Considerable evidence has accumulated to indicate that suboptimal intakes of calcium coupled with abnormalities in calcium metabolism may play a role in the genesis and maintenance of low-renin, salt-sensitive hypertension such as exists in American blacks. Although data from NHANES I and II were originally interpreted as indicating an inverse relationship between dietary calcium and blood pressure in the U.S. population, subsequent analysis of the data indicated that this relationship is only evident in black males (91), further suggesting a role for dietary calcium deficiency in the pathophysiology of hypertension in blacks. Several other epidemiological studies also indicate an inverse relationship between blood pressure and calcium intake (1,29,38,52, 106,114,118), and data from the 60,000 women participating in the 4-year prospective Nurses Health Study indicate a 23% reduction in the risk of hypertension associated with a calcium intake greater than 800 mg/day when compared with calcium intakes less than 400 mg/day (128).

The low-renin, salt-sensitive state that characterizes hypertension in blacks is accompanied by decreases in serum ionized calcium levels (84). Similarly, a number of animal models of hypertension exhibit decreased serum ionized or total calcium levels (63,73,129). A relative state of calcium deficiency in low-renin hypertension is further suggested by observed alterations in calcium regulatory hormones, with parathyroid hormone (PTH) and 1,25-(OH)$_2$-D levels being elevated and calcitonin suppressed in comparison with either normotensives or high-renin hypertensives (84). This relative calcium deficiency may be contributed to both by the aforementioned decrease in calcium intake in blacks compared with whites as well as by an increase in urinary calcium. Indeed, increased calcium excretion has been consistently observed in hypertensive individuals as well as in animal models of hypertension (110,122,130,133), and it has been observed that black hypertensives exhibit increased urinary calcium compared with black normotensives [Table 8.2; (103,132)].

Increased calcium excretion in salt-sensitive states may result from alterations in the renal handling of sodium. A relationship between renal tubular handling of sodium and calcium has been demonstrated in several studies (51,112). Relationships between urinary sodium and calcium excretion have subsequently been reported in hypertensive rats (110,122) as well as in elderly hypertensives (32). Similarly, significant, sustained calciuresis has been observed to accompany salt-induced increases in blood pressure in black hypertensives on low calcium diets (132,133). Thus, in salt-sensitive blacks, salt-induced increases in urinary calcium excretion coupled with a suboptimal calcium intake are likely to contribute to a relative state of "calcium deficiency." Consistent with this concept is the observation that blacks have higher blood levels of PTH and 1,25 dihydroxyvitamin D than whites (10), perhaps in compensation for this calcium deficiency. This relative calcium deficiency is likely limited to the extracellular fluid compartment, as bone mineral mass is generally increased in blacks compared with whites (15). There is accumulating evidence to suggest that correction of this calcium deficiency is likely to reduce blood pressure in this population by several mechanisms, discussed later.

Dietary calcium restriction causes vasoconstriction in both spontaneously hypertensive rats and their normotensive controls (9,48,62), while calcium supplementation lowers blood pressure in hypertensive rats (7). A number of dietary calcium intervention trials have been conducted in humans using intervention periods ranging from 5 days to 4 years (64,100,104). These studies have employed a variety of study designs, calcium levels, and calcium sources, and although some studies have not found an antihypertensive effect of calcium, a pattern emerges when evaluating these trials that indicates that there is a consistent antihypertensive effect of calcium supplementation in some populations, while others exhibit little or no effect. Specifically, there appears to be a consistent blood pressure–lowering effect of dietary calcium supplementation in hypertensive individuals who are likely to be salt sensitive by virtue of being black, elderly, or exhibiting a low plasma renin activity (84, 100,104).

Unfortunately, many calcium intervention trials have not included careful evaluations of baseline dietary calcium intakes. Since there appears to be a threshold effect of dietary calcium on blood pressure, with increased blood pressure associated with calcium intakes less than 400–500 mg/day (104,128), little or no blood pressure reduction would be expected from supplementing the diets of individuals with adequate calcium intake. For example, Grobbee and Hofman (35) noted that patients with elevated PTH levels, suggestive of suboptimal calcium intake, exhibit greater antihypertensive responses to calcium supplementation than patients with low to normal PTH levels. Similarly, we have consistently observed significant antihypertensive effects of calcium supplementation in both normotensive and hypertensive blacks in the Detroit area (133,135) with baseline calcium intakes of 300–500 mg/day (137). Since the elderly also generally exhibit salt sensitivity and inadequate dietary calcium intakes (134), it is noteworthy that calcium supplementation trials in the elderly have also consistently produced an antihypertensive effect (32,46,113). For example, in a randomized, placebo-controlled double-blind trial, Johnson et al. (44) reported that a 1,500 mg/day calcium supplement caused a 13 mm Hg reduction in systolic pressure in 16 hypertensive postmenopausal women studied over a 4-year period of supplementation, while the placebo-treated group of 18 women exhibited a 7 mm Hg increase. Thus, it appears that calcium supplementation is effective in reducing blood pressure in individuals consuming suboptimal levels of calcium, while those consuming adequate levels of calcium (>800–1000 mg/day) are unlikely to benefit from additional supplementation.

There are several possible mechanisms whereby correction of a subtle calcium deficiency may reduce blood pressure (Table 8.3). The renal handling of calcium and sodium exhibit a mutual interdependence, and an increase in the filtered load of either cation can increase the renal excretion of the other (51,112). Sodium loading increases urinary calcium excretion, as discussed earlier, while increasing dietary calcium has also been shown to cause a natriuretic and diuretic effect (130,131). Thus, calcium supplementation in volume expanded individuals, such as blacks, appears to be particularly effective in lowering blood pressure (132,133). Calcium supplementation in blacks has been reported to increase erythrocyte Na^+/K^+-ATPase activity and reduce intracellular sodium in salt-sensitive blacks [Table 8.3; (132)].

Low intakes of calcium have also been suggested to depress Ca^{2+}-ATPase-mediated calcium efflux and thereby increase intracellular calcium and vascular resistance (64,124); conversely, increasing dietary calcium intake would be expected to increase the activity of this pump, resulting in a decrease in intracellular calcium and vascular resistance. Erythrocyte Ca^{2+}-ATPase activity has been observed to be about 30% lower in black patients in comparison with whites (134). A significant impairment in calcium pump activity has also been noted in non-insulin-dependent diabetic hypertensive blacks (136), as well as in an animal model of insulin resistance and hypertension (94), which

TABLE 8.3. Postulated Mechanism of Action of Dietary Calcium, Magnesium, and Potassium in Hypertension

Calcium
Decreased vascular resistance

Natriuresis and reduced intravascular volume

Activation of the sodium-potassium membrane pump and the calcium extrusion pump

Suppression of circulating levels of 1,25 $(OH)_2$ D

Suppression of circulating parathyroid hypertensive factor and parathyroid hormone levels

Magnesium
Decreased vascular resistance

Inhibition of cellular calcium influx

Inhibition of calcium release from the sarcoplasmic reticulum

Activation of the sodium-potassium membrane pump

Activation of the cell membrane and the sarcoplasmic reticulum calcium pump

Potassium
Decreased vascular resistance

Natriuresis

Protection of vascular endothelium and preservation of endothelium-dependent vascular relaxation

is partially corrected by dietary calcium supplementation (136). Thus, although the mechanism whereby dietary calcium increases the activity of the
calcium pump is not known, this stimulation may contribute to the antihypertensive effect of calcium supplementation in some blacks with hypertension
(Table 8.3).

Increases in PTH and $1,25(OH)_2$ vitamin D in dietary calcium deficiency
may contribute to increases in peripheral vascular resistance, as both increase
cellular calcium influx in a variety of tissues, including vascular smooth muscle (84,131). Accordingly, it may be expected that dietary calcium supplementation of calcium-deficient individuals will reduce circulating levels of these
hormones and thereby reduce peripheral vascular resistance (Table 8.3). Consistent with this concept, Resnick and Laragh (84,86) reported that low-renin
hypertensives exhibited a hypotensive response to oral calcium supplementation in the absence of supplemental vitamin D, but that the addition of sup-
plementary $1,25(OH)_2$ D resulted in a pressor response instead.

The role of PTH in hypertension is unclear. Although PTH does stimulate
calcium influx in a variety of tissues, it has also been clearly demonstrated to
exert vasodilatory and hypotensive effects (18,76). However, Lewanczuk and
Pang (56,57,75) have described a new circulating hypertensive factor of parathyroid origin but distinct from parathyroid hormone, termed parathyroid hypertensive factor (PHF). PHF stimulates vascular smooth muscle calcium uptake, increases blood pressure, and potentiates vasoconstrictor responses to other
agonists (57). Like PTH, PHF levels are increased in spontaneously hypertensive rats on a low calcium diet and suppressed on a high calcium diet (56).
Thus, although the effects of dietary calcium on PHF levels in humans have
not yet been reported, it is possible that the antihypertensive effects of calcium
may be attributed, in part, to suppression of circulating PHF (Table 8.3).

MAGNESIUM

African Americans have been reported to ingest less magnesium than whites
(137), and this relative magnesium deficiency may also contribute to the increased prevalence of hypertension among blacks (see Table 8.1). Resnick et
al. (85) have reported that untreated hypertensives exhibited significantly
lower levels of free intracellular magnesium than either normotensive individuals or successfully treated hypertensive patients. Further, strong negative
correlations were found between intracellular free magnesium and both systolic and diastolic blood pressure (85). These observations are consistent with
a role for magnesium in mediating vascular relaxation (3). Magnesium partic-
ipates in regulation of vascular tone by several mechanisms (Table 8.3). Magnesium inhibits cellular calcium influx by competition for a calcium receptor
on a calcium-regulated efflux channel (108). Magnesium can also stimulate sarcoplasmic reticulum Ca^{2+}-ATPase (25,108), plasma membrane Ca^{2+}-ATPase and
Na^+/K^+-ATPase activity (108,125). Magnesium also inhibits the release of calcium from the sarcoplasmic reticulum (108).

Magnesium supplementation of diuretic-treated hypertensives has been
reported to correct diuretic-induced decreases in intracellular magnesium and

Na$^+$/K$^+$-ATPase activity and associated increases in intracellular calcium (135) and to reduce blood pressure (20). In contrast, magnesium does not lower blood pressure or affect intracellular magnesium, calcium, or cation pump activities in patients who were not receiving diuretics and who were therefore probably not magnesium depleted (14,138). However, the effects of magnesium supplementation, specifically in salt-sensitive individuals, have not yet been reported, and it is possible that these individuals may exhibit a sufficient degree of magnesium depletion, possibly by virtue of salt-induced increases in magnesium excretion, to benefit from magnesium supplementation.

POTASSIUM

African Americans also exhibit lower intakes of potassium than whites, and an inverse relationship between blood pressure and potassium intake has been reported [Table 8.1; (34,53,137)]. Potassium may exert its effects on blood pressure, in part, by increasing renal production of natriuretic substances, thereby enhancing sodium excretion [Table 8.3; (41,127)]. Indeed, increasing dietary consumption of potassium was observed to produced natriuresis and a negative sodium balance in black children but not white children (125,126). In addition, potassium supplementation reduces the incidence of stroke in stroke-prone, spontaneously hypertensive rats (98,115–117), and epidemiological data indicate that a 40% decrease in the incidence of stroke-related mortality is associated with a 10 mmol increase in the daily potassium intake of elderly individuals (50). Further, these effects appear to be independent of potassium-induced decreases in blood pressure (50,117). Although the mechanism of this protection against stroke is not clear, it appears to be related to protection of the vascular endothelium against salt-induced damage (79,111). Potassium may also exert its effects on blood pressure, in part, by helping to preserve vascular endothelial functional integrity [Table 8.3; (79)]. Thus, although the effects of increasing potassium intake on blood pressure reductions are generally modest, maintaining higher levels of dietary potassium may yield some protection against stroke in the black salt-sensitive population, although definitive long-term prospective clinical trials to test this concept have not yet been conducted.

REFERENCES

1. Ackley, S., E. Barret-Connor, and L. Suarez. Dairy products, calcium and blood pressure. *Am. J. Clin. Nutr. 38:* 457–461, 1983.
2. Akinkugbe, O. O. World epidemiology of hypertension in blacks. In: *Hypertension in Blacks: Epidemiology, Pathophysiology and Treatment,* edited by W. D. Hall, E. Saunders, and N. B. Shulman. Year Book Medical Publishers, Chicago, 1985, pp. 3–16.
3. Altura, B. M., and B. T. Altura. Magnesium ions and contraction of vascular smooth muscle. Relation to some vascular diseases. *Fed. Proc. 40:* 2672–2676, 1981.
4. Anderson, N. B., J. D. Lane, R. Muranaba, R. B. Williams, and S. J. Honseworth. Racial differences in blood pressure and forearm vascular responses to the cold face stimulus. *Psychosom. Med. 50:* 57–63, 1988.
5. Aristimuno, G. G., R. A. Foster, A. W. Voors, S. R. Srinivasan, and G. S. Berenson. Influence of persistent obesity in children on cardiovascular risk factors: the Bogalusa heart study. *Circulation 69:* 895–904, 1984.

6. Aschrof, M. T. Prevalence of hypertension and associated EKG abnormalities in Jamaica and the West Indies. *West Indian Med. J. 24:* 24–33, 1977.

7. Ayachi, S. Increased dietary calcium lowers blood pressure in the spontaneously hypertensive rat. *Metabolism 28:* 1234–1238, 1979.

8. Baird, D., H. A. Tyroler, G. Heiss, L. E. Chambless, and C. G. Hames. Menopausal change in serum cholesterol: black/white differences in Evans County, Georgia. *Am. J. Epidemiol. 122:* 982–993, 1985.

9. Belizan, J. M., O. Pineda, S. Sainz, L. A. Mendez, and R. J. Vill. Rise of blood pressure in calcium-deprived pregnant rats. *Am. J. Obstet. Gynecol. 141:* 163–169, 1981.

10. Bell, N. H., A. Greene, S. Epstein, M. J. Oexmann, S. Shaw, and J. Shary. Evidence for alteration of the vitamin D-endocrine system in blacks. *J. Clin. Invest. 75:* 1083–1086, 1985.

11. Blair, D., J-P. Habicht, E. A. H. Sims, D. Sylvester, and S. Abraham. Evidence for an increased risk for hypertension with centrally located body fat and the effect of race and sex on this risk. *Am. J. Epidemiol. 119:* 526–540, 1989.

12. Canessa, M., A. Spalvins, N. Adrugna, and B. Falkner. Red cell sodium countertransport and cotransport in normotensive and hypertensive blacks. *Hypertension 6:* 344–351, 1984.

13. Canessa, M., J. Bize, A. Spalvins, B. Falkner, and E. Katz. Na-K-Cl cotransport and Na pump in red cells of young blacks and blood pressure response to salt loading. *J. Clin. Hypertens. 2:* 101–108, 1986.

14. Cappucci, O., N. D. Markandu, G. W. Beynon, A. C. Shore, B. Sampson, and G. A. McGregor. Lack of effect of oral magnesium on high blood pressure. A double blind study. *Br. Med. J. 291:* 235–238, 1985.

15. Cohn, S. H., C. Abesamis, S. Yasamura, J. F. Aloia, F. Zanzi, and K. J. Ellis. Comparative skeletal mass and radial bone mineral content in black and white women. *Metab. Clin. Exp. 26:* 171–178, 1975.

16. Cooper, R. S., N. Shamsi, and S. Katz. Intracellular calcium and sodium in hypertensive patients. *Hypertension 9:* 224–229, 1987.

17. Critchley, J. A., K. Sriwatanakul, M. Balali-Mood, G. L. Boye, T. Y. Chan, N. C. Brocklesby, and M. R. Lee. Ethnic differences in the renal dopamine response to an oral salt load. Abstracts of the Fourth International Interdisciplinary Conference on Hypertension in Blacks, p. 17, 1989. *J. Hum. Hypertens. 4(2):* 91–93, 1990.

18. Cross, M. F., and P. K. T. Pang. Parathyroid hormone: a coronary artery vasodilator. *Science 217:* 1087–1089, 1980.

19. Dimsdale, J. E., R. Graham, M. G. Ziegler, R. Zusman, and C. C. Berry. Age, race, diagnosis and sodium effects on the pressor responses to infused norepinephrine. *Hypertension 10:* 564–569, 1987.

20. Dychner, T., and P. O. Wester. Effect of magnesium on blood pressure. *Br. Med. J. 286:* 1847–1849, 1983.

21. Falkner, B., S. Hulman, J. Tannenbaum, and H. Kushner. Insulin resistance and blood pressure in young black men. *Hypertension 16:* 706–711, 1990.

22. Feldman, R., A. J. Sender, and M. S. Siegelaub. Difference in diabetic and non-diabetic fat distribution patterns by skinfold measurements. *Diabetes 18:* 478–486, 1969.

23. Ferdinand, K. C. Hypertension in blacks: controversies, current concepts, and practical applications. *Intern. Med. 10(8):* 62–79, 1989.

24. Ferrannini, E., G. Buzzigoli, and R. Bonadona. Insulin resistance in essential hypertension. *N. Engl. J. Med. 317:* 350–357, 1987.

25. Flatman, P. W., and V. L. Lew. The magnesium dependence of sodium-pump mediated sodium-potassium and sodium-sodium exchange in intact human red cells. *J. Physiol. 315:* 421–426, 1981.

26. Fredickson, M. Racial differences in cardiovascular reactivity to mental stress in essential hypertension. *J. Hypertens. 4:* 321–331, 1986.

27. Frohlick, E. D. Hemodynamic differences between black patients and white patients with essential hypertension. *Hypertension 15:* 675–680, 1990.

28. Fuh, M. M-T., S-M. Shieh, D-A. Wu, Y-DI. Chen, and G. M. Reaven. Abnormalities of carbohydrate and lipid metabolism in patients with hypertension. *Arch. Intern. Med. 147:* 1035–1038, 1987.

29. Garcia-Palmer, M. R., R. Costas, Jr., and M. Cruz-Vidal. Milk consumption, calcium intake and decreased hypertension in Puerto Rico. *Hypertension 6:* 322–328, 1984.

30. Garn, S. M., S. M. Bailey, P. E. Cole, et al. Level of education, level of income, and level of fatness in adults. *Am. J. Clin. Nutr. 30:* 721–725, 1977.

31. Gill, J. R., H. G. Gullner, C. R. Lake, D. J. Lakatua, and G. Lan. Plasma and urinary

catecholamines in salt-sensitive idiopathic hypertension. *Hypertension 11:* 312–319, 1988.

32. Gilliland, M., E. T. Zawada, D. McClung, and J. TerWee. Preliminary report: natriuretic effect of calcium supplementation in hypertensives over forty. *J. Am. Coll. Nutr. 6:* 139–143, 1987.

33. Gordon, M. S., C. A. Steunkel, P. R. Conlin, N. K. Hollenberg, and G. H. Williams. The role of dopamine in nonmodulating hypertension. *J. Clin. Endocrinol. Metab. 69*(2): 426–432, 1989.

34. Grim, C. E., F. C. Luft, J. Z. Miller, G. R. Meneety, H. D. Battarbee, C. G. Hames, and L. K. Dahl. Racial differences in blood pressure in Evans County, Georgia: relationship to sodium and potassium intake and plasma renin activity. *J. Chronic Dis. 33:* 87–94, 1980.

35. Grobbee, D. E., and E. Hofman. Effect of calcium supplementation on diastolic blood pressure in young people with mild hypertension. *Lancet 2:* 703–707, 1986.

36. Haffner, S. M., M. P. Stern, H. P. Hazuda, J. Pugh, and J. K. Patterson. The role of behavioral variables and fat patterning in explaining ethnic differences in serum lipids and lipoproteins. *Am. J. Epidemiol. 123:* 830–839, 1986.

37. Haigh, N. Z., K. M. Salz, G. A. Chase, et al. The East Baltimore study: the relationship of lipids and lipoproteins to selected cardiovascular risk factors in an inner city black adult population. *Am. J. Clin. Nutr. 38:* 320–326, 1983.

38. Harlan, W. R., and L. C. Harlan. An epidemiological perspective on dietary electrolytes and hypertension. *J. Hypertens.* 4(Suppl. 5): S334–S339, 1986.

39. Hartz, A. J., D. C. Rupley, and A. A. Rimm. The association of girth measurements with disease in 32,856 women. *Am. J. Epidemiol. 119:* 71–80, 1984.

40. Hatori, N., H. Tomonari, B. P. Fine, and A. Aviv. Racial differences in fibroblast Na^+/H^+ antiport (abst). *Kidney Int. 33:* 297, 1988.

41. Horwitz, D., H. S. Margolius, and H. R. Keiser. Effects of dietary potassium and race on urinary excretion of kallikrein and aldosterone in man. *J. Clin. Endocrinol. Metab. 47:* 296–299, 1978.

42. Hutchinson, J. Relation between African admixture and blood pressure variation in the Caribbean. *Hum. Hered. 36:* 12–18, 1986.

43. Hypertension Detection and Follow-up Program Cooperative Group. Blood pressure studies in 14 communities: a two-stage screen for hypertension. *J.A.M.A. 237:* 2391, 1977.

44. Johnson, A. L., J. C. Cornoni, J. C. Cassel, H. A. Tyroler, S. Heyden, and C. G. Hames. Influence of race, sex and weight on blood pressure behavior in young adults. *Am. J. Cardiol. 35:* 523–530, 1975.

45. Johnson, J. L., E. F. Heineman, G. Heiss, C. G. Hames, and H. A. Tyroler. Cardiovascular disease risk factors and mortality among black women and white women aged 40–64 years in Evans County, Georgia. *Am. J. Epidemiol. 123*(2): 209–220, 1986.

46. Johnson, N. E., I. L. Smith, and J. L. Freudenhim. Effects on blood pressure of calcium supplementation of women. *Am. J. Clin. Nutr. 42:* 12–17, 1985.

47. Kannel, W. B., N. Brand, J. J. Skinner, Jr., T. R. Dawber, and P. M. McNamar. The relation of adiposity to blood pressure and development of hypertension: the Framingham Study. *Ann. Intern. Med. 67:* 48–59, 1967.

48. Karanja, N., J. Metz, D. Lee, T. Phanouvang, and D. A. McCarron. Effects of Ca^{2+} and Na^+ on blood pressure, food consumption and weight in the spontaneously hypertensive rat. *Kidney Int. 27:* 193, 1985.

49. Khaw, K. T., and G. Rose. Population study of blood pressure and associated factors in St. Lucia, West Indies. *Int. J. Epidemiol. 11*(4): 372–377, 1982.

50. Khaw, K. T., and E. Barrett-Connor. Dietary potassium and stroke-associated mortality. A 12 year prospective population study. *N. Engl. J. Med. 316:* 235–240, 1987.

51. Kleeman, C. R., J. Bohamman, D. Bernstein, S. Ling, and M. H. Maxwell. Effect of variations in sodium intake on calcium excretion in normal humans. *Proc. Soc. Exp. Biol. Med. 115:* 29–32, 1964.

52. Kromhaut, D., E. B. Bosschieter, and C de L. Coulander. Potassium, calcium, alcohol intake and blood pressure: the Zutphen Study. *Am. J. Clin. Nutr. 41:* 1299–1304, 1985.

53. Langford, H. G., F. P. J. Langford, and M. Tyler. Dietary profile of sodium, potassium, and calcium in U.S. blacks. In: Hypertension in Blacks: Epidemiology, Pathophysiology and Treatment, edited by W. D. Hall, E. Saunders, and N. B. Shulman. Year Book Medical Publishers, Chicago, 1985, pp. 49–57.

54. Lasker, N., L. Hopp, S. E. Grossman, R. Banforth, and A. Aviv. Race and sex differences in erythrocyte Na, K and Na-K adenosine triphosphatase. *J. Clin. Invest. 74:* 1813, 1985.

55. Levy, S. B., J. J. Lilley, R. P. Frigon, et al. Urinary kallikrein and plasma renin activity

as determinants of renal blood flow. The influence of race and dietary sodium intake. *J. Clin. Invest. 60:* 129–138, 1977.

56. Lewanczuk, R. Z., and P. K. T. Pang. In vivo potentiation of vasopressors by spontaneously hypertensive rat plasma. *Clin. Exp. Hypertens. 11:* 1471–1485, 1989.

57. Lewanczuk, R. Z., A. Chen, and P. K. T. Pang. The effects of dietary calcium on blood pressure in spontaneously hypertensive rats may be mediated by parathyroid hypertensive factors. *Am. J. Hypertens. 3:* 349–353, 1990.

58. Light, K. C., P. A. Obrist, A. Sherwood, S. A. James, and D. S. Strogatz. Effects of race and marginally elevated blood pressure on response to stress. *Hypertension 10:* 555–563, 1987.

59. Love, W. D., and G. E. Burch. Plasma and erythrocyte sodium and potassium in a group of southern white and Negro blood donors. *J. Lab. Clin. Med. 41:* 258–267, 1953.

60. Luft, F. C., N. S. Fineberg, J. Z. Miller, L. I. Rankin, C. E. Grim, and M. H. Weinberger. The effects of age, race and heredity on glomerular filtration rate following volume expansion and contraction in normal man. *Am. J. Med. Sci. 279:* 15–24, 1980.

61. Luft, F. C., L. I. Rankin, R. Bloch, A. E. Weyman, L. R. Willis, R. H. Murray, C. E. Grim, and M. H. Weinberger. Cardiovascular and humoral responses to extremes of sodium intake in normal black and white man. *Circulation 60*(3): 697–706, 1979.

62. McCarron, D. A., P. A. Lucas, R. S. Schneidman, R. LaCour, and T. Druke. Blood pressure development of the spontaneously hypertensive rat after concurrent manipulations of Ca^{2+} and Na^+ in relation to intestinal fluxes. *J. Clin. Invest. 76:* 1147–1154, 1985.

63. McCarron, D. A., N. N. Yung, B. A. Ugoretz, and S. Krutzik. Disturbances of calcium metabolism in the spontaneously hypertensive rat. *Hypertension 3:* I-162–167, 1981.

64. McCarron, D. A., C. D. Morris, and R. Bukoski. The calcium paradox of essential hypertension. *Am. J. Med. 82*(Suppl 1B): 27–33, 1987.

65. Mueller, W. H. The changes with age of the anatomical distribution of fat. *Soc. Sci. Med. 16:* 191–196, 1982.

66. Munro-Faure, A. D., D. M., Hill, and J. Anderson. Ethnic differences in human red blood cell sodium concentration. *Nature 231:* 457–458, 1971.

67. Nakamura, A., J. Gardner, N. Hatori, M. Nakamura, B. P. Fine, and A. Aviv. Differences in Ca^{2+} regulation in skin fibroblasts from blacks and whites. *J. Cell Physiol. 138:* 367–374, 1989.

68. National Center for Health Statistics. Health, United States, 1986. DHHS 87-1232, U.S. Government Printing Office, Washington, D.C., 1986.

69. National Center for Health Statistics. "Plan and Operation of the National Health and Nutrition Examination Survey, 1976-80," no. 15, DHHS publication no. (PHS) 81-1317 (U.S. Public Health Service, Washington, D.C., 1981).

70. National Diabetes Data Group. Classification and diagnosis of diabetes mellitus and other categories of glucose intolerance. *Diabetes 28:* 1039–1057, 1979.

71. Neser, W. B., J. Thomas, K. Semenya, et al. Obesity and hypertension in a longitudinal study of black physicians: the Meharry Cohort Study. *J. Chronic Dis. 39*(2): 105–113, 1986.

72. Oken, B., A. Hartz, E. Giefer, et al. Relation between socioeconomic status and obesity changes in 9046 women. *Prev. Med. 6:* 447–453, 1977.

73. Overbeck, H. W. Attenuated arteriolar dilator responses to calcium in genetically hypertensive rats. *Hypertension 6:* 647–653, 1984.

74. Paffenberger, R. S., M. C. Thorne, and A. L. Wing. Chronic disease in former college students. VIII. Characteristics in youth predisposing to hypertension in later years. *Am. J. Epidemiol. 88:* 25–32, 1968.

75. Pang, P. K. T., and R. Z. Lewanczuk. Parathyroid origin of a new circulating hypertensive factor in spontaneously hypertensive rats. *Am. J. Hypertens. 2:* 898–902, 1989.

76. Pang, P. K. I., M. C. M. Vang, K. T. Kautmann, and A. D. Kenny. Structure activity relationship of parathyroid hormone: separation of hypotensive and hypercalcemic properties. *Endocrinology 112:* 284–289, 1983.

77. Pobee, J. O. M., E. B. Larbi, D. W. Belcher, F. K. Wurapa, and S. R. A. Dodu. Blood pressure distribution in a rural Ghanian population. *Trans. R. Soc. Trop. Med. Hyg. 71:* 66–72, 1977.

78. Pratt, J. H., J. J. Jones, J. Z. Miller, M. A. Wagner, and N. S. Fineberg. Racial differences in aldosterone excretion and plasma aldosterone concentrations in children. *N. Engl. J. Med. 321:* 1152–1157, 1989.

79. Raij, L., T. F. Luscher, and P. M. Vanhoutte. High potassium diet augments endothelium-dependent relaxations in the Dahl rat. *Hypertension 12:* 562–567, 1988.

80. Ramsay, L. E., M. H. Ramsay, J. Hettiarachchi, D. L. Davies, and J. Winchester. Weight reduction in a blood pressure clinic. *Br. Med. J. 2:* 244–245, 1978.

81. Reaven, G. M., and B. B. Hoffman. Hypertension as a disease of carbohydrate and lipo-
    protein metabolism. *Am. J. Med. 87*(Suppl 6A): 2S–6S, 1989.
82. Reisin, E., R. Abel, M. Modan, D. S. Silverberg, H. E. Eliahou, and B. Modan. Effect of
    weight loss without salt restriction on the reduction of blood pressure in overweight
    hypertensive patients. *N. Engl. J. Med. 298:* 1–6, 1978.
83. Report of the Secretaries Task Force on Black and Minority Health, Vol. IV. Cardiovas-
    cular and cerebral disease. U.S. Department of Health and Human Services, January
    1986.
84. Resnick, L. M. Uniformity and diversity of calcium metabolism in hypertension. A con-
    ceptual framework. *Am. J. Med. 82*(Suppl 11B): 16–26, 1987.
85. Resnick, L. M., R. K. Gupta, and J. H. Laragh. Intracellular free magnesium in erythro-
    cytes of essential hypertensives: relation to blood pressure and serum divalent cation.
    Proc. Natl. Acad. Sci. U.S.A. 81: 6511–6515, 1984.
86. Resnick, L. M., and J. H. Laragh. Does dihydroxyvitamin D(1,25 D) cause low renin hy-
    pertension. *Hypertension 6:* 792, 1984.
87. Rimm, I. J., and A. A. Rimm. Association between socioeconomic status and obesity in
    59,556 women. *Prev. Med. 3:* 543–552, 1974.
88. Robinson, B. F. Altered calcium handling as a cause of primary hypertension. *J. Hyper-
    tens. 2:* 453–460, 1984.
89. Roseman, J. M. Diabetes in black Americans. In: *National Diabetes Data Group, Diabetes
    in America, Diabetes Data Compiled 1984,* edited by M. I. Harris and R. F. Hamman.
    U.S. Department of Health and Human Services, Public Health Services, NIH Pub-
    lication No. 85-1468, 1985, pp. 1–24.
90. Savage, D. D., L. O. Watkins, C. E. Grim, and S. K. Kumanyika. Hypertension in black
    populations. In: *Hypertension: Pathophysiology, Diagnosis, and Management,* edited
    by J. H. Laragh and B. M. Brenner. Raven Press, New York, 1990, pp. 1837–1852.
91. Sempos, C., R. Cooper, M. G. Kovar, C. Johnson, T. Drizd, and E. Yettey. Dietary calcium
    and blood pressure in National Health and Nutritional Examination Surveys I and
    II. *Hypertension 8:* 1067–1074, 1986.
92. Shaper, A. G., and G. A. Saxton. Blood pressure and body build in a rural community in
    Uganda. *East Afr. Med. J. 46:* 228–245, 1969.
93. Shaper, A. G., P. J. Leonard, K. W. Jones, and M. Jones. Environmental effects on the
    body build, blood pressure and blood chemistry of nomadic warriors serving in the
    army in Kenya. *East Afr. Med. J. 46:* 282–289, 1969.
94. Shehin, S. E., J. R. Sowers, and M. B. Zemel. Impaired vascular smooth muscle ^{45}Ca efflux
    and hypertension in Zucker obese rats. *J. Vasc. Med. Biol. 1:* 278–282, 1989.
95. Shen, D-C., S-M. Shieh, M. Fuh, D-A. Wu, Y-DI. Chen, and G. M. Reaven. Resistance to
    insulin-stimulated glucose uptake in patients with hypertension. *J. Clin. Endocrinol.
    Metab. 66:* 580–583, 1988.
96. Simons, F. J. Primary adult lactose intolerance and the milking habit: a problem in bio-
    logic and cultural interrelation. *Am. J. Dig. Dis. 14:* 819–824, 1969.
97. Singer, P., W. Godick, S. Voigt, I. Hajdu, and M. Weiss. Postprandial hyperinsulinemia in
    patients with mild essential hypertension. *Hypertension 7:* 182–186, 1985.
98. Smeda, J. S. Hemorrhagic stroke development in spontaneously hypertensive rats fed a
    North American, Japanese-style diet. *Stroke 20:* 1212–1218, 1989.
99. Society of Actuaries and Association of Life Insurance Medical Directors of America. Build
    Study 1979. Recording and Statistical Corporation, Chicago, 1980, pp. 43–45.
100. Sowers, J. R. Dietary calcium effects in salt-sensitive hypertension. *Clin. Nutr. 8*(4): 158–
    163, 1989.
101. Sowers, J. R., M. Nyby, and K. Jasberg. Dopaminergic control of prolactin and blood pres-
    sure: altered control in essential hypertension. *Hypertension 4:* 431–437, 1982.
102. Sowers, J. R., M. S. Golub, M. E. Berger, and L. A. Whitfield. Dopaminergic modulation
    of pressor and hormonal responses in essential hypertension. *Hypertension 4:* 424–
    430, 1982.
103. Sowers, J. R., M. B. Zemel, P. Zemel, F. W. J. Beck, M. F. Walsh, and E. T. Zawada. Salt
    sensitivity in blacks: salt intake and natriuretic substances. *Hypertension 12:* 485–
    490, 1988.
104. Sowers, J. R., M. B. Zemel, P. R. Standley, and P. C. Zemel. Calcium and hypertension. *J.
    Lab. Clin. Med. 114:* 338–348, 1989.
105. Sowers, J. R., S. Khoury, P. Standley, P. Zemel, and M. Zemel. Mechanisms of hyperten-
    sion in diabetes. *Am. J. Hypertens. 4:* 177–182, 1991.
106. Sowers, M. F., R. B. Wallace, and J. H. Lemke. The association of intakes of vitamin D
    and calcium with blood pressure among women. *Am. J. Clin. Nutr. 42:* 135–142, 1985.
107. Stallones, R. A. Epidemiologic studies of obesity. *Ann. Intern. Med. 103:* 1003–1005, 1985.

108. Stephenson, E. W. E., and R. J. Podolsky. Regulation by magnesium of intracellular calcium movement in skinned muscle fibers. *J. Gen. Physiol. 69:* 17–35, 1977.

109. Stern, M. P., and S. M. Haffner. Body fat distribution and hyperinsulinemia as risk factors for diabetes and cardiovascular disease. *Arteriosclerosis 6:* 123–130, 1986.

110. Stern, N., D. Lee, V. Silis, F. Beck, L. Deftos, S. Monolagas, and J. R. Sowers. The effects of high calcium intake on blood pressure and calcium metabolism in the young spontaneously hypertensive rat. *Hypertension 6:* 639–646, 1984.

111. Sugimoto, T., L. Tobian, and M. C. Ganguli. High potassium diets protect against dysfunction of endothelial cells in stroke-prone spontaneously hypertensive rats. *Hypertension 11:* 579–585, 1988.

112. Suki, W. N. Calcium transport in the nephron. *Am. J. Physiol. 237* (Renal Fluid Electrolyte Physiol. 6): F1–F6, 1979.

113. Tabuchi, Y., T. Ogihara, K. Hashizume, H. Saito, and Y. Kumahar. Hypotensive effect of long-term oral calcium supplementation in elderly patients with essential hypertension. *J. Clin. Hypertens. 3:* 254–262, 1986.

114. Tillotson, J., and R. J. Havlik. Milk consumption, calcium intake and decreased hypertension in Puerto Rico: Puerto Rico Heart Health Program Study. *Hypertension 6:* 322–328, 1984.

115. Tobian, L. High-potassium diets markedly protect against stroke deaths and kidney disease in hypertensive rats, an echo from prehistoric days. *J. Hypertens. 4:* S67–S76, 1986.

116. Tobian, L., J. M. Lange, M. A. Johnson, D. A. MacNeill, T. J. Wilke, K. M. Ulm, and L. J. Wold. High-K diets markedly reduce brain hemorrhage and infarcts, death rate and mesenteric arteriolar hypertrophy in stroke-prone spontaneously hypertensive rats. *J. Hypertens. 4*(5): S205–S207, 1986.

117. Tobian, L., J. Lange, K. Ulm, L. Wold, and J. Iwai. Potassium reduces cerebral hemorrhage and death rate in hypertensive rats, even when blood pressure is not lowered. *Hypertension 7:* I-110–I-114, 1985.

118. Trevisan, M., V. Krogh, E. Farinaro, S. Panico, and M. Mancini. Calcium-rich foods and blood pressure: findings from the Italian National Research Council study (the nine communities study). *Am. J. Epidemiol. 127:* 115–116, 1988.

119. Tuck, M. L., J. R. Sowers, L. Dornfeld, G. Kledzik, and M. Maxwell. The effect of weight reduction on blood plasma renin activity and plasma aldosterone levels in obese patients. *N. Engl. J. Med. 304:* 930–933, 1981.

120. Tuck, M. L., D. B. Corry, M. Maxwell, and N. Stern. Kinetic analysis of erythrocyte Na^+-K^+ pump and co-transport in essential hypertension. *Hypertension 10:* 204–211, 1987.

121. Tyroler, H. A., S. Heyden, and C. G. Hames. Weight and hypertension: Evans County studies of blacks and whites. In: *Epidemiology and Control of Hypertension,* edited by O. Paul. Stratton Intercontinental, New York, 1975, pp. 177–201.

122. Umemura, S., D. D. Smuth, M. Nicar, J. P. Rapp, and W. A. Pettinger. Altered calcium homeostasis in Dahl hypertensive rats: physiological and biochemical studies. *J. Hypertens. 4:* 19–26, 1986.

123. Vaughan, G. P. Blood pressure and heart murmurs in a rural population in the United Republic of Tanzania. *Bull. W. H. O. 57:* 89–97, 1979.

124. Vincenzi, F. F., C. D. Morris, L. B. Kinsel, M. Kenny, and D. A. McCaron. Decreased calcium pump adenosine triphosphatase in red blood cells of hypertensive subjects. *Hypertension 8:* 1058–1066, 1986.

125. Voors, A. W., E. R. Dalferes, G. C. Frank, G. C. Aristimuno, and G. S. Berenson. Relation between ingested potassium and socium balance in young blacks and whites. *Am. J. Clin. Nutr. 37:* 583–594, 1983.

126. Watson, R. L., H. G. Langford, J. Abernathy, T. Y. Barnes, and M. J. Watson. Urinary electrolytes, body weight, and blood pressure: pooled cross-sectional results four groups of adolescent females. *Hypertension 2*(Suppl I): 93–98, 1980.

127. Weinberger, M. H., F. C. Luft, R. Block, D. P. Henry, J. H. Pratt, A. E. Weyman, L. I. Rankin, R. H. Murray, L. R. Willis, and C. E. Grim. The blood pressure-raising effects of high dietary sodium intake: racial differences and the role of potassium. *J. Am. Coll. Nutr. 1:* 139–148, 1982.

128. Witteman, J. C. M., W. C. Willett, M. J. Stampfer, G. A. Colditz, F. M. Sacks, B. Rosner, F. E. Speizer, and C. H. Hennekens. Dietary calcium and magnesium and hypertension: a prospective study (abstract). *Circulation 76*(Suppl IV): 35, 1987.

129. Wright, G. L., and G. O. Rankin. Concentrations of ionic and total calcium in plasma of four models of hypertension. *Am. J. Physiol. 243* (Heart Circ. Physiol. 12): H365–370, 1982.

130. Zemel, M. B., and J. R. Sowers. Salt sensitivity and systemic hypertension in the elderly. *Am. J. Cardiol. 61:* 7H–12H, 1988.
131. Zemel, M. B., and J. R. Sowers. Calcium regulating hormones in hypertension. In: *Hypertension: Pathophysiology, Diagnosis and Management,* edited by J. H. Laragh and B. M. Brenner. Raven Press, New York, 1990.
132. Zemel, M. B., S. M. Gualdoni, and J. R. Sowers. Sodium excretion and plasma renin activity in normotensive and hypertensive black adults as affected by dietary calcium and sodium. *J. Hypertens. 4*(Suppl 6): S343–S345, 1986.
133. Zemel, M. B., S. M. Gualdoni, and J. R. Sowers. Reductions in total and extracellular water associated with calcium-induced natriuresis and the antihypertensive effect of calcium in blacks. *Am. J. Hypertens. 1:* 70–72, 1988.
134. Zemel, M. B., J. Kraniak, P. R. Standley, and J. R. Sowers. Erythrocyte cation metabolism in salt-sensitive blacks as affected by dietary sodium and calcium. *Am. J. Hypertens. 1:* 380–392, 1988.
135. Zemel, M. B., J. Greene, P. C. Zemel, F. Douglas, R. Geiser, and J. R. Sowers. Effects of magnesium supplementation on erythrocyte cation transport in diuretic-treated hypertensives. *Nutr. Res. 9:* 1285–1292, 1989.
136. Zemel, M. B., B. A. Bedford, P. C. Zemel, O. Marwah, and J. R. Sowers. Altered cation transport in non-insulin dependent diabetic hypertension: effects of dietary calcium. *J. Hypertens. 6:* S228–S230, 1988.
137. Zemel, P. C., S. Gualdoni, and J. R. Sowers. Racial differences in mineral intake in ambulatory normotensives and hypertensives. *Am. J. Hypertens. 1:* 1465–1485, 1988.
138. Zemel, P. C., M. B. Zemel, M. Urberg, F. Douglas, R. Geiser, and J. R. Sowers. Effect of oral magnesium supplementation on blood pressure and cellular cation metabolism in patients with essential hypertension. *Am. J. Clin. Nutr. 51:* 665–669, 1990.

9

Intracellular Ions and Hypertension in Blacks

RICHARD S. COOPER AND JAMES L. BORKE

In large part because of increased risk of hypertension observed among blacks compared with whites, considerable attention has been focused on possible racial differences in ion metabolism. There are at least two reasons that these differences might be important. First, etiologic research in most disciplines relies heavily on the investigation of high-risk subgroups. If we knew why the risk of hypertension among blacks is twice that found among whites we would know a great deal more about what causes this disease than we do today. Second, cardiovascular diseases continue to be the primary cause of higher death rates experienced by black adult Americans. Approximately half of the higher mortality among blacks compared with whites can be accounted for by the complications of high blood pressure (77). We urgently need effective strategies for primary prevention of this disease; to achieve that goal a better understanding of the etiologic process is required. Whether the excess risk of hypertension among U.S. blacks is conferred by their genetic heritage or exposure to high levels of environmental risk factors remains undetermined. Observed phenotypic alternations in ion metabolism could result from either genetic predisposition or exposures to external causes. A distinction between a finding that reflects special or unique characteristics of the black population, or a universal human trait that is simply exaggerated in this group, is crucial when the data collected on ion metabolism are being used to construct a theory of the pathophysiology of hypertension. Is the pathophysiology of hypertension essentially the same in blacks and whites, or can we expect to find consistent differences at a basic level? There is evidence, for example, that among the various hypertensive strains of rats, different alterations in ion transport systems exist (28,35). Are there comparable differences among "strains" of humans? Before reviewing the primary reports in this field we will attempt to address the implications of these questions.

Classification of ethnicity is used with imprecision in biomedical research (15). Clearly the race category is most often employed with the intent to designate genetic likeness. This apparently straightforward goal is difficult to achieve, however. Significant admixture has occurred among all immigrants to the United States, including blacks (42,76), and ongoing evolutionary change separates migrants from those who remained behind. From an anthropological perspective, there is reason to doubt whether subspecies or races actually exist among humans (15,73). While human populations clearly vary on

181

a wide range of traits, our recent common origin has made us more alike than different (60). There is no a priori reason, therefore, to assume that control mechanisms for a fundamental physiological process, like blood pressure regulation, would be different between Africans and Europeans. In a recent extensive review of the genetics of hypertension, Ward (116) has persuasively argued that the pattern of inheritance of blood pressure is similar in the various ethnic groups that have been studied to date. This inference is based in large part on the observation of a unimodal blood pressure distribution curve in all population samples, and the consistent interactive effect of age with environmental factors. Ward further argues that "studies of genetically admixed populations point to the pervasive effect of the sociocultural environment . . . with little evidence that genetic heterogeneity plays a role" (116, p. 84). While frequencies of some of the genes contributing to hypertension may vary, these differences do not contribute substantially to aggregate risk for the entire group.

Although it may not be possible to estimate precisely the distribution of hypertension genes in blacks and whites (52,67,72,78), either for the population or the individuals within it, we do know that large social differences exist between these ethnic groups. Taking into account the two most rudimentary risk factors for hypertension, namely obesity and education, the black–white blood pressure difference is eliminated for women, and greatly narrowed for men (54). Unequal exposure to risk factors thus accounts for a sizable proportion of the racial differentials in this disease. Physiological markers of hypertension risk that are identified in adulthood may be a result of these exposures, just as low serum cholesterol levels among the Japanese reflect dietary patterns rather than genetic factors. The opposite form of the genotype–phenotype interaction can also occur. For example, much has been made over the years of low-renin levels among blacks as a marker of volume expanded or "salt-sensitive" hypertension. Recent evidence suggests that the differences in renin levels between blacks and whites may simply result from different distributions of the allele regulating renin production (8). Whether an individual has a high or low plasma renin concentration may have nothing to do with hypertension risk, reflecting instead only a different genetic set point.

Comparison of physiological traits across racial groups is therefore a complex process. We would propose four criteria for successful studies of this character. First, we should have reliable laboratory methods to identify the biochemical or physiological traits—the "intermediate phenotype" proposed by Sing et al. (97). Second, the important environmental factors that modify the trait of interest should be understood. Third, stable quantitative estimates of the relationship between the trait and the outcome measure, such as blood pressure, should be available. Fourth, a gene marker for the trait should be available. If this last condition cannot be satisfied, an estimate of heritability derived from family or twin studies would be helpful (116). Unfortunately, these conditions cannot be satisfied in their entirety for any of the transport systems studied to date.

Because of these limitations, it is premature, in our view, to propose a coherent theoretical explanation of racial patterns in blood pressure based on differences in ion transport. Sufficient data do exist, however, to provide the outline of such a theory. The continued rapid development of research techniques in this field holds forth the promise of a parallel growth in new knowledge. This promise will only be realized, however, if the experimental research is based on an understanding of the epidemiological questions.

Comprehensive reviews on the potential role of alterations in ion metabolism in the pathogenesis of hypertension have been published in recent years (7,29,79,97,101); we will only describe the basic aspects of this theory. The underlying physiological abnormality of hypertension is increased peripheral resistance, mediated by excessive vascular smooth muscle tone. Given the role of intracellular calcium (Ca_i) as a second messenger in coupling the excitation–contraction process, increases in the availability of Ca_i could be the final pathway through which environmental exposures lead to high blood pressure in susceptible individuals. Cytosolic free Ca_i could be increased by a number of processes. A 10,000-fold gradient in Ca^{2+} concentration exists between the intracellular and extracellular environment, and greater membrane permeability could lead to higher intracellular levels. Efficient systems exist to extrude calcium from the cell, however, and a defect in the plasma membrane Ca^{2+} pump, or a reduced activity level, is more likely to result in net higher Ca_i levels. Ca_i levels are influenced by the concentration of other intracellular ions, most notably, sodium (Na). An increase in intracellular sodium (Na_i) enhances contractility, which is the basis of the well-described inotropic effect of the digitalis compounds. This process could be mediated through the sodium-calcium exchange mechanism; higher levels of Na_i result in a reduced Na_o-Na_i gradient, and less outward movement of calcium. Increased sodium permeability, or reduced sodium pump activity, should thus secondarily result in higher Ca_i. It has also been suggested that agonist-mediated elevations in Ca_i are associated with increased sodium-hydrogen antiport activity, providing another potential link between the cellular control of these two ions (7). Little experimental evidence exists to support this link, however. The ubiquitous role of calcium as second messenger for a variety of secretory functions could also affect other components of the blood pressure control system, such as renin and neurotransmitters.

While many investigators argue that these abnormalities in ion transport arise from genetic defects in transport activity or membrane function (7,79), an important variant of this theory postulates the presence of circulating sodium pump inhibitors (54). According to this theory, a habitual diet high in sodium results in the elaboration of a natriuretic substance in the kidney. While promoting diuresis, and reducing volume overload, this substance selectively inhibits the sodium-potassium pump in vascular smooth muscle raising cell sodium and calcium (29). This form of volume-expanded or salt-sensitive hypertension is thought to be more common in blacks (66).

It can thus be seen that all of the common versions of the ion transport theory of the pathophysiology of hypertension relate to alterations in the cellular handling of sodium and calcium. These ions, of course, are of fundamental importance in cell metabolism, and are regulated by a series of interrelated membrane transport processes, not all of which may be known. Specific tissues have developed specialized adaptations of ion transport; for example, the sodium-potassium pump is very inactive in red cells, and platelets are highly impermeable to the passive entry of calcium.

It is not surprising, therefore, given the variety of cell lines studied, the differences in sampling schemes, and the lack of standardization of laboratory procedures, that consistent findings are the exception. Some investigators even question whether useful links between ion metabolism and hypertension have been demonstrated at all (100). The need for reliable physiological markers of hypertension to classify distinct subgroups and test controlled interventions, in combination with the rapid advances being made in the development of molecular probes, however, provide sufficient rationale for continuing to pursue this important line of investigation.

In addition to the contribution of research in this field to our general knowledge about the etiology of hypertension, these data are also of potential significance in understanding the pathophysiology of hypertension in blacks. We will therefore review areas of research where sufficient data exist to draw some conclusions on the relevance of transport systems to high blood pressure among blacks, regardless of whether parallel data exist that permit comparison with whites. These areas of research are listed in Table 9.1.

Two methodological challenges confront the reviewer in this field. First, the laboratory techniques used in the studies that we have reviewed vary considerably and may estimate the underlying physiological phenomena with varying accuracy. We have consciously not attempted to evaluate the physiological meaning of each assay reported, nor have we made a judgment on the relative merit of the techniques applied in individual laboratories. Although these issues are of vital importance, a review of this depth would require considerably more space than available. We have therefore only summarized the data as reported by the investigators.

Second, a subject overview, or meta-analysis, should be grounded in accepted statistical procedures. These techniques have been most extensively developed for pooling data from clinical trials, and we are unaware of procedures designed for reviewing a literature comprising mainly small case-control studies. Meta-analysis generally requires assumptions regarding the design of the studies examined, for example, random assignment to treatment group. None of the studies in this literature are randomized trials, and no consistent sampling procedures were used. Each study varies in the age, sex, and race composition of the participants, as well as other key factors, such as current treatment for hypertension. Because the assumptions about comparability of design cannot be met, and laboratory procedures were not standardized across studies, pooling of the data is unjustified and could be misleading.

TABLE 9.1. Ion Concentrations and Exchange Systems
Investigated among Blacks

Intracellular sodium

Sodium-potassium ATPase

Sodium-lithium countertransport

Intracellular calcium

Membrane-bound calcium

Sodium-hydrogen exchange

Sodium-potassium cotransport

At the same time, it is not appropriate simply to count "positive" and "negative" studies based on statistical significance derived from comparisons between cases and controls. Since sample size strongly influences significance tests, not all studies are equal. In fact, with small studies, type II statistical error—not finding a true difference when one exists—is more common than concluding one exists when it does not—type I error. In balance, therefore, "positive" studies count more heavily in the final judgment. We have chosen, with one exception, to display the original data from the published reports and examine the overall trends for consistency without overly emphasizing results of significance testing. Our primary goal was to determine whether these trends confirm the prior hypotheses.

When they were available, we also summarized correlation and regression coefficients from published studies. It should be recognized that the numerical strength of these relationships is not the sole, or even crucial, measure of their importance. Measurement error, intrinsic physiological variability, and a variety of other factors tend to weaken true relationships. In addition, small differences in a physiological trait, such as observed for the coronary risk factors, can have a major influence over the course of a lifetime.

While it is difficult to assess the presence or absence of general relationships in this data set, it is even more difficult to detect differences in the strength of these relationships between groups. This difficulty can be demonstrated through two straightforward sample size calculations. Thus, a correlation of 0.10 between a given trait and blood pressure may be detectable with 80% certainty in a sample of 778 persons. (As discussed subsequently, a correlation of this magnitude is the current estimate of the association between the best studied transport system—sodium-lithium countertransport—and blood pressure.) At the same time, detection of a significant difference between a correlation of 0.10 in group A compared with a correlation of 0.20 in group B (i.e., a 100% difference) would require a sample of 1,498 in each of the two groups (67). (These calculations are based on two-tailed tests, with 1-beta = 0.80 and alpha = 0.05.) Because studies on blacks to date are small, many of the apparent differences in the relationships between a given cation parameter and hypertension across the race groups may be due to chance alone. None of the studies reported permit a formal statistical test of this question.

The effect of sample size on the validity of conclusions about differences between groups can further be appreciated when one examines the variation in reported relationships by sex. There is clearly no reason to suspect that sex-related effects should vary from sample to sample; in fact, associations are often reported as stronger in one sex than the other in different studies. This inconsistency can serve as a proxy for the variability one might anticipate by race, assuming in fact the relationship being studied is real. To restate this proposition in a different way, relationships between cation measures and blood pressure should have similar relative strength in white men compared with white women in different samples; this, however, is not the empirical observation. Based on the statistical considerations described before, one can assume that this variability is primarily due to chance, that is, sampling variability. Observed variability in the observed relationships of the same order of magnitude between blacks and whites is equally likely to be due to chance alone. These considerations should be kept in mind when evaluating the cautious tone of the conclusions advanced in this review.

INTRACELLULAR SODIUM CONCENTRATION

Data on Na_i from meaningful human populations are available only on circulating blood cells—with a single exception (57). The erythrocyte is an attractive cell to study because of its abundance and relatively robust character. On the other hand, it has several atypical features that limit its potential usefulness as a model cell line. Compared with most other body cells, active sodium transport and membrane permeability are very low in the red blood cell (RBC) (49). White cells, on the other hand, provide lower yields from equivalent blood samples and represent a mixture to varying extent of leukocytes and lymphocytes. Measurement of Na_i in platelets is technically difficult because of the problem of trapped plasma. To our knowledge, only data on RBC Na_i have been reported on blacks.

Na_i is the balanced result of all membrane exchange processes; the physiology of these systems has been extensively reviewed elsewhere (102,104). Six principal transport systems are known to exchange sodium across the cell membrane (Table 9.2). Sodium-hydrogen exchange may play a role in the pathophysiology of hypertension, and will be discussed in this review, but its role in red cells is uncertain. Influx of sodium occurs down its concentration gradient by way of membrane channels. The Na^+-K^+-ATPase pump is the principal cellular mechanism for maintaining the electrochemical gradient and accounts for 90% of the net sodium extrusion. The linked sodium-potassium cotransport system effects simultaneous movement of sodium and potassium either into or out of the cell, depending on their concentration gradients. Sodium-lithium countertransport operates as a sodium exchanger and does not result in net transfer under normal physiological conditions, although it may reflect activity of the sodium-hydrogen antiporter (36,38).

Based on data from a large pedigree study, it has been estimated that RBC Na_i concentration is 84% heritable, of which 29% can be attributed to the effect of a major gene and 55% to polygenic heritability (122). Four alleles are present at the major gene locus, although the "very high" and "very low" alleles are

TABLE 9.2. Sodium Transport Pathways in Red Blood Cell Membranes

Pathway	Ion	Transport protein
Na^+–K^+ pump	Na, K	Na^+–K^+-ATPase
Na^+–Li^+ exchange	Na, Li	Unknown
Na^+–K^+ cotransport	Na, K	Unknown
$LiCO_3$–$NaCO_3$ exchange	Na, Li	Band 3
Choline transport	Na, K, Li	Unknown
Membrane leak	Na, K, Li	Unknown

Adapted from Tosteson (104).

uncommon (122). Only 10% of the population in this study was homozygous for the high Na_i allele; this pattern was more common in families of hypertensive probands (122). The largely polygenic nature of this trait suggests that the phenotypic concentrations of Na_i are most likely a result of the contribution of several different membrane transport systems (74).

The concentration of RBC Na_i is remarkably stable in the same individual over time; however, it has been shown to be influenced by dietary intake of sodium (5,11,24). In a small randomized trial of adolescents we detected a significant 10% fall in Na_i with a reduction in dietary sodium from 200 to 70 mEq/day (5). Blood pressure reduction was also observed in this trial. A recent study reported in abstract form suggested that sodium sensitivity is closely related to Na_i (83). Na_i is similar in boys and in girls before menarche but falls among females 10% below levels of men until menopause is reached; subsequently Na_i rises to the average observed for men (107). No important changes with increasing age have been described for males (107,108).

In 1952 Tobian and Binion (103) reported increased sodium content of renal arteries obtained at autopsy among hypertensives. This study has never been replicated, and the findings are hard to interpret given the difficulty estimating the contribution of sodium in the extracellular space in solid tissues. Utilizing the red cell, Losse et al. (64) first described increased Na_i in 1960. By 1986 Hilton was able to identify 20 papers reporting on 965 hypertensives and 1,857 controls that included data on RBC Na_i (49). Based on this literature, he concluded that an average increase in Na_i of 13% exists among the hypertensives, and this difference was highly significant statistically ($p < 0.001$). Since Hilton's review, two major new studies have been published. A group of Japanese investigators reported findings on 1,445 men, detecting a significant difference in Na_i between the 81 hypertensives and the remaining normotensives (9.00 ± 1.17 vs. 8.58 ± 1.10, mmol/liter, $p < 0.05$) (69). In a regression model including adiposity, heart rate, age, uric acid, and family history of hypertension, the relationship between Na_i and BP persisted (beta coefficient = 0.08, $p < 0.01$). Additional findings are available from the Gubbio Study, a large population-based survey performed in central Italy (83). RBC Na_i was not significantly related to BP in multivariate analysis among men across the age range 25–74 in this study (coefficient = 0.06, Na_i and systolic BP; $p > 0.05$), although among older men increased Na_i was found among hypertensives. A significant association did appear for women (coefficient = 0.24, Na_i and systolic BP, $p < 0.01$), which was also stronger in the older age group.

Taken together these data suggest that a weak positive association between BP and RBC Na_i has been demonstrated among nonblack population groups. The limited strength of this association, if one accepts a multivariate coefficient in the range of 0.10 as the best estimate of the true relationship, would often be unapparent in studies with fewer than 1,000 participants. While it is possible, as has recently been suggested, that this relationship is obscured by the admixture of several phenotypic alterations in ion transport in the hypertensive group, no methods currently exist to identify the "high Na_i" genotype. Gene markers for the relevant alleles would make such discrimination feasible. It may be possible, for example, that the Na_i-BP association is accounted for primarily by the 10% of persons who are homozygous for the

TABLE 9.3. Reported Studies on RBC Sodium in Blacks and Whites by Hypertension Status (x, sd; mmol/liter)

Study	Hypertension status	Whites Men/women[a]	Blacks Men/women
A. *Sexes combined*			
Aderounmu et al. (1)[b]	(+)	—	13.6 ± 5.9 (100)
	(−)	6.7 ± 2.2 (7)	9.7 ± 3.9 (908)
Ryzielksi et al. (87)	(−)	6.70 ± 1.24 (127)	7.63 ± 2.08 (120)
Ringel et al. (85)	(+)	—	9.66 ± 3.02 (56)
	(−)	—	8.87 ± 2.50 (32)
Weissberg et al. (121)[c]	(+)	20.7 ± 7.7 (32)	27.3 ± 9.7 (17)
	(−)	19.0 ± 3.4 (57)	22.1 ± 6.4 (13)
Forrester et al. (34)[c]	(+)	—	47.4 ± 17.4[d] (20)
	(−)	—	39.4 ± 19.8 (14)
Weder et al. (119)	(+)	2.3 ± 0.5[e] (29)	3.0 ± 1.31 (11)
	(−)	2.8 ± 1.5 (57)	3.6 ± 1.4 (23)
Linjen et al. (62)	(−)	7.3 ± 1.1 (43)	13.4 ± 4.1 (12)
Tuck et al. (111)	(+)	8.3 ± 0.5 (29)	8.7 ± 0.4 (18)
	(−)	8.4 ± 0.5 (38)	9.2 ± 0.6 (20)

	Hypertension status	Whites		Blacks	
Study		Men	Women	Men	Women
B. By sex					
Trevisan et al. (108)	(−)	6.69 ± 1.15 (229)	6.33 ± 1.23 (97)	8.36 ± 2.07 (33)	7.92 ± 2.26 (58)
Love et al. (65)	(−)	7.0[f] (30)	6.3 (18)	8.7 (32)	8.1 (25)
Munro-Faure et al. (75)	(+)	7.73[f] (38)[g]	7.44 (29)	9.03 (7)	9.48 (8)
	(−)	7.25 (37)	—	9.05 (9)	—
Lasker et al. (57)	(−)	8.63 ± 1.38 (10)	7.59 ± 1.20 (9)	10.19 ± 3.00 (9)	8.89 ± 1.56 (9)
Smith et al. (98)	(−)	6.80 ± 1.58 (23)	5.87 ± 1.46 (26)	7.18 ± 2.34 (13)	7.15 ± 1.72 (18)
	(+)	6.25 ± 1.14 (134)	6.01 ± 1.03 (11)	8.54 ± 1.70 (10)	6.95 ± 2 (19)
Sharma et al. (93)	(NA)	5.2 ± 2.5 (8)	7.6 ± 3.6 (11)	7.1 ± 3.4 (23)	7.0 ± 3.6 (11)
Trevisan et al. (106) (children)[h]	(NA)	6.75 ± 0.88 (18)	6.13 ± 1.19 (23)	8.71 ± 1.36 (10)	8.79 ± 2.07 (19)

[a]Sex composition not stated.
[b]Blacks were Nigerian.
[c]Blacks were West Indian.
[d]Leukocytes, Na/mmol/liter cell water.
[e]Lithium loaded RBCs.
[f]sd not reported.
[g](N).
[h]Age range 11–15 years.
NA, not applicable.

189

major gene related to high Na_i and at increased risk of hypertension (122). If the relationship is restricted to this subgroup, then of course the causal theory linking increased Na_i and Ca_i to hypertension would not be universally applicable.

Abundant data now exist demonstrating higher mean Na_i among persons with ties to the African gene pool (Table 9.3). Over the last 10 years a number of reports have been published that permit biracial comparisons of cell Na_i and the association with hypertension. The studies from the United States that included adults have likewise reported 10%–20% higher Na_i among blacks without exception (58,85,87,93,98,111,119). Trevisan et al. (106) recruited a sample of black and white children with a mean age of 12 from parochial schools in Chicago. RBC Na_i was significantly higher among the black children of both sexes compared with whites; there was no association with BP in either ethnic group, however. Forrester and Alleyne (34) reported this same racial pattern among Jamaicans, and Weissberg et al. (121) found significantly higher RBC Na_i among Afro-Caribbeans living in Birmingham, England. Females of both races had lower Na_i than men in all studies where data were provided. No consistent racial pattern emerges for potassium or cell water, although data for cell water are available from only two reports (75,119).

U.S. blacks have experienced significant European gene admixture, estimated to vary from 15% to 40% (42,52,68,73,79), and it would be anticipated that this would dilute the importance of cell Na_i as a racial trait. In fact, data are available that provide direct comparisons between individuals from West Africa and Europeans. Aderounmu and Salako (1) studied a sample of 1,008 Nigerians in Ibadan and compared them with 7 Europeans, and found approximately 30% higher Na_i among the Africans. Twelve men from Zaire resident in Belgium were also compared with 43 Europeans; the black participants in this study had RBC Na_i levels almost twice those of the whites (62). Our group recently completed a triethnic study comparing West Africans, U.S. blacks, and U.S. whites of similar age (17). All participants were normotensive and taking no medications. Detailed data on diet, exercise, smoking, and other health-related characteristics suggested that these groups were very similar in their current lifestyle. A graded increase in cell sodium was noted across the three groups, paralleled by estimates of gene admixture derived from red cell antigens and serum proteins (Table 9.4).

As a purely descriptive finding these ethnic differences would be of little use. Further analysis suggests, however, that the relationship between Na_i and BP may also be different across races. This finding was clearly demonstrated in our triethnic study (17). Although no correlation was apparent between systolic BP and Na_i among the whites ($r = 0.07$), a strong association was observed among both groups of blacks ($r = 0.7$ and $r = 0.3$, systolic BP vs. Na_i, for U.S. and African blacks, respectively). In an entirely separate study of normotensive and untreated hypertensive blacks from Chicago, we earlier demonstrated a significant association between Na_i and blood pressure of similar magnitude (18). In this sample of 217 persons the correlation between systolic blood pressure and RBC Na_i was 0.4 ($p > 0.001$), and hypertensives had Na_i levels 11% higher than normotensives ($p = 0.02$). These samples were not population based, however, which in part limits their generalizability.

TABLE 9.4. Cellular Electrolytes and Genetic Markers in U.S. Whites, U.S. Blacks, and West African Blacks

A. RBC intracellular sodium

Variable	U.S. whites (N = 27)	U.S. blacks (N = 21)	West African blacks (N = 27)
RBS sodium (mEq/liter cells; x; SD)	7.72 ± 2.49	9.96 ± 2.35	10.7 ± 2.81

B. Genetic markers

Marker	U.S. whites (%)	U.S. blacks (%)	West African blacks (%)
ABO: A	44[a]	33	29
B	17	13	14
AB	11	—	—
O	28	53	59
Duffy a$^+$/b$^+$	56	7	—
a$^-$/b$^-$	—	53	100
Other	44	40	—
Rh: R^0/r	5	53	57
R^2/r and r/r	44	14	10
Other	51	33	33

C. Correlation between RBC sodium and systolic blood pressure

Variables	U.S. whites	U.S. blacks	West African blacks	Pooled
RBC Sodium-SBP	.069	.716*	.294	.378*

[a]Relative frequency per group.
Adapted from Cooper et al. (17).   *p<.01

In summary, it appears well established that increased RBC Na$_i$ is a trait characteristic of persons of West African origin. Based on the two large epidemiological studies published to date (69,83), the association between Na$_i$ and BP is weak and inconsistent among nonblacks. The Na$_i$-BP relationship appears to be stronger among blacks, and could explain as much as 15% of the interindividual variance in blood pressure (18). Given the strong evidence for the heritability of high cell Na$_i$, it is possible that the black populations that have been studied are enriched with persons homozygous for this trait. It should be recognized that this hypothesis is based on inferences from findings of family studies among whites in the United States (122), since no studies have investigated heritability of Na$_i$ concentration in black populations. At any rate, there is no direct evidence that the higher prevalence of the high Na$_i$ trait among blacks contributes to the overall increased risk of hypertension. Based on the findings of the studies of heritability and blood pressure in various populations, Ward (116) concluded that genetic factors contributed less among blacks than other groups, although this conclusion was based on the findings of a single survey.

The findings reviewed here are subject to several important limitations. Most investigators with an interest in cation transport metabolism share a primary interest in physiological mechanisms. All too often studies reported by these laboratories do not reflect collaboration with epidemiologists. Recruitment of participants from convenience samples may be appropriate for preliminary studies of a new laboratory assay, especially if the relationships being examined are thought to be strong. Definitive evidence can only be obtained from appropriately designed population-based studies, however, and true etiologic relationships must ultimately be established prospectively. Only a distinct minority of the studies reviewed here recruited participants from a defined sampling frame. In addition, the sample sizes of the studies among blacks are very limited, generally ranging from 5 to 20 participants. Only in three studies did the number of black participants exceed 100 in number (1,18,87). Given the relatively small magnitude of relationships being examined, sample sizes under 100 will be subject to beta statistical errors in the range of 50%. Finally, no systematic standardization has been attempted between laboratories. Some investigators have even suggested that all the findings on Na_i concentration are subject to bias because of systematic errors in measurement technique (96). At some point in the development of this area of research a decision must be made, based on the potential importance of the question posed, to commit adequate resources to overcome each of these shortcomings.

Two general conditions could result in higher Na_i among blacks than whites—an increased rate of membrane sodium leak, or a reduced rate of sodium efflux. Etkin et al. (33) reported that red cell permeability, as measured by influx of ^{22}Na in red cells in a medium containing ouabain, was slightly lower among whites than blacks (0.266 ± 0.044 vs. 0.216 ± 0.069, whites and blacks, respectively). Among the whites studied, sodium leak was significantly higher in the hypertensives than the normotensives; however, this was not the case among the blacks. Higher influx among whites than blacks was confirmed in a second study by this group, although the differences were not significant after adjustment for sex and body mass index (43). Other investigators studying Europeans have suggested that sodium leak is part of the pathophysiology of hypertension in a subgroup of patients (37), although to our knowledge no other studies have examined black–white differences in this trait. Similar rates of lithium leak have been reported in black and white children (106).

Thus there is no basis for concluding that increased sodium leak among blacks plays a role in maintaining higher Na_i. At the same time, a number of investigators have reported reduced active transport in blacks compared with whites (9,37,62,87); this issue will be discussed in greater detail subsequently. These studies, therefore, suggest that differences in the sodium pump are the only likely candidate to explain higher Na_i in blacks as described previously.

SODIUM-LITHIUM COUNTERTRANSPORT

As reviewed by Tosteson (104), the countertransport exchange system is an example of transcoupling of exchanged ions. This phloretin-sensitive sodium-sodium exchange system will accept lithium, as well as some other cations depending on the intra- and extracellular conditions. Tosteson (104) has suggested in general that coupled ion exchange may be a "device for the regulated dissipation of free energy made available from metabolic reactions." The physiological function of sodium-lithium countertransport (Na^+-Li^+ CT) is obscure, however, since no net sodium exchange is accomplished. Some investigators have pointed out the similarity between this transporter and another electroneutral monovalent cation exchanger, the sodium-hydrogen antiporter (36,68). Unlike all other transport systems studied in circulating blood cells, there is good evidence that the rates of Na^+-Li^+ CT reflect activity of this system in one of the tissues involved in blood pressure regulation, since there are some data suggesting that a negative correlation exists between renal clearance of lithium and red cell Na^+-Li^+ CT (117).

Attention was initially focused on the possible role of Na^+-Li^+ CT by the report of Canessa et al. (12) demonstrating higher exchange rates of Na^+-Li^+ CT in hypertensives, as well as normotensive offspring of patients with high blood pressure. Over the last decade, considerable evidence has continued to accumulate in support of the positive association between Na^+-Li^+ CT and blood pressure (2,19,21,23,58,92,105,109,112). Although sample sizes for several of these studies have exceeded 1,000, only two were population based (58,109), and no prospective data have yet been reported. The most extensive findings again come from the Gubbio Study (23). Based on a cross-sectional survey of 2,748 men and women aged 25–74 years, the correlation between systolic blood pressure and Na^+-Li^+ CT was 0.107 for men and 0.163 for women; both coefficients were significant at $p < 0.001$ (9). Although reduced considerably by adjustment for age, body mass index, and other blood pressure–related covariates, this relationship remained significant in multiple linear regression analysis. Persons with higher countertransport values were approximately 50% more likely to be hypertensive than persons with normal values. Turner et al. reported their findings on 1,475 white residents of Rochester, Minnesota, between the ages of 5 and 89 (112), largely confirming the results from the Gubbio Study. In combination with earlier data from the People's Gas Company study (58), these two large surveys have adequately established the consistency of the Na^+-Li^+ CT–blood pressure relationship in populations of European descent.

Mean values of Na^+-Li^+ CT are higher for men than women at all ages. In addition, the activity of this transport system is significantly correlated with several anthropometric and physiological variables, including cholesterol, triglycerides, uric acid, glucose, insulin, body mass index, and age (51,58,122). Pregnancy increases the rate of Na^+-Li^+ CT considerably (125). Based on likelihood analysis of the Utah pedigree data, total heritability of this trait was 80%, with 34% ascribed to a major gene and 46% to polygenic effects (122). Lewitter (61) found a high degree of concordance among adult monozygotic compared with dizygotic twins and estimated heritability of Na^+-Li^+ CT at 98%. It has been reported that Na^+-Li^+ CT may be aggregated in families with hypertension (74). Family history of hypertension itself is a weak marker for increased Na^+-Li^+ CT, although this is likely to result from methodological problems (21,92).

Sodium-lithium countertransport has been reported to be approximately 30% lower among blacks than whites in virtually every study published to date

TABLE 9.5. Reported Studies on RBC Sodium-Lithium Countertransport in Blacks and Whites by Hypertension Status (x; sd)

Study	Hypertension status	Whites Men/women[a]	Blacks Men/women
A. Sexes combined			
Weder et al. (119)	(+)	0.37 ± 0.05[b] (29)[c]	0.27 ± 0.10 (11)
	(−)	0.27 ± 0.15 (57)	0.21 ± 0.10 (23)
Canessa et al. (13)	(+)	0.51 ± 0.14[b] (23)	0.18 ± 0.02 (18)
	(−)	0.28 ± 0.12 (14)	0.18 ± 0.05 (18)
Weinberger et al. (120)	(+)	0.308 ± 0.107 (23)	0.225 ± 0.116 (9)
	(−)	0.212 ± 0.096 (21)	0.115 ± 0.049 (9)

Study	Hypertension status	Whites Men	Whites Women	Blacks Men	Blacks Women
B. By sex					
McDonald et al. (70)	(−)	0.26[c] ± 0.12 (103)	0.16 ± 0.09 (116)	0.19 ± 0.12 (112)	0.09 ± 0.16 (150)
Trevisan et al. (108)	(NA)	5.38 ± 1.94[c] (229)	4.36 ± 1.47 (97)	3.91 ± 1.27 (33)	3.47 ± 1.49 (58)
Smith et al. (98)	(+)	0.352 ± 0.116 (34)	0.318 ± 0.119 (11)	0.226 ± 0.115 (10)	0.236 ± 0.136 (9)
	(−)	0.225 ± 0.081 (23)	0.209 ± 0.087 (26)	0.173 ± 0.092 (13)	0.143 ± 0.092 (18)
Sharma et al. (93)	(NA)	0.16 ± 0.11 (8)	0.14 ± 0.10 (11)	0.16 ± 0.19 (23)	0.16 ± 0.13 (11)
Trevisan et al. (106) (children)[d]	(NA)	4.84 ± 1.44[c] (18)	4.26 ± 1.20 (23)	3.41 ± 0.99 (10)	3.02 ± 0.90 (19)

[a]Sex-specific data not given.
[b]mmol/liter RBC/h.
[c]mmol/liter RBC/min.
[d]Age range 11–15.
NA, not applicable.

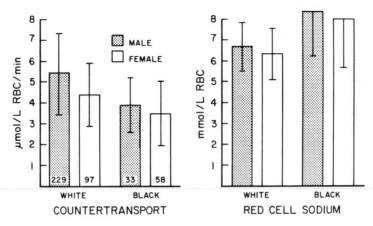

FIGURE 9.1. Sodium-lithium countertransport and red cell sodium concentration by sex and race.

(Table 9.5; Fig. 9.1). The relationship between Na^+-Li^+ CT and blood pressure in this ethnic group is somewhat inconsistent, however. Three studies have reported higher Na^+-Li^+ CT in hypertensive compared with normotensive blacks (98,119,120), while in one investigation this finding was not apparent (13). In total, only 177 hypertensives and 222 normotensives were represented in the studies providing mean values displayed in Table 9.5 (261 whites and 138 blacks). An unweighted mean percentage difference (hypertensives—normotensives/hypertensives) was calculated for each race group. Among hypertensive whites, mean levels were 54% higher (95% confidence intervals [CI] = ± 8), while the corresponding value for blacks was 44% (95% CI = 8); this difference is not significant. Because of varying laboratory techniques and sex composition of the samples, however, this is not an ideal summary statistic and should be regarded as an approximate comparison. Nonetheless it is curious to note that although Na^+-Li^+ CT levels are one-third lower among blacks, the same relative difference between hypertensives and normotensives exists in each race group.

The Coronary Artery Risk Development in Young Adults (CARDIA) study, which examined men and women between the ages of 20 and 32, noted a significant correlation between Na^+-Li^+ CT and blood pressure among white men and white women (partial correlation, systolic blood pressure and Na^+-Li^+ CT, adjusted for serum lipids, obesity, insulin, pulse, and uric acid: white men = 0.16, white women = 0.25, black men = 0.12, black women = 0.05; $p < 0.01$ for white women; a significant correlation of 0.18 was noted for diastolic blood pressure for white men) (70; A. McDonald, personal communication). The actual difference in the r values for men of the two races is quite small, of course. Significant correlations were also absent for blacks in two other studies (93,119). On the other hand, Trevisan et al. (106) reported a significant correlation between blood pressure and Na^+-Li^+ CT among 29 black children ages 12 and 13, while finding none among a comparable white sample. It should be recognized that small sample sizes systematically bias the outcome toward the null, so studies where the relationship is present or absent cannot be simply weighed one against the other. If the true correlation between countertransport and blood pressure is around 0.1, as suggested by the Gubbio Study, then a sample of at least 780 is required to achieve a significance level less than or equal to 0.05. In balance, therefore, it would appear that the relationship between Na^+-Li^+ CT and blood pressure is similar in blacks and whites, although more work is needed to define any special meaning among blacks.

SODIUM-POTASSIUM PUMP ACTIVITY

A classic form of carrier-mediated, energy-requiring ion exchange, the Na^+-K^+-ATPase pump is ubiquitously distributed throughout body tissues, although the level of activity may vary (102). A wide range of studies have examined the relationship between ouabain-sensitive sodium transport in blood cells and hypertension, as reviewed by others (10,49,87). Based on current theories relating cellular ion metabolism to hypertension, decreased Na^+-K^+-ATPase activity could be a cause of raised Na_i or Ca_i—failing to balance net influx. On the other hand, activity could be higher as a result of increased cell sodium attempting to return Na_i to normal. Reports of both positive and negative associations with blood pressure have in fact appeared, without the emergence of any consistent pattern (21,49). Laboratory techniques have been more varied in this area, and none of the large population-based epidemiological studies have examined the role of this transport system.

The most recent findings relating Na^+-K^+-ATPase and blood pressure are derived from the work by Rygielski et al. (87). Based on a sample of 247 individuals, a negative correlation of 0.240 was noted between systolic blood pressure and RBC ghost Na^+-K^+-ATPase activity ($p < 0.001$). Consistent correlations between Na_i and blood pressure were also observed in this data set. Although not presented separately, this finding appeared to be consistent for men and women, and blacks as well as whites. A negative correlation of 0.144 was reported between Na_i and ATPase activity ($p < 0.025$), providing support for a causal connection between Na_i, pump activity, and blood pressure elevation. Although the sample size in this study is sufficiently large to provide reasonable estimates of the observed relationships, participants were recruited for this study from a convenience sample, and the findings have not been supported by independent replication, to our knowledge. A subsequent study from France, for example, found no correlation at all between sodium pump activity and blood pressure (37). The relationship between reduced Na^+-K^+-ATPase activity and risk of high blood pressure can therefore be accepted with less confidence than applies to Na_i and Na^+-Li^+ CT.

Lower levels of sodium pump activity have been reported among nonwhites by most but not all investigators (Table 9.6). The most extensive data among blacks are derived from the work by investigators at the New Jersey College of Medicine (87). In this study, both sexes combined, Na^+-K^+-ATPase activity was 140.3 ± 4.2 compared with 167.3 ± 4.7 in 120 blacks compared with 127 whites (units as nmol P_i/ protein/h; $p = 0.0002$). These investigators have also reported lower sodium-potassium pump density in blacks (50). Sig-

Table 9.6. Reported Studies of RBC Sodium-Potassium Pump Activity in Blacks and Whites by Hypertension Status (x; sd)

Study	Hypertension status	Whites Men/women[a]	Blacks Men/women
A. Sexes combined			
Rygielski et al. (87)	(NA)	167.3 ± 53.0[a] (127)[b]	140.3 ± 46.0 (120)
Lijnen et al. (62)	(NA)	2.16 ± 0.46[c] (43)	1.80 ± 0.55 (12)
Tuck et al. (111)[d]	(+)	5.0[e] (38)	5.9 (20)
	(−)	5.4 (29)	5.4 (18)
Woods et al. (123)[d]	(+)	2.9[c] (16)	2.3 (10)
	(−)	2.4 (22)	2.2 (23)
Aderounmu et al. (1)	(+)	—	4.2 ± 1.3[f]
	(−)	—	5.7 ± 2.0

Study	Hypertension status	Whites Men	Whites Women	Blacks Men	Blacks Women
B. By sex					
Smith et al. (98)	(+)	1.66 ± 0.16[d] (34)	1.57 ± 0.17 (11)	1.72 ± 0.22 (10)	1.42 ± 0.19 (9)
	(−)	1.60 ± 0.17 (23)	1.48 ± 0.22 (26)	1.50 ± 0.17 (13)	1.47 ± 0.16 (18)
Sharma et al. (93)	(NA)	3.8[g]	3.8	3.3	3.4

[a] nmol P_i/mg protein/h given.
[b] N.
[c] ^{86}Rb uptake μmol/L cells/h.
[d] Estimated from figure.
[e] Stimulated Na efflux.
[f] Na efflux/L cells/h.
[g] ^{86}Rb influx/L cells/h.

nificantly lower active transport in blacks compared with whites was found by
Sharma et al. (93) ($p < 0.003$). Reporting on 12 persons from Zaire living in
Belgium, Lijnen et al. (62) reported Na^+-K^+-ATPase activity decreased compared with Europeans when estimated by ouabain-sensitive-^{86}Rb uptake
(1.80 ± 0.16 vs. 2.16 ± 0.07, blacks vs. whites, respectively). A similar contrast has been noted between a small sample of whites in England and immigrants from India (3). On the other hand, Woods et al. (124) found racial differences in Rb uptake, but not in the ouabain-sensitive fraction. Smith et al.
(98) likewise found no race difference in ouabain-sensitive sodium efflux.
Other investigators have recently reported a lower density of ouabain binding
sites in red cells of black children, and have suggested this might provide a
decreased "sink" for a circulating ATPase inhibitor (99).

Studies from another cell line—skin fibroblasts—make the interpretation
of racial differences in sodium pump activity more complicated (56). In serially
passed cultures, fibroblasts from black patients (n = 15) exhibited accelerated
sodium turnover rates compared with cells from whites (n = 15). This difference was accounted for by increased activity of the sodium-potassium pump
(ouabain-sensitive sodium washout rate, 3.46 ± 0.22 vs. 1.84 ± 0.28 mEq/
liter/min, blacks and whites, respectively; $p = 0.0006$) (57). Influx rates and
initial Na_i were also higher in blacks. No consistent relationship was noted
between the study variables and blood pressure, however. While interesting,
particularly because they extend observations on cation transport to cell lines
other than the hematopoietic system, on the surface the findings with fibroblasts are inconsistent with previous results with RBCs. It is possible that
tissue-to-tissue differences exist, or, as suggested by Kuriyama et al. (57),
other transport systems determine net exchange.

Unlike the findings with Na_i and Na^+-Li^+ CT, only one published report
directly addresses the issue of the relative strength of the relationship between
blood pressure and sodium-potassium pump activity in blacks and whites (93).
While noting a significant correlation between ouabain-sensitive transport
and systolic blood pressure among black men ($r = 0.4$, $p = 0.02$) in a study
with 34 participants, no association was noted in the much smaller sample of
whites (n = 12 and 13 for white men and white women, respectively). Inex-
plicably a borderline significant negative correlation was noted with active
transport and blood pressure among black women. These differences are likely
due to chance. On inspection of the scattergrams provided in the paper by
Rygielski et al. (87), no strong race effect is apparent, but this visual estimate
is not sufficiently reliable. In the Nigerian study by Aderounmu (1), active
sodium efflux was significantly lower in hypertensives (n = 16) than normotensives (n = 14) (0.31 ± 0.02 vs. 0.49 ± 0.05, mmol/liter/hr).

In summary, although intriguing, the data sat currently available on the
relationship between the sodium-potassium pump and blood pressure is insufficient to serve as the basis for firm conclusions. Given the low mean levels of
ouabain-insensitive transport observed among blacks, Hennesy et al. (48) estimated that 85% of net exchange is ouabain sensitive among blacks, compared
with 77% among whites. Lower *net* transport by ouabain-sensitive and insensitive mechanisms thus could contribute to the higher observed Na_i concentrations among blacks.

SODIUM-HYDROGEN EXCHANGE

A potential role for the sodium-hydrogen (Na^+-H^+) antiporter in hypertension has only recently been proposed (6). Driven by the sodium and hydrogen gradients, this exchange system is activated by a variety of agonists and mediates cell functions such as vascular contractility, platelet activation, mitogenic responses, and sodium reabsorption by renal proximal tubules (46,90,127). This exchange is thought by some investigators to be the physiological equivalent of Na^+-Li^+ CT, although recent evidence suggests a poor correlation of the activity of the two systems (91). It is possible that the antiporter can operate in more than one mode and exchange both lithium-sodium and sodium-hydrogen. Higher rates of sodium-hydrogen exchange could increase cell sodium flux, or lead to pH changes; on the other hand, greater activity of this system could be a result of higher cell Ca_i. A cDNA probe for the fibroblast antiporter has been cloned (88) and used in linkage analysis in a pedigree where hypertension appeared to be segregating (30). This study suggested an odds against linkage between the sodium-hydrogen antiporter and essential hypertension of between 10:1 and 110:1, depending on the assumptions about penetrance and mode of inheritance. Based on this preliminary report it is unlikely that variants of the sodium-hydrogen antiporter are candidate genes for risk of hypertension.

Interest in the relation between sodium-hydrogen exchange and high blood pressure was prompted initially by the report from Livne et al. (63). Utilizing volume change of platelets induced by propionate, these investigators noted higher exchange rates in platelets of hypertensives compared with normotensives (63), and these findings have since been confirmed (94,98). Resting pH is not different in platelets of hypertensives and normotensives, suggesting that chronic acidification of the cytosol does not drive the sodium-hydrogen exchanger in these patients (94,118).

Using the double beam spectrophotometer, we estimated volume change in platelets treated with propionate in a subsample of the participants in our triethnic study discussed earlier (17). Contrary to the report by the New Jersey group (47), we noted lower rates in both African and U.S. blacks compared with whites, although the differences were not significant (7.3 ± 1.8, 8.2 ± 2.0 and 9.0 ± 2.1, in U.S. blacks, African blacks, and U.S. whites, respectively; 28 individuals were studied) (17). Based on a relatively small sample, Schmouder and Weder also concluded that no important differences in mean sodium-hydrogen exchange rates in platelets existed between blacks and whites (Table 9.7) (89). Similar hypertensive–normotensive contrasts were noted in the two races (89). On the other hand, Gretler et al. (44) found significantly lower rates of maximal amiloride-sensitive swelling in platelets of black compared with white normotensives (14.4 ± 0.8 vs. 17.3 ± 0.7 [per cent increase between 5 and 60 sec] $p = 0.02$, n = 12 in each race group) (44; D. Gretler, personal communication).

Too little empirical data exist to warrant substantive conclusions regarding sodium-hydrogen exchange among blacks, and additional work is required to develop more reliable laboratory procedures. Studies that provide confirmatory measures of intracellular pH would be helpful in evaluating the sig-

TABLE 9.7. Platelet Sodium-Hydrogen Exchange Among Hypertensives Compared with
Normotensives by Race (x; SEM)

	Whites		Blacks	
	Hypertensive	Normotensive	Hypertensive	Normotensive
N	12	17	8	7
Age	29 ± 2	44 ± 3	29 ± 2	37 ± 3
Systolic BP	121 ± 2	157 ± 7	128 ± 6	140 ± 5
Platelet Na$^+$-H$^+$ exchange[a]	2.28 + 0.18	2.83 ± 0.16*	2.15 ± 0.25	3.30 ± 0.39**

[a]Percentage volume change at 10 min.
Adapted from Schmouder and Weder (90).
*$p = 0.03$, white hypertensives vs. normotensives.
**$p = 0.02$, black hypertensives vs. normotensives.

nificance of the estimates inferred from volume changes. Lower rates of sodium-hydrogen exchange, as noted by our group (17) and Gretler et al. (44),
are consistent with the established finding of lower Na$^+$-Li$^+$ CT in blacks.
Contrary to Na$^+$-Li$^+$ CT, there also appears to be more reason to expect that
sodium-hydrogen exchange could have a meaningful influence on cellular
physiology.

CELL CALCIUM

Investigators have suggested that increased basal Ca$_i$ might serve as a common pathway between vasopressor insults and sustained hypertension
(7,29,97). To study this question, research teams have examined a variety of
physiological measures of cell calcium metabolism in hypertension, including
ionized plasma calcium, free cytosolic calcium, calcium transport, and membrane-bound calcium. In fact, relatively little is known about the relationship
between cytosolic calcium and either resting tone or increased agonist-induced
responses of vascular smooth muscle (32,66). In the face of this limited background of basic physiological knowledge, it is perhaps surprising that published reports have been consistently positive (22,32,53,71,82). Although no
reports have corroborated the extraordinarily high correlation of 0.9 between
Ca$_i$ and blood pressure found in the original report by Erne et al. (91), r values
have generally been in the range of 0.3–0.4 (22,32,53,71,82). This association
translates into 10%–30% higher resting concentrations of Ca$_i$ in hypertensives
than in normotensives. Although this work was all based on platelets (22,32,
53,71,82,91), this finding has been replicated in red cells (84,114).
    As is apparent from the earlier discussion on sodium that consistency of
this degree is unusual in this literature. It is reasonable to assume, therefore,
that the underlying association is fairly strong. Alternatively it is also possible
that a publication bias favors only positive reports. This bias may be a particular problem with small studies, since the investment required for population

studies is likely to result in publication of the results no matter what the outcome. We suspect, for example, that this bias may in part explain the discrepancy between the 40%–50% difference in Na^+-Li^+ CT reported between hypertensives and normotensives in clinical series (see Table 9.5) and the more modest correlations observed in population-based studies (58). It would be prudent, therefore, to wait for larger population studies before reaching a final verdict on the strength of the relationship between Ca_i and blood pressure.

Additional reports have demonstrated changes in membrane calcium transport that might be predicted from the current ion theory of the pathophysiology of hypertension. Thus, Vincenzi et al. found lower calcium pump ATPase activity in red cells of hypertensives than in controls (115), while other workers have reported increased membrane permeability, with reduced calcium pump activity (27,80,86). The role of calcium in hypertension is discussed in detail in Chapter 8.

Utilizing the membrane permanent dye "fura 2" we demonstrated significantly higher resting Ca_i in platelets of untreated black hypertensives (Table 9.8) (22). Participants for this study were recruited from a screening clinic and matched in age to normotensives attending the same facility for minor illness. In this study we were also able to show for the first time a positive correlation between cell Ca_i and Na_i ($r = 0.3$, $p < 0.05$). In the triethnic study of U.S. whites, blacks, and African blacks described earlier, platelet Ca_i was also measured (17). Significantly lower Ca_i was noted in U.S. blacks compared with whites (75.7 ± 16.5 vs. 89.6 ± 26.6, respectively; $p < 0.05$). Among these same individuals, it should be noted, Na_i was 30% higher among the blacks than the whites, suggesting different internal ratios between these two ions in the two ethnic groups. Levels of Ca_i among the Africans were intermediate between the other two groups; no associations with blood pressure were seen in this small sample.

In an additional study, based on the clinic sampling scheme just described,

TABLE 9.8. Blood Pressure, Intracellular Electrolytes, and Related Variables in Hypertensive and Normotensive Blacks, Chicago, Illinois (x; sd)

Variable	Normotensive (n = 38)	Hypertensive (n = 19)
Systolic BP (mm Hg)	113.1 ± 12.5	153.8 ± 19.5*
Diastolic BP (mm Hg)	75.8 ± 7.1	101.9 ± 6.0*
Pulse (beats/min)	75.8 ± 10.6	76.2 ± 11.0
Intracellular electrolytes		
Ca^{2+} (nmol)[a]	98.4 ± 28.0	118.6 ± 29.2*
Na^+ (mmol)[b]	8.6 ± 2.1	9.4 ± 2.3**
K^+ (mmol)[b]	85.7 ± 10.9	88.4 ± 9.2

[a]Assayed in platelets.

[b]Assayed in red blood cells (per liter of red blood cells) of hypertensive (n = 55) and normotensive (n = 67) subjects. Adapted from Cooper et al. (22).

*$p < 0.02$

**$p < 0.05$.

we examined membrane-bound calcium with chlortetracycline and an epifluorescence technique (Table 9.9) (20). Significantly higher levels of calcium were bound to membranes of platelets from hypertensives; blood pressure was correlated with bound calcium at the level of 0.213 ($p = 0.58$). In separate experiments utilizing radiolabeled chlortetracycline and adding EGTA to the medium, we excluded the possibility that this finding could be attributed to differential binding properties of platelets from hypertensives or solely to external calcium on the plasma membrane. These experiments therefore allow us to conclude that these patients had a higher cell burden of calcium, implying greater potential responsiveness. No differences were noted after stimulation of platelets with PGI_2, suggesting that platelets from both groups sequestered calcium in response to agonists at similar rates. These experiments have not been replicated by others, and we know of no similar data from whites. Contrary to most—but not all—published reports among whites, we were unable to confirm an association between ionized serum calcium and blood pressure among blacks (16).

Based on the relatively limited data base summarized here, the relationship between cell calcium metabolism and hypertension appears to be no different in blacks than whites, with the possible exception of the ratio between Na_i and Ca_i.

SODIUM-POTASSIUM COTRANSPORT

Sodium-potassium cotransport (Na^+-K^+ CoT) is a ouabain-insensitive, furosemide-sensitive outward exchange system described as cis-coupling by Tosteson (38,104). In a ratio of 1:1, sodium and potassium are transported uphill

TABLE 9.9. Cellular Electrolytes in Hypertensive and Normotensive Blacks, Chicago, Illinois (x; sd)

Variable	Normotensive (n = 42)	Hypertensive (n = 39)
Platelet assays		
Membrane-bound Ca^{2+}[a]		
30-min	529 ± 106	564 ± 86*
45-min	512 ± 99	558 ± 93**
Tritiated tetracycline	620 ± 142	618 ± 188
	(n = 31)	(n = 27)
Red blood cell assays		
Intracellular Na (mmol/liter cells)	6.70 ± 1.97	7.88 ± 2.24[b]
Intracellular K (mmol/liter cells)	72.9 ± 14.0	74.3 ± 12.4

[a]Units reported in counts per second normalized to a uranium glass standard.
[b]Units reported as counts per minute normalized to 10^8 platelets.
Adapted from Cooper et al. (20).
*$p < 0.05$.
**$p < 0.02$.

against the sodium gradient independent of ATP. Activity of this system appears to be equally influenced by hereditary and environmental factors (122), and the laboratory assay is associated with a high coefficient of variation. Most investigators have relied on the measurement of V_{max} for this exchange system (39). Initial interest in the relationship of this exchange system to hypertension was stimulated by the report from Garay et al. (39,40) of reduced levels in patients with elevated blood pressure. Subsequent reports in whites have not uniformly confirmed these early findings, with some reports showing higher levels in hypertensives (2,111). There appears to be little evidence at the present time of a consistent association between this transport system and blood pressure in nonblack populations, although again the data base is limited.

Several studies have examined the role of Na^+-K^+ CoT in blacks (Table 9.10), and uniformly suggest markedly reduced levels in blacks compared with

TABLE 9.10. Reported Studies on RBC Sodium-Potassium Cotransport in Blacks and Whites by Hypertension Status (x; sd)

Study	Hypertension status	White Men/women	Black Men/women
A. Sexes combined			
Weder et al. (119)	(+)	0.30 ± 0.16^b (29)[c]	0.08 ± 0.07 (11)
	(−)	0.32 ± 0.30 (57)	0.10 ± 0.14 (23)
Adragna et al. (23)	(+)	0.51 ± 0.20^b (23)	0.25 ± 0.17 (18)
	(−)	0.31 ± 0.12 (14)	0.38 ± 0.24 (18)
Tuck et al. (111)	(+)	0.39 (38)	0.15 (30)
	(−)	0.28 (29)	0.23 (18)

Study	Hypertension status	White Men	White Women	Black Men	Black Women
B. By sex					
Smith et al. (99)	(+)	10.6 ± 5.0^e (34)	6.9 ± 3.8 (11)	6.0 ± 4.9 (10)	4.1 ± 2.1 (9)
	(−)	8.9 ± 5.0 (23)	7.4 ± 3.7 (26)	5.7 ± 3.5 (13)	4.5 ± 2.6 (18)
Ringel et al. (186)	(+)	—	—	0.66 ± 0.41 (53)	
	(−)	—	—	0.62 ± 0.28 (20)	

[a]Sex-specific data not given.
[b]mmol/L cells/h; Na efflux.
[c]SD not given.
[d]Estimated from figure.
[e]Li^+-K^+ cotransport.

whites. Based on an unweighted mean, levels are 45% lower in blacks. In addition, at least two groups have reported that the efflux ratio for sodium to potassium is greater than 1:1 in blacks. Both Tuck et al. (111) and Canessa et al. (12) have reported significantly reduced V_{max} for Na^+-K^+ CoT in small groups of black hypertensives compared with normotensives of the same race ($p < 0.05$). There is no real trend to be evaluated in these data. Garay (41) reported reduced Na^+-K^+ CoT in black hypertensives from the Ivory Coast compared with normotensives, and a similar finding expressed as the average of sodium plus potassium efflux was noted in South Africa (26).

Low mean levels of cotransport could play a role in group susceptibility to hypertension among blacks. Thus, it has been suggested that "hypertension among black subjects may be associated with an inherited defect in the Na^+-K^+ CoT system that would impair sodium removal as a backup to the sodium pump" (122). Although an attractive hypothesis, it would be helpful to have better evidence of an association between Na^+-K^+ CoT and blood pressure among blacks before making firm conclusions about between-group differences.

CONCLUSIONS

Is it reasonable to conclude that alterations in ion metabolism are part of the basic pathophysiology of hypertension? Considering the entire body of data available from all ethnic groups, several measures of cellular ions are different in hypertensives than in normotensives. None of these relationships are large quantitatively, although they are in the range found for other physiological risk factors for hypertension, such as uric acid and pulse rate. The strongest evidence for an association exists for Na^+-Li^+ CT. We conclude that higher mean levels of Na_i are also characteristic of persons with hypertension. The findings for Na^+-K^+-ATPase are suggestive but weighted by a single study (87). For Ca_i and membrane-bound calcium, published data are positive, but restricted to smaller samples that were not recruited to represent populations. Evidence is not sufficient to support any association between Na^+-K^+ CoT and hypertension.

Whether or not these associations have any causal meaning is an entirely different question, however. Given the enormously complex control mechanisms that regulate blood pressure, a single abnormality is perhaps more likely to be a secondary consequence of hypertension than a primary cause. It is entirely premature, in our view, to ascribe causal significance to any of the abnormalities in ion metabolism described to date, except perhaps Ca_i, since this ion is of fundamental importance in sustaining vascular smooth muscle contractility. Like the pattern of changes seen in serum lipids, insulin, renin, uric acid, and other physiological traits, these findings could all be simply epiphenomena (8,116). At the same time, hypertension is a polygenic disorder. If distinct subtypes do exist, then all phenotypes are being mixed together under our diagnostic rubric of essential hypertension (116). The high degree of heritability described for some of the transport systems does hold out the promise that gene markers can be identified that would greatly facilitate the study of separate phenotypes (36,116). For example, gene markers are now available for sodium-hydrogen exchange (88) and the plasma membrane calcium pump currently under investigation in our laboratory (11); strong evidence also exists for a major gene for high total urinary kallikrein (122). At the other extreme, population surveys are much more helpful in identifying polymodal distributions of a disease trait; small samples of convenience are not. Unless more precise laboratory markers are identified, considerable additional work in each of these areas will be necessary before a coherent theory can be constructed to explain cell ion transport in hypertension.

How reasonable is it to expect that genetic differences in ion metabolism account for the increased risk of hypertension in blacks compared with whites? The importance of proper function of the circulatory system under extremes of volume loading, physical activity, and other threats to whole body homeostasis have led to the evolution of highly sensitive and redundant control mechanisms for blood pressure. Many of these systems are shared in common with other species and are likely to have emerged early in our evolutionary history. All humans share a relatively recent common African ancestry (59). In preliterate society, where our species spent virtually all of its adaptive history, hypertension is essentially unknown; no selective pressure would therefore have existed for or against innate susceptibility to this disease. For large population differences to exist today, however, it would be necessary to postulate differential selection for a trait which at least cosegregated with hypertension risk. Humans are essentially tropical animals, relatively ill-adapted to other climatic extremes. When posing a contrast between Europeans and Africans, therefore, the evolutionary logic would suggest that Europeans have evolved away from the African norm.

At the present time, only one coherent theory has been proposed to link ion metabolism with increased risk of hypertension among blacks, namely, evolution of avid salt-retaining mechanisms among a tropical people that led to salt-sensitive, volume-expanded hypertension on adoption of the modern diet. Although this predisposition would explain the high frequency of the low-renin state among normotensive as well as hypertensive blacks, the underlying mechanism of renin hyporesponsivity may be more complex (see Chapter 10, this volume). A further refinement of this theory has been offered by Grim and Wilson (45), who postulate an evolutionary bottleneck created by the Atlantic slave trade. According to this theory, individuals with more highly developed salt-retention mechanisms had a greater chance of surviving the salt and water deprivation of the "middle passage."

Integrating this theory with findings on ion metabolism is difficult for several reasons. First, the evolutionary perspective would require a reason why Europeans evolved away from the supposed salt avidity that characterized early Africans. No such thesis has been proposed. Some non-African population groups have clearly not lost the extraordinary ability to retain salt that characterizes our species. The Yanomamo Indians of Brazil, who entered their current terrain as recently as 10,000 years ago, function successfully in a tropical rain forest with essentially no sodium intake (31). Second, there is firm evidence that hypertension among black populations in both East and West Africa is not as common as among U.S. blacks, despite nearly similar sodium intake (4,81,95). Third, in terms of the observed ion transport differences between blacks and whites, all the evidence suggests that blacks in the Western Hemisphere are genetically similar to West Africans, arguing against the notion of important selection during the slave trade. Fourth, no good evidence exists for a differential impact of genetics on blood pressure or different modes of inheritance of hypertension in distinct population groups (116).

In our view, there is no general conceptual precedent for genetically caused racial or population differences in diseases that result from disturbance of basic physiological control mechanisms. Some would argue these conditions have been met for anemia or low birth weight among U.S. blacks, diabetes among Amerindians, or coronary heart disease among persons from the Indian subcontinent (14,25,126). Important counterarguments apply in each of these examples, however, and the enormous impact of rapid modernization—along with persistent social disadvantage—cannot be discounted. Although space does not permit a full discussion of this question, each of these potential precedents has other differences with the paradigm posed for hypertension.

What patterns of ion transport have been demonstrated in blacks? The evidence suggests that at least four of the measures of ion metabolism described here are different between blacks and whites (Table 9.11). Na_i is clearly higher. Ouabain-insensitive transport (Na^+-Li^+ CT and Na^+-K^+ CoT) is clearly decreased, and sodium pump activity may be also lower. These findings are broadly consistent with the data showing a negative corelation between these transport systems and Na_i in the same individual (87,93,122). Na_i concentration appears to be positively associated with blood pressure among blacks, and the strength of the association is stronger than among whites. Increased countertransport is an equally strong marker of hypertension among blacks and whites. Based primarily on the reports from Rygielski et al. (87), reduced Na^+-K^+-ATPase also appears to be important in hypertension in both races, although it would be of interest to see a reexamination of their data by race as an estimate of a differential role for this transport system in blacks and whites. Insufficient published data exist to evaluate the sodium-hydrogen exchange system, although important differences have not been identified. The same conclusions apply to measures of cell calcium metabolism.

TABLE 9.11. Summary of Findings on Ion Transport and Hypertension among Blacks

Variable	Mean values Hypertensives vs. normotensives	Mean values Blacks vs. whites
1. Intracellular Na^+	↑ 12%	↑ 30%
2. Na^+-Li^+ countertransport	↑ 44%	↓ 30%
3. Na^+-K^+ pump	±[a]	±
4. Na^+-K^+ cotransport	±	↓ 50%
5. Intracellular Ca^{2+}	↑ 20%	No difference[b]
6. Na^+-H^+ exchange	↑ 45%	No difference[b]

[a]Reported findings inconsistent.
[b]Limited data available.

It would appear reasonable to conclude, therefore, that persons of African origin do function at higher levels of Na_i, and at the same time exhibit lower rates of ouabain-sensitive and insensitive membrane transport. At these different equilibrium points, however, the quantitative association with risk of hypertension is similar to whites. Since Na_i and Na^+-Li^+ CT appear to be influenced by changes in dietary intake of sodium, it is possible that this could provide a link to salt sensitivity (110,122). It should be noted, however, that in the studies cited, lower dietary sodium reduced Na_i, but there was no direct evidence that blood pressure was correspondingly changed in these same individuals (110,122). Black–white differences in this phenomenon have not yet been studied, to our knowledge, and this could represent a fruitful area for future research.

Whether any of these differences contribute to the increased risk of hypertension among blacks is also unknown. It is plausible, for example, that the high Na_i phenotype is more common among blacks. Lower rates of both ouabain-sensitive and insensitive transport systems could contribute to this phenotype. At most, however, this trait could account for only a fraction of the excess hypertension rates. If in fact, higher Na_i is a marker of hypertension risk, then higher mean levels among blacks could be the basis for greater genetic susceptibility to hypertension in this population. On the other hand, Na^+-Li^+ CT is higher in hypertensives, yet lower in blacks. If this cation–blood pressure relationship is causal (higher Na^+-Li^+ CT exchange rates = higher risk of hypertension) then this trait should confer *lower* risk to the black population. On balance, therefore, evidence on the two cation measures that have been most closely associated with hypertension risk essentially cancel out the possibility of genetic predisposition among the black population. As noted elsewhere, obesity and psychocultural factors already account for most of the excess black risk of hypertension (54); no pressing need remains to identify inherited metabolic causes.

It may be, as demonstrated in the cross-racial studies of renin (8), that a different set point for a physiological trait confers no risk of the disease outcome whatsoever. In different environments the same gene may yield different phenotypes; recent data demonstrate that changes in sodium balance can change the expression of mRNA for renin (55). An interaction between psychocultural factors and high dietary sodium may occur, for example. Finally, in the absence of reliable genetic markers, we still do not know with certainty if the observed phenotypic ion transport abnormalities described here reflect differential exposures, or different distributions of the genes.

Subtypes of hypertension may well exist, and certain subtypes may be more common among blacks (116). In this context the analogy between varied patterns of ion metabolism in different ethnic groups and the specific cation transport patterns seen in various strains of hypertensive rats, as posed in the introductory section, may be overstretched. All of the animal experimental models are highly inbred, in contrast to the broad diversity in gene composition among members of our species. The recent report of a complete cure of hypertension in the spontaneously hypertensive rat with a single dose of interleukin-2 suggests that this form of hypertension may have resulted from a unique mutation, having nothing to do with essential hypertension in humans (113).

It is more likely that various subtypes only differ in frequency between ethnic groups and that hypertension as a whole is the same disease (116).

Much has been learned in the last decade about alterations in ion metabolism in hypertension. The data base regarding black–white differences in ion metabolism remains relatively modest but permits an increasingly clear description of the overall pattern. Substantial new experimental work on cell calcium is currently in progress and should prove extremely valuable. While it seems doubtful that research in this area will demonstrate a metabolic basis for the increased susceptibility of U.S. blacks to hypertension, it may help in understanding the heterogeneity of this disease in the species as a whole.

REFERENCES

1. Aderounmu, A. F., and L. A. Salako. Abnormal cation composition and transport in erythrocytes from hypertensive patients. *Eur. J. Clin. Invest. 9:* 369–375, 1979.
2. Adragna, N., M. Canessa, H. Solomon, E. Slater, and D. C. Tosteson. Red cell lithium-sodium countertransport and sodium-potassium cotransport in patients with essential hypertension. *Hypertension 4:* 795–804, 1982.
3. Ahmad, M. N., and A. R. Leeds. More on sodium-potassium-ATPase and obesity. *N. Engl. J. Med. 310:* 1390–1391, 1984.
4. Akinkugbe, O. O., and O. A. Ojo. Arterial pressures in rural and urban populations in Nigeria. *Br. Med. J. 2:* 222–224, 1969.
5. Allen, A., J. Stamler, R. Stamler, F. Gosch, R. Cooper, M. Trevisan, and V. Persky. Observational and interventional experiences on dietary sodium intake and blood pressure. In: *The Role of Salt in Cardiovascular Hypertension,* edited by M. R. Kare and M. J. Fregly. Academic Press, New York, 1981, pp. 63–68.
6. Aviv, A. The link between cytosolic Ca^{2+} and the $Na+ -H^+$ antiport: a unifying factor for essential hypertension. *J. Hypertens. 6:* 685–691, 1988.
7. Aviv, A., and A. Livne. The Na/H antiport, cytosolic free Ca, and essential hypertension: a hypothesis. *Am. J. Hypertens. 1:* 410–413, 1988.
8. Barley, J., J. K. Cruickshank, N. D. Carter, S. Jefery, A. Smith, A. Charlett, and D. J. Webb. Renin and ANP RFLPs, plasma renin and blood pressure in black and white population samples. In preparation.
9. Beutler, E., W. Kuhl, and P. Sachs. Sodium-potassium ATPase activity is influenced by ethnic origin and not by obesity. *N. Engl. J. Med. 309:* 756–760, 1983.
10. Blaustein, M. P. Sodium transport and hypertension: where are we going? *Hypertension 6:* 445–453, 1984.
11. Borke, J., J. T. Penniston, and R. Kuman. Recent advances in calcium transport by the kidney. *Semin. Nephrol. 10:* 15–23, 1990.
12. Canessa, M., N. Adragna, H. S. Solomon, T. M. Connolly, and D. C. Tosteson. Increased sodium-lithium countertransport in red cells of patients with essential hypertension. *N. Engl. J. Med. 302:* 772–776, 1980.
13. Canessa, M., A. Spalvins, N. Adragna, an B. Falkner. Red cell sodium countertransport and cotransport in normotensive and hypertensive blacks. *Hypertension 6:* 344–351, 1984.
14. Chakraborty, R., R. E. Ferrell, M. P. Stern, S. M. Haffner, H. P. Hazuda, and M. Rosenthal. Relationship of prevalence of non-insulin-dependent diabetes mellitus to Amerindian admixture in the Mexican Americans of San Antonio, Texas. *Genet. Epidemiol. 3:* 435–454, 1986.
15. Cooper, R., and R. David. The biological concept of race and its application in epidemiology and public health. *J. Health Polit. Policy Law 11:* 97–116, 1986.
16. Cooper, R., and N. Shamsi. Ionized serum calcium in black hypertensives. *J. Clin. Hypertens. 3:* 514–519, 1987.
17. Cooper, R., O. Aina, L. Chaco, A. Achilihu, and H. Feinberg. Cell cations and blood pressure in U.S. whites, U.S. blacks and West African blacks. *J. Hum. Hypertens. 4:* 477–484, 1990.
18. Cooper, R., O. Aina, L. Chaco, A. Achilihu, N. Shamsi, and E. Ford. Red cell sodium and potassium in hypertension among blacks. *J. Natl. Med. Assoc. 81:* 365–370, 1989.
19. Cooper, R., D. LeGrady, S. Nanas, M. Trevisan, M. Mansour, P. Histand, D. Ostrow, and

J. Stamler. Increased sodium-lithium countertransport in college students with elevated blood pressure. *J.A.M.A. 249:* 1030–1034, 1983.

20. Cooper, R., J. Lipowski, E. Ford, N. Shamsi, H. Feinberg, and G. Le Breton. Increased membrane-bound calcium in platelets of hypertensive patients. *Hypertension 13:* 139–144, 1989.

21. Cooper, R., K. Miller, M. Trevisan, C. Sempos, E. Larbi, H. Ueshima, D. Ostrow, J. Stamler, A. Spalvins, and M. Canessa. Family history of hypertension and red cell cation transport in high school students. *J. Hypertens. 1:* 145–152, 1983.

22. Cooper, R., N. Shamsi, and S. Katz. Increased intracellular calcium and sodium in hypertensive patients compared to normotensives. *Hypertension 9:* 224–229, 1987.

23. Cooper, R., M. Trevisan, D. Ostrow, C. Sempos, and J. Stamler. Blood pressure and sodium-lithium countertransport: findings in population-based surveys. *J. Hypertens. 2:* 467–471, 1984.

24. Cooper, R., L. Van Horn, K. Liu, M. Trevisan, S. Nanas, and J. Stamler. The effect of dietary sodium reduction on red blood cell sodium concentration and sodium-lithium countertransport. *Hypertension 6:* 731–735, 1984.

25. Cruickshank, J. K., and D. G. Beevers, eds. *Ethnic Factors in Health and Disease.* Butterworth and Co., London, 1989.

26. Davidson, J. S., L. H. Opie, and B. Keding. Sodium-potassium cotransport activity as a genetic marker in essential hypertension. *Br. Med. J. 224:* 539–541, 1982.

27. De la Sierra, A., P. Hannaert, J-P. Ollivier, N. Senn, and R. Garay. Kinetic study of the Ca^{2+} pump in erythrocytes from essential hypertensive patients. *J. Hypertens. 8:* 285–293, 1990.

28. DeMendonca, M., A. Knorr, M. L. Grichois, D. Ben-Ishay, R. P. Garay, and P. Member. Erythrocytic ion transport systems in primary and secondary hypertension of the rat. *Kidney Int. 21*(Suppl 11): S69–S75, 1982.

29. deWardner, H. E., and G. A. MacGregor. Dahl's hypothesis that a saluretic substance may be responsible for a sustained rise in arterial pressure: its possible role in essential hypertension. *Kidney Int. 18:* 1–18, 1980.

30. Dudlye, C., L. Giuffra, P. Tippett, A. E. G. Raine, and S. T. Reeders. Genetic linkage analysis of a Na-H antiporter in essential hypertension. Program and Abstracts, American Society of Nephrology, 1989, 196A.

31. Elliot, P., ed. The Intersalt Cooperative Group. The Intersalt Study. *J. Hum. Hypertens. 3:* 331–407, 1989.

32. Erne, P., P. Bolli, E. Burgisser, and F. R. Buhler. Correlation of platelet calcium with blood pressure. *N. Engl. J. Med. 310:* 1084–1088, 1984.

33. Etkin, N. L., J. R. Mahoney, M. W. Forsthoefel, J. R. Eckman, J. D. McSwigan, R. F. Gillum, and J. W. Eaton. Racial differences in hypertension-associated red cell sodium permeability. *Nature 297:* 588–589, 1982.

34. Forrester, T. E., and G. A. O. Alleyne. Sodium, potassium and rate constants for sodium efflux in leukocytes from hypertensive Jamaicans. *Br. Med. J. 283:* 5–7, 1981.

35. Friedman, S. M., M. Nakashima, R. A. McIndoe, and C. L. Friedman. Increased erythrocyte permeability to Li and Na in the spontaneously hypertensive rat. *Experientia 32:* 476–478, 1976.

36. Funder, J., J. O. Wieth, H. E. Jensen, and K. K. Ibsen. The sodium/lithium exchange mechanism in essential hypertension: is it a sodium/proton exchanger? In: *Topics in Pathophysiology of Hypertension,* edited by H. Villarreal and M. P. Sambhi. Martinus Nijhoff, The Hague, 1984, pp. 147–161.

37. Garay, R. P., and C. Nazaret. Na^+ leak in erythrocytes from essential hypertensive patients. *Clin. Sci. 69:* 613–624, 1985.

38. Garay, R., N. Adragna, M. Canessa, and D. Tosteson. Outward sodium potassium cotransport in human red cells. *J. Membr. Biol. 62:* 169–174, 1981.

39. Garay, R. P., G. Dagher, M. Pernollet, M. Devynck, and P. Meyer. Inherited defect in a Na-K cotransport system in erythrocytes from essential hypertensive patients. *Nature 284:* 281–283, 1980.

40. Garay, R. P., P. Hyannaert, G. Dagher, C. Nazaret, Y. Maridonneau, and P. Meyer. Abnormal erythrocyte Na-K cotransport system: a proposed genetic marker of essential hypertension. *Clin. Exp. Hypertens. 3:* 861–870, 1981.

41. Garay, R. P., C. Nazaret, G. Dagher, E. Bertrand, and P. Meyer. A genetic approach to the geography of hypertension: examination of the Na-K cotransport in Ivory Coast Africans. *Clin. Exp. Hypertens. 3:* 861–870, 1981.

42. Glass, B., and C. Li. The dynamics of racial intermixture: an analysis based on the American Negro. *Am. J. Hum. Genet. 5:* 1–20, 1953.

43. Gomez-Marin, O., R. J. Prineas, R. F. Gillum, N. L. Etkin, and J. W. Eaton. Red blood cell

sodium permeability and blood pressure: the Minneapolis children's blood pressure study. The CVD Newsletter, AHA, Dallas, April 1985.

44. Gretler, D. D., K. C. Jones, and M. B. Murphy. Blood platelet sodium hydrogen exchange in black vs. white normotensive subjects. *Am. J. Hypertens. 3*(No. 5, Part 2): 54A, 1990.

45. Grim, C., and P. Wilson. The slavery hypothesis of hypertension among blacks. In: *Pathophysiology of Hypertension in Blacks,* edited by J. C. S. Fray and J. Douglas. Oxford University Press, New York, 1992.

46. Grinstein, S., and A. Rothstein. Mechanisms of regulation of the Na$^+$/H$^+$ exchanger. *J. Membr. Biol. 90:* 1–12, 1986.

47. Hatori, N., J. P. Gardner, H. Tomonari, B. P. Fine, and A. Aviv. Na+-H+ antiport activity in skin fibroblasts from blacks and whites. *Hypertension 15:* 140–145, 1990.

48. Hennessy, J. F., and K. P. Ober. Racial differences in intact erythrocyte ion transport. *Ann. Clin. Lab. Sci. 12:* 35–41, 1982.

49. Hilton, M. D. Cellular sodium transport in essential hypertension. *N. Engl. J. Med. 314:* 222–228, 1986.

50. Hopp, L., N. Lasker, S. Grossman, R. Bamforth, and A. Aviv. [^{3}H]ouabain binding of red blood cells in whites and blacks. *Hypertension 8:* 1050–1057, 1986.

51. Hunt, S. C., R. R. Williams, J. B. Smith, and K. O. Ash. Associations of three erythrocyte cation transport systems with plasma lipids in Utah subjects. *Hypertension 8:* 30–36, 1986.

52. Hutchinson, J., and M. H. Crawford. Genetic determinants of blood pressure level among the black caribs of St. Vincent. *Hum. Biol. 53:* 453–466, 1981.

53. Hvarfner, A., R. Larsson, C. Morlin, J. Rastad, L. Wide, G. Akerstrom, and Ljunghall. Cytosolic free calcium in platelets: relationships to blood pressure and indices of systemic calcium metabolism. *J. Hypertens. 6:* 71–77, 1988.

54. Hypertension Detection and Follow-up Program Cooperative Group. Race, education and prevalence of hypertension. *Am. J. Epidemiol. 107:* 351–361, 1977.

55. Iwao, H., K. Fukui, S. Kim, K. Nakayama, H. Ohkubo, S. Hakanishi, and Abe. Effect of changes in sodium balance on renin, angiotensinogen and atrial natriuretic factor messenger RNA levels in rats. *J. Hypertens. 6*(Suppl 4): S297–299, 1988.

56. Kuriyama, S., L. Hopp, H. Tamura, N. Lasker, and A. Aviv. A higher cellular sodium turnover rate in cultured skin fibroblasts from blacks. *Hypertension 11:* 301–307, 1988.

57. Lasker, J., L. Hopp, S. Grossman, R. Bamforth, and A. Aviv. Race and sex differences in erythrocyte Na$^+$, K$^+$ adenosine triphosphatase. *J. Clin. Invest. 75:* 1813–1820, 1985.

58. Laurenzi, M., and M. Trevisan. Sodium-lithium countertransport and blood pressure: the Gubbio Population Study. *Hypertension 13:* 408–415, 1989.

59. Leakey, R. Review of the evidence for our African origins. *Ethnicity and Disease, 1:* 8–20, 1991.

60. Lewin, R. Africa: cradle of modern humans. *Science 237:* 1292–1295, 1987.

61. Lewitter, F. Red cell sodium transport studies in adult twins. *Am. J. Hum. Genet. 36*(Suppl): 172s, 1984.

62. Lijnen, P., J. R. M'Buyamba-Kabangu, R. Fagard, J. Staessen, and A. Amery. More on sodium-potassium ATPase and obesity. *N. Engl. J. Med. 310:* 1390, 1984.

63. Livne, A., R. Veitch, S. Grinstein, J. W. Balfe, A. Marquez-Julio, and A. Rothstein. Increased platelet Na$^+$-H$^+$ exchange rates in essential hypertension. Application of a novel test. *Lancet 1:* 533–536, 1987.

64. Losse, H., W. Zidek, H. Zumkley, F. Wessels, and H. Vetter. Intracellular Na$^+$ as a genetic marker of essential hypertension. *Clin. Exp. Hypertens. 3*(4): 627–640, 1981.

65. Love, W. D., and G. E. Burch. Plasma and erythrocyte Na$^+$ and K$^+$ concentrations in a group of southern white and negro blood donors. *J. Lab. Clin. Med. 53:* 258–267, 1953.

66. Machin, D., and M. J. Campbell. *Statistical Table for the Design of Clinical Trials.* Blackwell Scientific Publication, Boston, 1987, pp. 89–92.

67. Maclean, C. J., M. S. Adams, W. C. Leysohn, P. L. Workman, R. E. Reed, H. Gershowitz, and L. R. Weitkamp. Genetic studies on hybrid populations. III. Blood pressure in an American black community. *Am. J. Hum. Genet. 26:* 614–626, 1974.

68. Mahnensmith, R. L., and P. S. Aronson. The plasma membrane sodium hydrogen exchanger and its role in physiological and pathophysiological processes. *Circ. Res. 57:* 773–788, 1985.

69. Matsumoto, K., I. Matsura, T. Oshima, H. Fujii, K. Kido, and G. Kajiyama. The significance of erythrocyte sodium contents on blood pressure: evaluation by multivariate analysis (abstract). *Circulation 74*(SupplII4):II488, 1986.

70. McDonald, A., K. Liu, J. Stamler, and D. Battle. Race-sex comparisons of Na-Li counter-transport in CARDIA (abstract). *Circulation 80*(Suppl II): II-301, 1989.
71. McVeigh, G. E., S. Copeland, J. McKellar, and D. Johnston. Effect of low versus conventional dose cyclopenthiazide on platelet intracellular calcium in mild essential hypertension. *J. Hypertens. 6:* 337–341, 1988.
72. Miller, J. M., and J. M. Miller. Duffy antigens and hypertension in a black population. *Am. J. Public Health 75:* 558–559, 1985.
73. Montagu, A., ed. *The Concept of Race.* Collier Macmillan, Canada, Toronto, 1964.
74. Motulsky, A. G., W. Burke, P. R. Billings, and R. H. Ward. Hypertension and the genetics of red cell membrane abnormalities. In: *Molecular Approaches to Human Polygenic Disease,* edited by G. Bock and G. Collings. Wiley, Ciba Symposium 130, Chichester, 150–166, 1987.
75. Munro-Faure, A. D., D. M. Hill, and J. Anderson. Ethnic differences in human blood cell sodium concentration. *Nature 231:* 457–458, 1971.
76. Nei, L. Genetic distance between populations. *Am. Naturalist 105:* 385–398, 1972.
77. Otten, M. W., S. M. Teutsch, D. F. Williamson, and J. S. Marks. The effect of known risk factors on the excess mortality of black adults in the United States. *J.A.M.A. 263:* 845–850, 1990.
78. Patel, R., and J. Johnson. Histocompatibility antigens in black patients with essential hypertension. *Circulation 64:* 1042–1044, 1981.
79. Postnov, Y. V., and S. N. Orlov. Cell membrane alteration as a source of primary hypertension. *J. Hypertens. 2:* 1–6, 1984.
80. Postnov, Y. V., S. H. Orlov, M. B. Rfeznikova, G. G. Rjazhsky, and N. I. Pokudin. Calmodulin distribution and Ca transport in the erythrocytes of patients with essential hypertension. *Clin. Sci. 66:* 459–463, 1984.
81. Poulter, N., K. T. Khaw, B. E. C. Hopwood, M. Mugambi, W. S. Peart, G. Rose, and P. S. Sever. Blood pressure and associated variables in a rural Kenyan community. *Hypertension 6:* 810–813, 1984.
82. Pritchard, K., A. E. G. Raine, C. C. Ashley, L. M. Castell, V. Somers, C. Osborn, J. G. G. Ledingham, and J. Conway. Correlation of blood pressure in normotensive and hypertensive individuals with platelet but not lymphocyte intracellular free calcium concentrations. *Clin. Sci. 76:* 631–635, 1989.
83. Resnick, L. M., R. K. Gupta, B. Di Fabio, R. M. Marion, and J. H. Laragh. Role of intracellular cations in dietary salt sensitivity. 13th Scientific Meeting of the International Society of Hypertension, Abstracts, Montreal, June, 1990, S53.
84. Resnick, L. M., R. K. Gupta, J. H. Laragh. Intracellular sodium in hypertension: relation to salt sensitivity and plasma renin activity. *Am. J. Hypertens. 3*(No. 5, Part 2): 52A, 1990.
85. Ringel, R. E., J. M. Hamlyn, J. Schaeffer, B. P. Hamilton, A. A. Kowarski, M. P. Blaustein, and M. A. Berman. Red cell cotransport activity and sodium content in black men. *Hypertension 6:* 724–730, 1984.
86. Rounquist, G., and G. Frithz. Decreased ^{45}calcium uptake in red cells of patients with essential hypertension. *Acta Med. Scand. 224:* 445–449, 1988.
87. Rygielski, D., A. Reddi, S. Kuriyama, N. Lasker, and A. Aviv. Erythrocyte ghost Na^+, K^+-ATPase and blood pressure. *Hypertension 10:* 259–266, 1987.
88. Sardet, C., A. Franchi, and J. Pouyssegur. Molecular cloning, primary structure, and expression of the human growth factor-activatable Na^+/H^+ antiporter. *Cell 56:* 371–280, 1989.
89. Schmouder, R. L., and A. B. Weder. Platelet sodium-proton exchange in increased in essential hypertension. *J. Hypertens. 7:* 325–330, 1989.
90. Seifter, J. L., and P. S. Aronson. Properties and physiologic roles of plasma membrane sodium-hydrogen exchange. *J. Clin. Invest. 78:* 859–864, 1986.
91. Semplicini, A., M. Canessa, M. G. Mozzato, G. Ceolotto, A. C. Marzola Pessina, D. Dal Palu. Red blood cell Na/H and Li/Na exchange in subjects with essential hypertension (abstract). *Am. J. Hypertens. 1*(No. 3, Part 2): 61A, 1988.
92. Sempos, C., R. Cooper, M. Trevisan, and J. Stamler. Red cell sodium-lithium countertransport and family history of hypertension. *Clin. Exp. Hypertens. A6:* 1379–1393, 1984.
93. Sharma, C., E. R. Dalferes, D. S. Freedman, A. Asamoah, and G. S. Berenson. Use of 86Rb and 22Na in assaying active and cotransport activities human erythrocytes in a biracial population. *Clin. Chim. Acta 176:* 133–142, 1988.
94. Siffert, W., D. Rosskopf, and U. Osswald. Overexpression of platelet Na+/H+ exchange activity in essential hypertension (abstract). *Am. J. Hypertens. 3:* 58A, 1990.
95. Simmon, D., G. Barbour, J. Congleton, J. Levy, and P. Meacher. Blood pressure and salt

intake in Malawi: an urban-rural study. *J. Epidemiol. Community Health 40:* 188–192, 1986.

96. Simon, G., and D. J. Conklin. In vivo erythrocyte sodium concentration in human hypertension is reduced, not increased. *J. Hypertens. 4:* 71–75, 1986.

97. Sing, C. F., E. Boerwinkle, and S. T. Turner. Genetics of primary hypertension. *Clin. Exp. Hypertens. [A]A8:* 623–651, 1986.

98. Smith, J. B., M. B. Wade, N. S. Feinberg, and M. H. Weinberger. Influence of race, sex and blood pressure on erythrocyte sodium transport in humans. *Hypertension 12:* 251–258, 1988.

99. Songu-Mize, E., B. S. Alpert, and E. S. Willey. Race, sex, and family history of hypertension and erythrocyte sodium pump 3[H]ouabain binding. *Hypertension 15:* 146–151, 1990.

100. Sowers, J. R., M. B. Zemel, P. Zemel, F. W. J. Beck, M. F. Walsh, and E. T. Zawada. Salt sensitivity in blacks. Salt intake and natriuretic substances. *Hypertension 12:* 485–490, 1988.

101. Swales, J. D. Ion transport in hypertension. *Biosci. Rep. 2:* 967–990, 1982.

102. Sweadner, K. J., and S. M. Goldin. Active transport of sodium and potassium ions. *N. Engl. J. Med. 302:* 777–783, 1980.

103. Tobian, I. Jr., and J. T. Binion. Tissue cations and water in arterial hypertension. *Circulation 5:* 754–758, 1952.

104. Tosteson, D. C. Cation countertransport and cotransport in human red cells. *Fed. Proc. 40:* 1429–1433, 1981.

105. Trevisan, M., R. Cooper, D. Ostrow, C. Sempos, and J. Stamler. Red cell cation transport in white and black essential hypertensives. *J. Hypertens. 1:* 245–249, 1983.

106. Trevisan, M., R. Cooper, D. Ostrow, C. Sempos, S. Sparks, and J. Stamler. Red cell cation transport: racial differences between black and white school children. *J. Hypertens. 1:* 245–249, 1983.

107. Trevisan, M., V. Krogh, and the Gubbio Collaborative Study Group. Erythrocyte sodium and potassium content and blood pressure. *Am. J. Hypertens. 2:* 54A, 1989.

108. Trevisan, M., D. Ostrow, R. Cooper, C. Sempos, and J. Stamler. Sex and race differences in sodium-lithium countertransport and red cell sodium concentration. *Am. J. Epidemiol. 120:* 537–541, 1984.

109. Trevisan, M., D. Ostrow, R. Cooper, K. Liu, S. Sparks, A. Okopnek, E. Stevens, J. Marquardt, and J. Stamler. Abnormal red blood cell ion transport and hypertension. The People's Gas Company Study. *Hypertension 5:* 363–367, 1983.

110. Trevisan, M., D. Ostrow, R. Cooper, K. Liu, S. Sparks, and J. Stamler. Methodological assessment of assays for red cell sodium concentration and sodium-dependent lithium efflux. *Clin. Chim. Acta 116:* 319–329, 1981.

111. Tuck, M. L., C. Gross, M. H. Maxwell, A. S. Brickman, G. Krasnoshtein, and D. Mayes. Erythrocyte Na$^+$, K$^+$ cotransport and the Na$^+$, K$^+$ pump in black and Caucasian hypertensive patients. *Hypertension 6:* 536–544, 1984.

112. Turner, S. T., W. H. Weidman, V. V. Michels, T. J. Reed, C. L. Ormson, T. Fuller, and C. F. Sing. Distribution of sodium-lithium countertransport and blood pressure in Caucasians five to eighty-nine years of age. *Hypertension 13:* 378–391, 1989.

113. Tuttle, R. S., and D. P. Boppana. Antihypertensive effect of interleukin-2. *Hypertension 15: 89–94, 1990.*

114. Vincenzi, F. F., A. Lindern, and T. R. Hinds. Elevated intracellular free calcium in red blood cells of human hypertensives: signal of a change in the calcium pump and leak system? *Am. J. Hypertens. 3*(No. 5, Part 2): 52A, 1990.

115. Vincenzi, F. F., C. D. Morris, L. B. Kinsel, M. Kenny, and D. A. McCarron. Decreased calcium pump adenosine triphosphatase in red blood cells of hypertensive subjects. *Hypertension 8:* 1058–1066, 1986.

116. Ward, R. Familial aggregation and genetic epidemiology of blood pressure. In: *Hypertension: Pathophysiology, Diagnosis, and Management,* edited by J. H. Laragh and B. M. Brenner. Raven Press, New York, 1990, pp. 81–100.

117. Weder, A. B. Red-cell lithium-sodium countertransport and renal lithium clearance in hypertension. *N. Engl. J. Med. 314:* 198–201, 1986.

118. Weder, A. B., S. E. Bahadosingh, and G. Heagos. Platelet intracellular pH in essential hypertensives and normotensives. *J. Hypertens. 7*(Suppl 6): S152–S153, 1989.

119. Weder, A. B., B. A. Torretti, and S. Julius. Racial differences in erythrocyte cation transport. *Hypertension 6:* 115–123, 1984.

120. Weinberger, M. H., J. B. Smith, N. S. Fineberg, and F. C. Luft. Red-cell sodium-lithium countertransport and fractional excretion of lithium in normal and hypertensive humans. *Hypertension 13:* 206–212, 1989.

121. Weissberg, P. L., K. L. Woods, M. J. West, and D. G. Beever. Genetic and ethnic influences on the distribution of Na^+ and K^+ in normotensive and hypertensive subjects. *J. Clin. Hypertens. 3:* 20–25, 1987.

122. Williams, R. R., S. C. Hunt, S. H. Hasstedt, P. N. Hopkins, L. L. Wu, T. D. Berry, B. M. Stults, G. K. Barlow, and H. Kuida. Inherited bimodal traits and susceptibility to hypertension in Utah pedigrees. In: *Salt and Hypertension,* edited by R. Rettig, D. Ganten and F. C. Luft. Springer-Verlag, Heidelberg, 1989, pp. 139–155.

123. Woods, K. L., D. G. Beevers, and M. J. West. Racial differences in the red cell cation transport in white and black hypertensives. *Postgrad. Med. J. 57:* 769–771, 1981.

124. Woods, K. L., D. G. Beevers, and M. J. West. Racial differences in red cell cation transport and their relationship to essential hypertension. *Clin. Exp. Hypertens. 3:* 655–662, 1981.

125. Worley, R. J., W. M. Mentscled, Cormier, S. Nutting, G. Pead, K. Zelenov, J. M. Smith, K. O. Ash, and R. R. Williams. Increased sodium-lithium countertransport in erythrocytes of pregnant women. *N. Engl. J. Med. 307:* 412–416, 1982.

126. Wilcox, A. J., and I. T. Russell. Perinatal mortality: standardizing for birth weight is biased. *Am. J. Epidemiol. 118:* 857–864, 1983.

127. Zavoico, G. B., E. J. Cragoe, Jr., and M. B. Feinstein. Regulation of intracellular pH in human platelets. *J. Biol. Chem. 261:* 13160–13167, 1986.

10

(pro)Renin Processing and Secretion in Black Essential Hypertension and Other Low-Renin Syndromes

J.C.S. FRAY

Renin, it is now certain, plays an important role in a significant number of disorders, such as essential hypertension and diabetic hypertension in blacks. These disorders have been categorized along sharp renin lines: high, normal, and low renin subgroups (11,54). Renin initiates the cleavage of angiotensin I, which is subsequently converted to angiotensin II, a potent vasoconstrictor molecule that stimulates aldosterone and vasopressin secretion and salt and water retention. By initiating the cascade, renin is therefore a significant factor in the physiological manifestation of the renin–angiotensin–aldosterone system (RAAS). RAAS plays an important role in cardiovascular homeostasis and chemiosmotic (*salt and water* coupled to proton movement) balance, but renin secretion from the kidney is a key step in the system. There is general agreement that renin physiological inhibition (or its equivalent) provides rational therapeutic efficacy for high-renin essential hypertension (106). Calcium channel blockade has also been shown to provide satisfactory results, even in the low-renin subgroup where earlier therapeutic strategies have proven largely ineffective. In low-renin hypertension (LRH) and diabetic low-renin hypertension (dLRH), characteristic of an increasing number of blacks, only recently has sufficient evidence been accumulated to target specific molecules controlling renin secretion at the cellular level, thereby opening the way for novel approaches to drug development. It is clear that calcium and chemiosmotic forces are central to the control of renin secretion and that the renin profiles observed in some renin disorders may reflect abnormal control at specific sites along the secretory cascade (33). This chapter surveys briefly the current state of knowledge in the low-renin subgroup, as it relates to *renin and prorenin* [(pro)Renin] processing, storage, and secretion. We also focus on theories of (pro)Renin secretion in an attempt to describe the sites of control (and thereby prime targets of abnormal function as evidenced by examples of low-renin syndromes [LRS]) (27), and consider briefly the prospects and sites of action of the most successful therapeutic agents used to address LRH and dLRH.

RENIN PROFILING IN ESSENTIAL AND DIABETIC HYPERTENSION

Renin profiling has played an important role in defining hypertensive humans in general (54). Upwards of 25% of all hypertensives have a low plasma renin activity (PRA) and relative hyporesponsiveness to stimulation (22). Renin profiling has been used as a successful tool in selecting antihypertensive therapy, particularly with regard to calcium and chemiosmotic forces (106). "Varieties" of LRH and dLRH exist (67), and issues of age and sex have some influence, but "race" has been one of the most well discussed characteristics in assessing and targeting low-renin hypertensives.

A greater prevalence of hypertension has long been recognized in human diabetics compared with the nondiabetic population. Christlieb (11) reviewed the epidemiological evidence and concluded that hypertension occurs in 41%–80% of diabetics. Diabetic hypertension falls into one of three types: essential hypertension, which generally complicates late onset diabetes; systolic hypertension secondary to atherosclerosis; and frank "diabetic hypertension," characterized as a form of renal hypertension accompanied by nephropathy. A substantial number of the latter have been termed dLRH and have commanded a fair amount of attention, since understanding the underlying mechanisms of renin hyporesponsiveness may be of importance not only to diabetics but also hypertensives in general (11).

But the renin status has been controversial in diabetics. For example, low (14,50), normal (10,15,35,61,98), and high PRA (5,8,50) have been reported. Responsiveness to relevant secretagogues has also been shown to be varied. To clarify these disparities, Christlieb et al. (15) postulated that in diabetes without nephropathy the renin responsiveness is normal, but with nephropathy it is subnormal. Specifically, diabetic patients with nephropathy are characterized as low renin on account of their low PRA and secretory hyporesponsiveness (11,75,101). The low PRA and renin hyporesponsiveness, it has been postulated, are consequences of decreased renal renin content (11). As will be demonstrated, these may be limited interpretations of the data. To begin with, LRH has been reported with or without diabetes (22) and low-renin diabetes has been observed in human hypertension with (and without) nephropathy, nephropathy with orthostatic hypotension and hypoaldosteronism, and in rodent alloxan diabetes (12). Direct measurements of renal renin content have revealed a remarkably high level, and this has provided the most compelling evidence to reopen the question of renin secretion in diabetes, particularly among blacks, in whom the incidence of this disorder is increasing.

LOW-RENIN HYPERTENSION IN BLACKS

Renin status has played a key role in defining blacks (40,87). Cases of hyperrenin states have been considered, but the majority of blacks are best described by low PRA and renin hyporesponsivity (Fig. 10.1). It is interesting, however, that even among the normotensive population, blacks generally have a lower PRA than whites (87). Even in children (up to 14 years), PRA is lower in blacks. Black hypertensives with lower PRA also have a lower renin secretory respon-

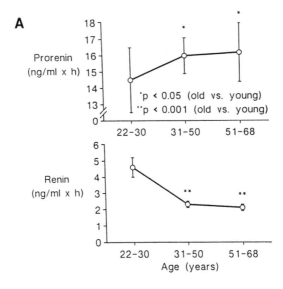

A

Prorenin (ng/ml x h)

*p < 0.05 (old vs. young)
**p < 0.001 (old vs. young)

22-30   31-50   51-68

Renin (ng/ml x h)

22-30   31-50   51-68
Age (years)

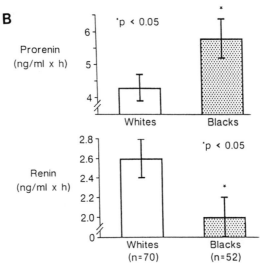

B

Prorenin (ng/ml x h)

*p < 0.05

Whites   Blacks

Renin (ng/ml x h)

*p < 0.05

Whites (n=70)   Blacks (n=52)

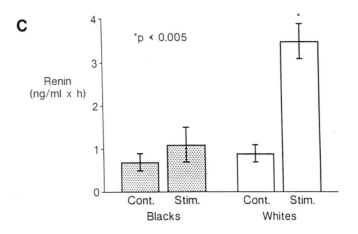

C

*p < 0.005

Renin (ng/ml x h)

Cont.   Stim.   Cont.   Stim.
Blacks   Whites

siveness than whites (Fig. 10.1), and this effect is also prevalent among children. Although some practitioners have called attention to the unwarranted classification of LRH in blacks [especially black women (41)], others have suggested that this form of hypertension, like the advanced stage of renal hypertension (1), is nothing more than a "stage" in the long-term course of essential hypertension. It has been argued that when PRA levels are adjusted for age and race, LRH in blacks (and the elderly) is less common than currently believed (36). The exact reason for the discrepancy is unclear, but whereas some practitioners have pointed to the arbitrariness of the demarcation, others have stressed the importance of accurate measuring technique (91). The majority view, however, is that LRH is a "distinct entity" (22,100), and a feature that best characterizes blacks in the literature and clinical practice.

Several theories have been advanced to explain low renin in black hypertensives. Genetic factors were postulated, but without support or confirmation. Overproduction of a salt-retaining hormone with a consequent plasma volume expansion was also suggested (9). Overproduction of salt-retaining hormones such as aldosterone has been observed in association with LRH, but also in hyperrenin states (4). Although the salt-retaining hormone was suggested to be some other than aldosterone (9), no such hormone has been identified. The presence of a salt-losing hormone has also been proposed (39), but not confirmed (73,74). Plasma volume expansion was predicted for blacks as a result of excess salt intake (9). But it has been shown that even when blacks and whites consume similar amounts of salt (as judged by urinary salt excretion), black hypertensives have a lower PRA (103).

It is generally believed that low PRA and renin hyporesponsivity in blacks is a consequence of volume expansion (9). It is also believed that the volume expansion is a result of chronic excessive salt consumption (9). But, as shown earlier, when blacks and whites are compared in terms of salt ingestion, blacks still have lower PRA (103), suggesting that salt intake alone is insufficient to explain the lower PRA. Furthermore, although plasma volume is demonstrably lower in white hypertensives, plasma volume was insignificantly different in white normotensives and blacks (hypertensive and normotensive) (56). Similar results have been reported for blacks (58). It has been demonstrated that a higher percentage of blacks (43%) than whites (21%) present with volume expansion, and a higher percentage of whites (79%) than blacks (57%) present with volume contraction, but there appears to be no significant difference in level of blood pressure and PRA between volume expanded and volume contracted blacks (16). A similar conclusion has been drawn for whites, providing strong support for the view that "reduction of renin in low-renin hypertension is not brought about by sodium retention with volume expansion" (88).

FIGURE 10.1. Plasma renin and prorenin activity profiles in normal subjects. Values are the mean ± SEM. Statistical significance was determined by unpaired Wilcoxon test. Renin enzymatic activity was measured by RIA and prorenin measured following cryoactivation. *Panel A* shows *renin and prorenin* [(pro)Renin] in a general population sample. *Panel B* shows the (pro)Renin difference in blacks and whites (all normotensives) [Adapted from Sealey et al. (100)]. *Panel C* shows basal PRA (Cont.) and the ineffectiveness of stimulation (Stim.) to raise plasma renin activity in blacks compared with whites.

Impairment at the juxtaglomerular (JG) apparatus has attracted much speculation to account for LRH in blacks. Increased pressure at the JG cells has been one suggestion (47,89). This proposal is in agreement with theory (30), but the predicted pressures have never been measured and the hyporesponsiveness has been demonstrated in isolated JG cells (33), suggesting that the impairment must be downstream from the "baroreceptor" sensor. A number of other factors bear on this proposal. Vascular resistance is inversely related to renin secretion (23,74,89), and black hypertensives have been observed with a markedly high renal resistance (55), in agreement with the biophysical observation that high resistance, low renal blood flow, and low renin secretion are all mediated by high intracellular calcium (Ca_i) (30). Thus, the high Ca_i observed in black hypertensives (19) may in part play a role in the secretory hyporesponsiveness. Another factor is that blacks have been known to have more extensive nephroscleroses than whites (55), and this disease was suggested to account for the impairment in LRH (99). It is true that reduced distensibility of the afferent arteriole reduces renin secretion (30), and it is true that thickening of the afferent arteriole has been demonstrated (97) and therefore may account for the reduced distensibility, but the impairment might be more complex, since it has been demonstrated in vitro without arteriolar integrity (33). Similar arguments may be advanced to disqualify increased salt load at the macula densa, "derangement" of the JG apparatus, decreased sympathetic nervous system activity, interference with generation of angiotensin II, and increased sensitivity to angiotensin II (47).

It is generally believed that the impairment is due to an inability of the JG cell to produce renin. No evidence has been presented to support this hypothesis, and several studies have shown that renin hyporesponsiveness is much more complex than the kidney's inability to "produce" renin (27). Hyporesponsiveness of the β-adrenergic mechanism for renin secretion has been advanced as another reason (57), but recent observations suggest that it is downstream from this mechanism (27). Finally, an endogenous sodium-potassium pump inhibitor has been advanced as a candidate (39), but recent studies failed to support this hypothesis (73,74). Thus, there is at present no confirmed extracellular explanation of LRH in the black population.

One possibility that has received support is that the impairment may be in the "release" mechanism (47). Unfortunately, details of the release mechanism itself were never provided nor did specific proposals for the site and nature of the impairment.

One striking observation in blacks in general is the disproportionately high concentration of prorenin in plasma (90). In blacks, over 74% of circulating total renin in plasma is prorenin (as judged by standards of cryoactivation) (90). Prorenin secretion may (or may not) be constitutive (and therefore unregulated) in blacks as it has been suggested for whites (77), but it is regulated by calcium in model studies (28,76). It is certain, however, that patterns of age and secretory inefficiency most severely attack blacks, such that between the ages of 22 and 68, blacks have a higher plasma prorenin, lower renin, and a more severe impairment in secretory responsiveness to conventional stimuli than whites (Fig. 10.1) and are therefore untreatable in terms of renin responsivity.

On account of their relatively untreatable renin status most patients go untreated. Thus there is now a staggeringly high morbidity and mortality rate in blacks compared with the general population (see Chapter 1, this volume). More refined knowledge of renin secretion, some practitioners argue (7), will hasten the discovery of better therapeutic strategies for blacks, since renin responsiveness is accepted as a basis of therapy choice. We will consider in detail the specific sites of the impairment in the context of the larger framework of generalized renin hyporesponsivity.

LOW-RENIN DIABETIC HYPERTENSION

Several studies have attempted to identify the locus of renin impairment in dLRH. Increased sodium retention (presumably at the macula densa) was suggested as an explanation (5), but this remains controversial because several workers have argued that it is chloride (51) or perhaps osmolality (95) that triggers macula densa control of renin secretion, not sodium. dLRH is also associated with a high exchangeable (or body) sodium, and this has been considered a candidate (5,10). Nevertheless, if sodium is the specific signal for renin secretion in diabetes, then additional evidence is required to assess its significance. Decreased afferent arteriolar distensibility has also been suggested as an explanation (62), since distensibility affects renin secretion (30). However, the magnitude of the effect of decreased distensibility is small compared with other factors (26) and may be insufficient to explain the powerful suppression seen in diabetes. Furthermore, the renin hyporesponsiveness is also observed in cases without alteration of afferent arteriolar distensibility (11). Lack of insulin was also suggested as an explanation for the renin impairment (48,78). In fact, it was suggested that insulin is necessary for the normal renin secretory response (78). This interpretation is at odds with all other studies showing excessive (or normal) renin secretion in diabetes in the absence of insulin (8,35,62). Furthermore, Cohen et al. (17) have shown an inhibitory effect of insulin on renin secretion, which raises serious difficulties for the "insulin-dependent" theory (48,78). Decreased sympathetic nervous system activity has also been postulated as the site of impairment (11,61), but even in isolated perfused kidneys an impairment in renin responsiveness to sympathomimetic agonist was observed (18). In the majority of studies, however, where the renin impairment has been observed, the sympathetic nervous system was normal (5,10,13) or could be activated (11), suggesting that depressed β-adrenergic responsiveness may be one manifestation of some forms of the disease but upstream from a more fundamental impairment. Finally, body fluid volume expansion was suggested as the signal for renin hyporesponsiveness in diabetes (11,12). Indeed, volume expansion has been observed with dLRH (11,13,50); but normal blood volume has also been observed (5,10). Thus, these disparities must be explained and a signal whereby a generalized blood volume expansion leads to renin suppression provided before this factor can be considered further as a serious candidate. Furthermore, the fact that the impairment remains in the isolated kidney weakens the argument for volume expansion to be a strong inhibitory signal (18). Thus, there remains no satisfactory extrarenal signal that accounts for the majority of the data of dLRH.

An intrarenal locus for the impairment has also been postulated. Christlieb (11) suggested that the defect was in renin production and storage (or content). To support this view he showed a decreased renal renin content in alloxan diabetes (11,13), and others have confirmed these findings in streptozotocin-induced diabetes (48). Renal renin content has not been reported in humans until recently, and the results are radically different from animal models, so the results of pharmacologically induced diabetes must be cautiously viewed, since the nephrotoxicity of these agents has been recognized (2,84). The renin profile in streptozotocin-induced diabetes has been shown to be biphasic: increase during the first week of treatment and decrease by the fourth week (50). More recent studies have shown an increased renal renin content with streptozotocin (86). Cohen et al. (18) have shown a striking increase in renal renin content in spontaneously diabetic rats (BioBreeding/ Worcester). Salt deprivation caused a further twofold increase in renal renin content in these rats (18). Thus, decreased renal renin content may not be a general phenomenon in diabetes. Furthermore, the fact that diabetic rats with excess renin are still hyporesponsive to secretagogues (18) suggests that the impairment may be at a step distal to synthesis. The currently available evidence, therefore, suggests that the site of the impairment must be somewhere along the secretory cascade.

The observation that diabetic kidneys secrete less renin per unit secretagogue than nondiabetic kidneys with less content suggests an impairment in the exocytic cascade. In fact, diabetic kidneys release half as much renin though they store twice as much as nondiabetics (18). It has been shown that renin-impaired JG cells engage in supergranular formation and export renin by a mechanism that leaves a large fraction of the renin trapped in the plasma membrane (33). It has been suggested that in this supergranular exocytosis a larger fraction of the exported renin reaches its destination as prorenin (27). It was postulated and subsequently demonstrated that an abundant amount of exported renin in diabetes may be in the proform (20,24,61,105).

Morphological evidence provides the best picture of the renin secretory process during diabetes. Rouiller and Orci (83) have conducted the most impressive series of investigations on intracellular trafficking. The JG cell during diabetes is primed for excess secretory activity (83). This priming includes supergranular formation (or granulopoiesis), renin-binding protein-renin complex in the cytosolic space, and migration to the plasma membrane for export (27). In diabetes, particularly in the spiny mouse where it has been well studied, supergranular formation is the most notable feature (83). Also observed are empty granules that released their secretory content, presumably intracellularly (83). We will focus on the (intra)cellular profile of (pro)Renin in the context of these morphological observations.

THEORIES OF (PRO)RENIN PROCESSING AND SECRETION: SITES OF CONTROL

Exocytosis, either by regulated degranulation (70) or constitutive vesiculation (49), is the conventional secretory theory. Except for a few polypeptide molecules (28), virtually all export is mediated by the exocytic secretory pathway

(49,70). Exocytic degranulation is characterized by injection into the rough endoplasmic reticulum (ER), migration to Golgi stacks, vesiculation at the transface of the Golgi, protogranulation and condensation into mature vesicles (or granules), and subsequent secretion triggered by increased Ca_i, cAMP, or protein kinase C or its intermediates. Constitutive vesiculation occurs by a similar process, except that vesiculation at the Golgi, it is believed, veers off into two separate pathways: one regulated *(exocytosis)* and the other *unregulated* (constitutive) (49). Processing therefore occurs in the rough ER, Golgi, condensation vesicles, and secretory granules to yield only mature secretory products in granules and extracellular environment. Except for a trace of basal precursors being shuttled through the secretory pathway, ER and Golgi do not store mature secretory products (70). The role of the plasma membrane is both transduction of secretory signal from the outside and fusion/fission of granules from inside. Cytosolic soluble space and plasma membrane subfractions are usually devoid of secretory products in conventional exocytic degranulation and constitutive vesiculation.

The renin secretory cascade may be more complex than that outlined in the conventional secretory pathway. The familiar omega images observed in other systems have also been observed in JG cells (83), but this represents only 10% of the chief exocytic feature, fusion (106). Calcium, it is now certain, is an inhibitory signal for renin secretion (32), whereas it is stimulatory in most other systems. The ER, Golgi, and granules are believed to be involved in renin secretion, but ER has been shown to be devoid of signs of heightened activity in hypersecretory states, Golgi has been bypassed in other instances, and the low renin storage in granules remain outstanding divergences from the conventional exocytic degranulation (27). Constitutive vesiculation has been suggested for prorenin (77), but (pro)Renin production (and export) has been shown to be regulated by a variety of factors, including calcium, cAMP, and sodium (34,72,76,82). Furthermore, the appearance of 50%–90% of the (pro)Renin in plasma in the proform represents a significant divergence from what is expected from the conventional secretory pathway (42,90). Taken together, these observations led to the suggestions that in addition to the conventional exocytic pathways, renin export may be by a novel pathway termed *divergence* translocation, the chief feature of which is translocation at the plasma membrane (27). Here we review the role of calcium and chemiosmotic forces in this process.

Signal transduction at the JG cell surface, chemiosmotic activation of secretory granules, and final expulsion at the plasma membrane have now been fairly well characterized (Fig. 10.2). The JG cell assesses its secretory mission by receiving and transducing a wide variety of extracellular signals by modulating Ca_i. These signals include the physical properties of the arteriole (such as stretch and compliance), circulating hormones (and neurohormones) and blood-borne factors, neurogenic inputs (mainly adrenergic, dopaminergic, opiate, and serotonergic systems), and by composition of the urinary fluid in the extracellular space at the level of the macula densa. Other intracellular messengers such as cAMP, cGMP, and prostaglandins have been suggested to be of significance, but where the evidence is available to make critical assessment, these messengers may also operate through calcium (52).

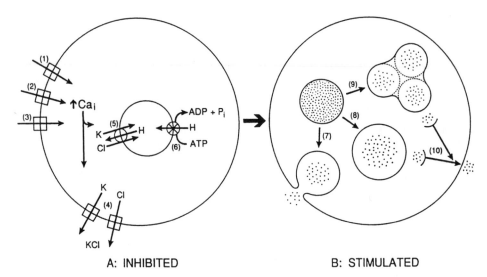

A: INHIBITED   B: STIMULATED

FIGURE 10.2. Calcium and chemiosmotic factors involved in controlling renin secretion from *inhibited* (A) and *stimulated* (B) juxtaglomerular (JG) cells. *Ten* chief features describe the components and the process. Although the presence of voltage-operated calcium channels have also been proposed and their functional features mimic the stretch-activated channels, their role has been questioned and their importance challenged in the context of transporting calcium into JG cells. *A* shows a sequence for inhibiting renin secretion. Ca_i may be increased by activating the *calcium receptor* (1) or by influx through the *stretch-activated* (2) or *receptor-operated* (3) calcium channels. Once Ca_i is elevated it inhibits the *chloride and potassium channels* (4) in the surface membrane and the *potassium chloride-hydrogen antiport-symport exchanger* (5) in the granular membrane. Elevated Ca_i therefore lowers cellular potassium chloride by promoting extrusion of potassium chloride and thereby deprives the granular membrane of the primary substrate and precursor for swelling. The granular membrane also has a *proton ATPase* (6) which is unaffected by Ca_i. *B* shows the two primary pathways effecting renin export. *Granular exocytosis* (7) has been observed, although neither fusion protein nor fusion-motive force has been identified. Both exocytic degranulation and constitutive vesiculation follow this granular exocytic pathway. *Granular swelling* (8) to form *supergranules* has been observed, but *granule-granule fusion* (9) also to form supergranules has been the most widely observed feature of JG cell during stimulation, except those instances of chronic heightened secretory activity where *8* and *9* are rapidly turning over to yield increased renin in cytosol and plasma membrane (10). The renin released from supergranules enters the cytosolic space and is translocated by a process termed *supergranular exocytosis*. The latter process diverges with conventional exocytosis in that both cytosol and plasma membrane play important roles in *divergence translocation*, a process whereby renin (or prorenin) on the cytosolic side is ejected to the extracellular space.

The presence of prorenin in all secretory components, including the plasma membrane, suggests that all considerations of renin secretion must be extended to prorenin, the immediate renin precursor. *Renin and prorenin* may be designated as *(pro)Renin* to highlight the precursor privilege enjoyed by prorenin (impaired processing) while at the same stroke calling attention to renin as the star participant in the renin–angiotensin–aldosterone system. (pro)Renin = total renin, renin + prorenin. This figural definition may also serve as a metaphor of origin in those cases of low-renin syndrome in which the dominant feature is impaired prorenin processing where we immediately see that prorenin is "closed off," *locked-out* (albeit artificially), diverted from complete processing, and thereby fails in its mission of liberating mature renin to the exterior, unless divergance has profound adaptive value. Under normal conditions prorenin is an intracellular operator, whereas renin is the extracellular messenger of the JG cell. Supergranular exocytosis is a divergance pathway. "*Diverge*-1. To go or extend in different directions from a common point [see *7, 8,* and *9*]; branch out. 2. To *differ*, as in opinion or manner. 3. To depart [see *8* and *9*] from a set course or norm [see *7*]; deviate." Thus for (pro)Renin secretion we see images of exocytic degranulation and constitutive vesiculation (7), but we also see confirmed demonstrative signs of supergranular formation (8 and 9) and divergance translocation (10). From Fray (27).

At least three calcium transporting systems have been identified in JG cell plasma membrane in regulating transduction (27). The first is a "calcium receptor" activated by calcium, barium, and strontium, but deactivated by magnesium, lanthanum, and manganese; second, stretch-activated calcium channels that are blocked by magnesium and verapamil; third, receptor-operated calcium channels responsible for transducing hormones and neurohormones. Voltage-operated calcium channels have also been suggested and functional studies have demonstrated their resemblance to stretch-activated calcium channels, but their role in renin secretion is uncertain (52). Entry of calcium through all three pathways leads to an elevation of Ca_i (27). Calcium outflow through a calcium-sodium exchanger and a calcium pump have been shown to be of importance (32).

Two primary targets have been identified for Ca_i inhibition of renin secretion (Fig. 10.2). The first is a potassium chloride translocating system in the plasma membrane (53). The system consists of a calcium-activated chloride channel that promotes the efflux of chloride in the presence of high Ca_i. Chloride outflow through the chloride channel causes membrane depolarization, which activates potassium efflux through an anomalous inward rectifying potassium channel (52). The second mechanism of action of Ca_i is a potassium chloride-hydrogen antiport-symport exchange system in the granular membrane (92). Deactivation of the potassium chloride-hydrogen exchanger requires calcium and a protein, probably calmodulin or protein kinase C, and is central to the renin secretion process (92). The exchange system may have a potassium channel, a chloride channel, a hydrogen channel, potassium-hydrogen exchange as well as a chloride-hydrogen exchanger as functional components (92). The granular membrane also contains a proton pump, but there is no evidence that calcium affects this component (92). Thus, both the cytosolic face of the plasma membrane and the granular membrane emerge as significant sites of control in renin secretion.

A renin translocating system has also been demonstrated in the plasma membrane (27). The system was functionally characterized using isolate preparations of plasma membrane vesicles of inside out orientation. The view is that the renin translocating system has many biochemical features in common with the protein channel in the ER membrane (94). The following summarizes the chief features of the renin translocating system in the JG cell plasma membrane (27,65,66): Renin cleavage is stimulated by trypsin, melittin, kallikrein, phospholipase A_2, lysolecithin, and high salt. The effect of melittin and kallikrein is modified by calcium (29). Calcium and barium increase cleavage, whereas magnesium and manganese decrease cleavage from inside out membrane vesicles. Translocation is affected by calmodulin (in the absence of calcium) and potassium chloride.

LOW-RENIN SYNDROMES AND SITES OF IMPAIRMENT

Low-renin syndrome (LRS) is a newly discovered syndrome, or clustering of syndromes, characterized most profoundly by renal renin hyporesponsivity (27). In some cases basal renin secretion may be normal, but in all cases *stimulated* renin secretion is impaired (27). It is this impairment in secretory responsiveness that best characterizes LRS. The syndrome is associated with renal hypertension (phase III), chronic salt excess, pheochromocytoma (late stages), pituitary deficiency, thyroid deficiency, diabetes mellitus with many of its nephropathies and neuropathies, primary aldosteronism, chronic stress, acromegaly, and an extensive list of other clinical disorders. It is also associated with a new form of hypertension termed Gordon's syndrome; New's syndrome, characterized by an "apparent mineralocorticoid excess" found most prevalently in children; and essential hypertension in blacks (27). LRS is extremely prevalent; one conservative projection is that over 72% of the American population suffers from at least one of the many manifestations of LRS, including hypertension, stroke, renal pathology and eventual failure, heart disease, and intellectual impairment. As demonstrated previously, the renin hyporesponsiveness does not always result from decreased renin production, because in cases such as pheochromocytoma (late stages), diabetes, thyroid deficiency, and pituitary deficiency, renin content is substantially above normal (see below), although secretion is impaired.

Several features characterize LRS at the level of the JG cell (27). The first is maldistribution of renin at the subcellular level. This abnormal subcellular renin profile is the hallmark of all cases of LRS. Second, prorenin is also abnormally distributed at the subcellular level, suggesting impairment in processing. Third, excess prorenin secretion is observed in most cases of LRS including human culture systems. Fourth, there may be defective "renin channels" in rough ER, similar to those for other secretory proteins (94), and in the granular and plasma membranes as well. Renin anchorage to these translocating systems may be peptidic, since cleavage is facilitated by cold stress, proteases, toxins, and ionic washes. Here we will briefly summarize the data supporting these characteristics as demonstrated in blacks and then show their generality in animal models of LRS.

Table 10.1 summarizes renin content in partially purified JG cells from blacks and whites. Renin content was lower in black normotensives than white normotensives, but insignificantly different from white hypertensives. Black hypertensives stored the lowest amount of renin in all groups. What is striking is that black normotensives, although they stored a comparable amount of total renin [(pro)Renin = renin + prorenin]), prorenin storage was 20-fold greater compared with white normotensives. The observation that blacks, at least in the prehypertensive stage, store a lower renin and higher prorenin than whites at a similar stage may explain the lower PRA and higher prorenin in plasma of blacks (see Fig. 10.1). It may be expected, therefore, that blacks, again in the prehypertensive stage, should store more prorenin in secretory granules than whites. Furthermore, blacks should have a different and significantly higher subcellular distribution of prorenin compared with whites, suggesting an impairment in prorenin processing in blacks, even before hypertension develops.

Table 10.1 also summarizes recent observations of renin profiling at the subcellular level in JG cells of whites and blacks. Black normotensives stored a significantly greater amount of (pro)Renin in plasma membrane and light microsomes than all other groups, and black hypertensives stored more in these compartments than whites. Black normotensives also stored a larger

TABLE 10.1. Subcellular Renin and Prorenin Profiles (μg/ml·h/mg protein) in Microsomes of Partially Purified Juxtaglomerular Cells from Kidneys of Whites and Blacks

Origin of kidneys	Crude homogenate		Plasma membrane and light microsomes		ER and Golgi and heavy microsomes		Vesicles and granules	
	Renin	Prorenin	Renin	Prorenin	Renin	Prorenin	Renin	Prorenin
Black normotensive (n = 14)	19.5 ± 3.0	21.9 ± 10.5	7.62 ± 0.14	7.36 ± 2.34	1.44 ± 0.01	7.69 ± 0.08	60.65 ± 5.09	169.02 ± 27.87
White normotensive (n = 4)	50.3 ± 2.9	1.0 ± 0.2	1.10 ± 0.10	1.60 ± 0.50	185.8 ± 6.40	6.70 ± 5.30	29.50 ± 0.60	10.10 ± 0.10
Black hypertensive (n = 4)	1.8 ± 0.2	0.9 ± 0.1	4.00 ± 0.40	3.50 ± 0.30	1.4 ± 0.10	1.50 ± 0.10	1.80 ± 0.10	1.80 ± 0.10
White hypertensive (n = 4)	26.7 ± 4.2	22.9 ± 3.0	1.70 ± 0.10	1.40 ± 0.70	134.4 ± 5.40	291.2 ± 41.8	41.00 ± 7.00	2.60 ± 1.00

Kidneys were supplied by the National Disease Research Interchange (Philadelphia) and processed to yield partially purified juxtaglomerular cells and subcellular microsomal fractions as described previously (92). Briefly, cells were washed in Krebs buffer supplemented with 50 mM KCl, pH 6.5, and then disrupted in a Waring blender for 20 sec and centrifuged at low speed (1000 rpm). The diluted crude homogenate was made isotonic with sucrose, and postnuclear supernatant was prepared by differential centrifugation (1400 × g) on continuous Percoll gradients. Plasma membrane and light microsomes, ER and Golgi and heavy microsomes, and vesicles and granules were all distinguished by density-specific marker beads and appropriate compartment-specific marker enzymes. The number of determinations (n) in this table was obtained from gradients using the pellet from the initial low speed centrifugation. Renin was determined by radioimmunoassay for angiotensin I per ml per hour of incubation per mg of protein. Prorenin was calculated as the difference between trypsin-activated renin and pretrypsinized renin determination.

amount of (pro)Renin in secretory vesicles and mature granules than all other groups, though black hypertensives stored less in these compartments than whites. White normotensives stored a higher renin specific activity in the ER, Golgi, and heavy microsomes than all other groups, though white hypertensives stored the largest (pro)Renin activity in these compartments. In fact, white hypertensives stored a twofold greater (pro)Renin in the ER, Golgi, and heavy microsomal compartment compared with white normotensives and severalfold greater compared with blacks. The data in Table 10.1 suggest that blacks (normotensive and hypertensive) may have a *secretory impairment* both at the level of the plasma membrane and secretory granules, because, at least in the prehypertensive cases, they store more renin in these compartments than other groups, though they secrete less. In the case of black hypertensives, there may be an additional impairment at the site of synthesis, since content was lower, whereas in the case of black normotensives, there may be an additional *impairment in prorenin processing,* since a greater than usual proportion (74%) of cellular prorenin was stored in granules. Unlike blacks in general, whites stored the greatest fraction of (pro)Renin in the ER, Golgi, and heavy microsomes. Secreted protein therefore originates from these compartments by conventional regulated exocytic degranulation and constitutive vesiculation in whites and from other compartments by divergance translocation in blacks. These secretory profiles are important characteristics of LRS (27).

LRS characteristics have also been demonstrated in several animal models (27). Table 10.2 summarizes recent demonstrations of the subcellular renin profiles in pituitary deficiency (surgical), diabetes mellitus (congenital), and thyroid deficiency (surgical). Plasma membrane and light microsomes, ER and Golgi and heavy microsomes, and vesicles and granules store 15%, 13%, and 72%, respectively, of the particulate renin in JG cells from normal rats. Whereas the 15% and 13% are substantially higher than what is expected from studies of other secretory proteins, the 72% in vesicles and granules is substantially lower than what is expected for either exocytic degranulation or constitutive vesiculation. All three models of LRS demonstrate significant renin content in all subcellular compartments (Table 10.2). The demonstrated in-

TABLE 10.2. Subcellular Renin Profile (ng/ml·h/mg protein) in Juxtaglomerular Cells of Rat Models of Low-Renin Syndrome

Condition[a]	Plasma membrane and light microsomes	ER and Golgi transport vesicles	Vesicles and granules
Normal (n = 5)	35 ± 4	29 ± 4	163 ± 5
Pituitary deficiency (n = 4)	1,090 ± 180	430 ± 20	5,783 ± 790
Diabetes mellitus (n = 4)	2,100 ± 23	714 ± 10	983 ± 9
Thyroid deficiency (n = 5)	330 ± 20	1,590 ± 100	4,820 ± 170

Values are mean ± SEM.

TABLE 10.3. Renin Production, Storage, and Export in Low-Renin Syndromes[a]

Condition	Synthesis	Storage	Secretion
Essential hypertension (blacks)	↓	↓	↓
Diabetes mellitus	↑	↑	↓
Thyroid deficiency	↑	↑	↓
Pituitary deficiency	↑	↑	↓
Pheochromocytoma (advanced stage)	↑	↑	↓
Renovascular hypertension (phase III)	↑	↑	↓
Chronic salt excess	↓	↓	↓

[a]Clinical disorders classified as low-renin syndromes and their status in terms of synthesis, storage, and secretion of renin. ↑, increase; ↓, decrease.

creased renin content in all secretory compartments and the associated low rate of secretion suggest significant impairment (27).

Three sites of potential impairment have now been identified in LRS (Table 10.3). The first is the secretory cascade, since renin secretion is reduced in all cases of LRS. Ca_i has been shown to be a universal intracellular messenger regulating renin secretion (32). It may not be unreasonable, therefore, to expect that disorders in cellular calcium metabolism should precipitate LRS. The three phases of renovascular hypertension have been shown to be functions of (intra)cellular calcium management (30; see Chapter 11, this volume), so impairment of any of these cellular components of calcium flux and storage is expected to alter renin secretion. Salt loading has been shown to raise Ca_i and precipitate LRS, whereas salt depletion lowers Ca_i (108) and restores renin secretory responsiveness (25). Essential hypertension in blacks has been characterized by a generalized increase in Ca_i (19), but the exact transport systems affected have not all been accounted for, though ionic sodium-hydrogen, sodium-calcium, sodium-lithium, sodium-potassium, etc. have been under investigation (19). Cellular control of renin secretion in model systems suggests that at the plasma membrane a calcium receptor, calcium channels, sodium-calcium, potassium-hydrogen, and chloride-hydrogen exchangers, calcium pump, potassium channel, and chloride channel may play significant roles, but the importance of these systems has not been explored in blacks. Some studies implicate impaired sodium transporting systems at the core of hypertension in blacks, but even at the genetic level the problem remains unresolved (37). Calcium-regulating hormones such as vitamin D, parathyroid hormone, and calcitonin have all been implicated and shown to affect renin secretion, but their role in LRS is uncertain (81). Thus, some site(s) along the secretory cascade is impaired in LRS, except where the impairment may be upstream at production.

Renin storage is the second site of potential impairment in LRS (Table 10.3). Granular storage (approximately 100% of cellular content) is usually expected in most conventional secretory systems. Calcium is known to play an important role in conventional exocytosis. In renin secretion, calcium also plays an important role at the (semi)final regulatory site in the cascade of supergranule exocytosis, the granular membrane (92). Calcium deactivates an ion exchanger in the granular membrane believed to exchange potassium chloride for protons (92). The exchanger is sensitive to subtle changes in potassium chloride, and acid-base balance. Thus disorders associated with (cellular) acidosis or alkalosis (some forms of diabetes mellitus, primary aldosteronism, and Cushing's syndrome) may be expected to precipitate LRS by affecting renin secretion at the level of the granular membrane. The potassium chloride-hydrogen exchange system in the granular membrane has been suggested to be one site of action of calcium-regulatory proteins such as protein kinase C and calmodulin (92). Unfortunately, not much is known of the renin secretory granule in disease, at least at a functional level. At an anatomical level, renin granules flourish in many different cases of LRS (3,83). At the granular membrane, several components may be targets of impairment: potassium-hydrogen, and chloride-hydrogen exchangers, hydrogen pump, potassium, chloride, and hydrogen channels (92). Research is now required to bring to light the biochemical features of these molecules in LRS, particularly in blacks, because, at least in the prehypertensive stage, blacks store an unusually large amount of (pro)Renin in granules, though they secrete less.

The molecular events from renin synthesis to storage may be sites of impairment, but only in a few restricted cases of LRS (Table 10.3). In Dahl's salt-sensitive rats, the impairment has been identified at the level of the renin genome (80). In experimental renovascular hypertension, where the contralateral kidney remains untouched, renin synthesis decreases in the kidney exposed to hypertension but increases in the kidney seeing hypotension (38). It is unclear whether renal perfusion pressure itself, or stretch of the JG cells, is a stimulus for renin synthesis, but it is certain that stretching the JG cells themselves controls secretion (29). It is unclear, however, whether renin hyporesponsiveness in renal ischemia may be explained solely on the basis of decreased renin synthesis, because an increased secretion of prorenin has been reported from this as well as other cases of LRS (20,21,43,68,69,77), suggesting an impairment in processing rather than synthesis. Indeed, a constitutive pathway where the impairment is in sorting at the Golgi, which diverts prorenin processing from supergranular formation to constitutive vesiculation, was proposed (77). That 50%–99% of the secreted renin in various cases of LRS is exported as prorenin suggests that exocytic constitutive vesiculation bypasses granulopoiesis (77). But in at least one case of LRS, granulopoiesis is a predominant feature of the JG cell (3,83). Furthermore, in cases such as hypothyroidism (6), pituitary deficiency (93), and diabetes mellitus (18), there is a demonstrative renin hyporesponsivity accompanied by an enhanced renin production. It is unlikely, therefore, that depressed renin synthesis is a generalized feature of LRS.

Chronic salt loading, and perhaps direct hypertension, is the only well-documented case of LRS where decreased synthesis is a significant site of impairment (Table 10.3). In salt loading in rats, LRS is associated with a decreased synthesis (25,63), but this decrease is insufficient to explain the complete impairment. For example, renin secretion is fixed at a basal level and secretory responsiveness is completely abolished in salt loading, despite only a moderate decrease in synthesis and storage (25). The lower renin storage in black hypertensives may be used as provisional evidence to conclude, at least tentatively, that synthesis is suppressed in this subgroup, though the possibility of increased degradation has not been excluded.

Renin release from granules and subsequent export across the plasma membrane remains the most likely pathway for significant impairment in LRS. In advanced renovascular hypertension (phase III of the clipped kidney), pheochromocytoma, pituitary deficiency, and diabetes mellitus where confirmed evidence has been provided, the steps leading to synthesis, sorting, targeting, and storage appear highly developed, and the morphological as well as functional picture support vigorous supergranular exocytosis, but the renin exported is far below that which is expected under normal conditions (3,18,31,33,38,83). Detailed studies in one case of LRS show the chronic nature of the impairment (33,93). Even in in vitro studies of isolated kidneys, isolated JG cells, isolated renin granules, and isolated plasma membrane vesicles, the impairment persists (33). These latter studies clearly identified the renin granule and the cytosolic face of the plasma membrane as key potential sites of impairment. Attacking the plasma membrane with growth hormone abolishes the impairment (93). In fact, growth hormone treatment renders the JG cell hyperresponsive to stimulation (93), although the specific component in the membrane activated by growth hormone remains unidentified.

The cytosol is of some significance in LRS. Since transporting molecules and certain renin convertases have been postulated in supergranular exocytosis (27), several studies have shown the presence of a renin binding protein (RnBP) in the cystolic space, and this RnBP has been suggested to be an important cellular protective measure in renin pathologies, although LRS was never mentioned specifically (44,60,85,102,107). Although the gene for at least one RnBP has been identified and cloned (52), there are still insufficient data to assess the importance of RnBP in LRS. A prorenin convertase has also been identified (46,79). The exact location and identity of the convertase remain uncertain, though kallikrein has been shown to be effective (21,79). The effect of kallikrein is calcium-dependent (29) and directed specifically to renin in the plasma membrane (65,66). Stroke-prone spontaneously hypertensive rats have been shown to be deficient in the convertase, and this has been advanced as the chief reason for the high prorenin in this model (46). The role of the convertase is to cleave the prosegment from the prorenin molecule (46). These isolated instances add to the growing body of evidence implicating sorting, targeting, and further processing as key sites of impairment in LRS. They also show that by developing an elaborate system of supergranular exocytosis, the JG cell supports a vigorous secretory repertoire during LRS. Morris (59) has considered the molecular steps involved in great detail.

Table 10.4 summarizes the possible sites of impairment that have so far been identified in LRS. In blacks with essential hypertension, storage and secretion are low, suggesting low synthesis as well, though direct measurements are unavailable with respect to synthesis. In diabetes, thyroid and pituitary deficiencies, pheochromocytoma, and the late stages of renovascular hypertension, both synthesis and storage are high, but secretion is low. Aside from es-

TABLE 10.4. Sites (Potential) of Impairment[a] in Juxtaglomerular Cells of Black Essential and Diabetic Hypertension

Transduction at the plasma membrane
1. Ca^{2+} receptor

2. Stretch-activated Ca^{2+} channels

3. Receptor-operated Ca^{2+} channels

4. Ca^{2+}-Na^+ exchanger

5. Ca^{2+} pump

6. K^+ channel

7. Cl^- channel

8. K^+-H^+ exchanger

9. Cl^--H^+ exchanger

Regulation at the renin granular membrane
1. K^+Cl^--H^+ exchanger

2. H^+ pump

3. K^+-H^+ exchanger

4. Cl^--H^+ exchanger

5. K^+ channel

6. Cl^- channel

7. H^+ channel

Regulation of processing (synthesis, targeting, and storage)
1. cDNA and mRNA

2. Signal receptor in ER and elsewhere

3. Prorenin convertase

4. Renin channel in ER and elsewhere

5. Renin binding protein

[a]The table shows at least 21 components subjected to potential impairment in the juxtaglomerular cells of blacks.
Modified from Fray (27).

sential hypertension in blacks, chronic salt loading is the only case where the impairment appears to be at the levels of synthesis, storage, and secretion (see Table 10.3). Biochemical characterization of the functional components summarized in Table 10.4 are now required for a more complete description of (pro)Renin impairment in blacks.

SUMMARY AND OUTLOOK

Analysis of low-renin hypertension and diabetic hypertension in blacks suggests several striking similarities with other low-renin syndromes. First, the low PRA signifies an impairment in renin secretion, which most likely results from abnormal JG cell secretory function. Second, the impairment is most likely of intracellular origin and is downstream from signal transduction at the JG cell plasma membrane, at least in most cases of LRS. Components of signal transduction such as calcium translocation systems may however, be impaired in blacks. Third, reduced cellular renin content is not responsible for the low PRA, because in most cases a significantly elevated renin content has been observed, although there may be a few exceptions. Blacks in the prehypertensive stage store a significant amount of renal renin, though secretion is generally lower. Fourth, cellular renin *redistribution and improper processing* may play a role, as evidenced by the disproportionately large amounts of (pro)Renin in granules and plasma membrane compartments of blacks, at least in the prehypertensive stage. Fifth, prorenin is the predominant species secreted in blacks, at least in the prehypertensive stage, and this species may originate from granules. Sixth, the unusually large fraction of prorenin presence in secretory granules and plasma membrane provides strong evidence favoring impaired prorenin processing in blacks, at least in the prehypertensive stage, and in other low-renin syndromes. Seventh, although constitutive vesiculation and exocytic degranulation may play important roles in some systems, divergence translocation may be of central importance in blacks, and perhaps other cases of LRS as well (27).

The following sites of the (pro)Renin secretory pathway may be impaired in blacks and in other cases of LRS (Table 10.4): transduction and translocation at the plasma membrane, chemiosmotic regulation at granular membrane, and regulation of production and processing. The plasma membrane's role in the transport of ions and transduction of secretory signals is well recognized. Abnormality in a variety of ion transport systems has been established in blacks (19). The significant amount of (pro)Renin in the plasma membrane of blacks and other cases of LRS suggests that this is a site of impairment in (pro)Renin translocation through the divergence secretory pathway (27). Granular storage appears intact in blacks (see Table 10.1). However, granular release of (pro)Renin may be severely impaired. Aside from the control of granular release by calcium, several chemiosmotic components may be impaired in the granular compartment to account for the excess storage and sparse secretion. Functional characteristics of these molecules have been described (27). Research is now necessary to characterize the biochemical features of the molecules responsible for the impairment. The (pro)Renin production system involves the ER and Golgi. These sites of synthesis, sorting, and segregating may be impaired in blacks, as evidenced by the unusually large amount of subcellular renin appearing in this subfraction (see Table 10.1), at least in the prehypertensive stage.

Sites of control are not unusually sites of impairment, and consequently sites of therapeutic attack. The key role of the plasma membrane, both in calcium signal transduction and renin divergence translocation, suggests that therapeutic agents such as "high-ceiling" loop diuretics (71), may attack at least one site of impairment. These as well as other therapeutic interventions in blacks have relied mainly on blood pressure as assay (106), rather than renin secretory responsiveness. The evidence presented in this chapter strongly suggests that renin secretory responsiveness should be a more accurate measure of the effectiveness of diuretics in blacks, because one mechanism of action is the plasma membrane of JG cells (71). The over nine specific sites of regulation at the plasma membrane of the JG cell, the over seven sites at the granular membrane, and the over five sites identified in the regulation of production and processing, suggest a broad spectrum for therapeutic attack, because some of these sites have already been identified as sites of impairment in blacks as well as other cases of LRS. The stage is now set for therapeutic intervention at several sites of (pro)Renin production, storage, and export in blacks as well as in other disorders classified as LRS.

REFERENCES

1. Abe, K., N. Irokawa, H. Aoyagi, M. Seino, M. Yasujima, K. Ritz, T. Ito, S. Chiba, Y. Sakurai, K. Saito, T. Kusaka, Y. Otsuka, S. Miyazaki, and K. Yoshinaga. Low renin hypertension: is it a stage of essential hypertension? *Tohoku J. Exp. Med. 121:* 347–354, 1977.
2. Bailey, C. C., O. T. Bailey, and R. S. Leech. Alloxan diabetes with diabetic complications. *N. Engl. J. Med. 230:* 533–536, 1944.
3. Barajas, L. The development and ultrastructure of the juxtaglomerular cell granule. *J. Ultrastruct. Res. 15:* 400–413, 1966.
4. Bartter, F. C., P. Pronoue, J. R. Gill, R. C. McCardle. Hyperplasia of the juxtaglonerular complex with hyperaldosteronism and hypokalemic alkalosis: a new syndrome. *Am. J. Med. 33:* 811–828, 1962.
5. Beretta-Picesli, C., P. Weidmann, W. Ziegler, Z. Gluck, and G. Kensch. Plasma catecholamines and renin in diabetes mellitus: relationships with posture, age, sodium, and blood pressure. *Klin. Wochenschr. 57:* 681–691, 1979.
6. Bouhnik, J., F. X. Galen, E. C. Clauser, J. Menard, and P. Corvol. The renin-angiotensin system in thyroidectomized rats. *Endocrinology 108:* 647–650, 1981.
7. Brunner, H. R., J. Nussberger, and B. Waeber. Responsiveness of renin secretion: a key mechanism in the maintenance of blood pressure. *J. Hypertens. 4*(Suppl. 4): S89–S94, 1986.
8. Burden, A. C., and H. Thurston. Plasma renin activity in diabetes mellitus. *Clin. Sci. 56:* 255–259, 1979.
9. Channick, B. J., E. V. Adlin, A. D. Marks. Suppressed plasma renin activity in hypertension. *Arch. Intern. Med. 123:* 131–140, 1969.
10. Chatel, R. D., P. Weidmann, J. Flammer, W. H. Ziegler, C. Beretta-Piccoli, W. Vetter, and F. C. Reubi. Sodium, renin, aldosterone, catecholamines, and blood pressure in diabetes mellitus. *Kidney Int. 12:* 412–421, 1977.
11. Christlieb, A. R. Diabetes and hypertensive vascular disease. *Am. J. Cardiol. 32:* 592–606, 1976.
12. Christlieb, A. R. Renin–angiotensin–aldosterone system in diabetes mellitus. *Diabetes 25* (Suppl. 2): 820–825, 1976.
13. Christlieb, A. R. Renin, angiotensin, and norepinephrine in alloxan diabetes. *Diabetes 23:* 962–970, 1974.
14. Christlieb, A. R., A. Kaldany, J. A. D'Elia. Plasma renin activity and hypertension in diabetes mellitus. *Diabetes 25:* 969–974, 1976.
15. Christlieb, A. R., A. Kaldany, J. A. D'Elia, and G. H. Williams. Aldosterone responsiveness in patients with diabetes mellitus. *Diabetes 27:* 732–737, 1978.
16. Chrysant, S. G., K. Danisa, D. C. Kem, B. L. Dillard, W. J. Smith, and E. D. Frohlich. Racial differences in pressure, volume and renin interrelationships in essential hypertension. *Hypertension 1:* 136–141, 1979.
17. Cohen, A. J., P. Laurens, and J. C. S. Fray. Suppression of renin secretion by insulin: dependence on extracellular calcium. *Am. J. Physiol 245 (Endocrinol Metab. 8):* E531–E534, 1983.
18. Cohen, A. J., K. McCarthy, R. R. Rossetti. Renin secretion by the spontaneously diabetic rat. *Diabetes 35:* 341–346, 1986.
19. Cooper, R. S., and J. L. Borke. Intracellular ions and hypertension in blacks. In: *Pathophysiology of Hypertension in Blacks*, edited by J. C. S. Fray and J. G. Douglas. Oxford University Press, New York, 1992.
20. Deleiva, A., A. R. Christlieb, J. C. Melby, C. A. Graham, R. P. Day, J. A. Luetscher, and R. G. Zager. Big renin and biosynthetic defect of aldosterone in diabetes mellitus. *N. Engl. J. Med. 295:* 639–643, 1976.
21. Derky, F. H. M., G. J. Wenting, A. J. Manl'TVeld, R. P. Verhoeven, and M. A. D. H. Schalekamp. Evidence for activation of circulating inactive renin by the human kidney. *Clin. Sci. 56:* 115–120, 1979.

22. Dunn, M. J., and R. L. Tannen. Low-renin hypertension. *Kidney Int. 5:* 317–325, 1974.
23. Fagard, R., A. Amery, T. Reybrouck, P. Lijnen, L. Billiet, and J. V. Jossens. Plasma renin levels and systemic haemodynamics in essential hypertension. *Clin. Sci. Molec. Med. 52:* 591–597, 1977.
24. Franken, A. A. M., F. H. M. Derky, A. J. ManI'tVeld, W. C. J. Hop, G. H. Rens, E. Peperkamp, P. T. V. M. Dejohn, and M. A. D. H. Schalekamp. High plasma prorenin in diabetes mellitus and its correlation with some complications. *J. Clin. Endocrinol. Metab. 71:* 1008–1015, 1990.
25. Fray, J. C. S. Mechanism of increased renin release during sodium deprivation. *Am. J. Physiol. 234 (Renal Fluid Electrolyte Physiol. 4):* F376–F380, 1978.
26. Fray, J. C. S. Stimulus-secretion coupling of renin: role of hemodynamic and other factors. *Circ. Res. 47:* 485–492, 1980.
27. Fray, J. C. S. Regulation of renin secretion by calcium and chemiosmotic forces: (patho) physiological considerations. *Biochim. Biophys. Acta* 1097: 243–262, 1991.
28. Fray, J. C. S. Subcellular dysregulation of renin and prorenin expression in black essential and diabetic hypertensives. *Ethnicity Dis. 2:* 142–157, 1992.
29. Fray, J. C. S., and D. J. Lush. Stretch receptor hypothesis for renin secretion: the role of calcium. *J. Hypertens.* 2(Suppl. 1): 19–23, 1984.
30. Fray, J. C. S., D. J. Lush, C. S. Park. Interrelationship of blood flow, juxtaglomerular cells, and hypertension: role of physical equilibrium and Ca. *Am. J. Physiol. 251 (Regulatory Fluid Electrolyte Physiol. 20):* R643–R662, 1986.
31. Fray, J. C. S., and P. V. H. Mayer. Decreased plasma renin activity and renin release in rats with phaeochromocytoma. *Clin. Sci. Molec. Med. 53:* 447–452, 1977.
32. Fray, J. C. S., C. S. Park, and A. N. D. Valentine. Calcium and the control of renin secretion. *Endocr. Rev. 8:* 53–93, 1987.
33. Fray, J. C. S., and S. M. Russo. Mechanism for low renin in blacks: studies in hypophysectomised rat model. *J. Hum. Hypertens. 4:* 160–162, 1990.
34. Ginesi, L. M., K. A. Munday, and A. R. Noble. Secretion control for active and inactive renin: effects of calcium and potassium on rabbit kidney cortex slices. *J. Physiol. 344:* 453–463, 1983.
35. Gossain, V. V., E. E. Werk, L. J. Sholiton, L. Srivastava, and H. C. Knowles. Plasma renin activity in juvenile diabetes mellitus and effect of diazoxide. *Diabetes 28:* 833–835, 1975.
36. Grim, C. E., F. C. Luft, N. S. Fineberg, and M. H. Weinberger. Responses to volume expansion and contraction in categorized hypertensive and normotensive man. *Hypertension 1:* 476–485, 1979.
37. Grim, C. E., and T. W. Wilson. Salt, slavery and survival: physiological principles underlying the evolutionary hypothesis of salt sensitive hypertension in Western Hemisphere blacks. In: *Pathophysiology of Hypertension in Blacks,* edited by J. C. S. Fray and J. G. Douglas. Oxford University Press, New York, 1992.
38. Gross, F., A. J. Vander, R. D. Bunag, and G. M. C. Masson. Renin content of kidneys. In: *Renal Hypertension,* edited by I. E. Page and J. W. McCubbin. Year Book Publishers, Chicago, 1968, pp. 118–133.
39. Haddy, F. J. Sodium-potassium pump in low-renin hypertension. *Ann. Intern. Med. 93* (part 2): 781–784, 1983.
40. Helmer, O. M. The renin-angiotensin system and its relation to hypertension. *Progr. Cardiovasc. Dis. 8:* 117–128, 1965.
41. Holland, O. B., C. Gomez-Sanchez, C. Fairchild, and N. M. Kaplan. Role of renin classification for diuretic treatment of black hypertensive patients. *Arch. Intern. Med. 139:* 1365–1370, 1979.
42. Hsueh, W. A. Potential effects of renin activation on the regulation of renin production. *Am. J. Physiol. 247 (Renal Fluid Electrolyte Physiol. 16):* F205–F212, 1984.
43. Hsueh, W. A., E. J. Carlson, and V. J. Dzau. Characterization of inactive renin from human kidney and plasma. *J. Clin. Invest. 71:* 506–517, 1983.
44. Ikemoto, F., K. Takaori, H. Iwao, and K. Yamamoto. Intrarenal localization of renin binding substance in rats. *Life Sci. 31:* 1011–1016, 1982.
45. Inoue, H., K. Fukui, S. Takahashi, and Y. Miyake. Molecular cloning and sequence analysis of a CDNA encoding a procine kidney renin-binding protein. *J. Biol. Chem. 265:* 6556–6561, 1990.
46. Itoh, S., M. Tanaka, F. Ikemoto, K. Yamamoto, N. Morita, and K. Okamoto. Renal high-molecular-weight renin: unusual formation in the aged stroke-prone spontaneously hypertensive rats. *Renal Physiol. 9:* 177–186, 1986.
47. Jose, A., J. R. Crout, and N. M. Kaplan. Suppressed plasma renin activity in essential hypertension. Roles of plasma volume, blood pressure, and sympathetic nervous system. *Ann. Intern. Med. 72:* 9–16, 1970.

48. Katayama, S., and J. B. Lee. Hypertension in experimental diabetes mellitus: renin-prostaglandin interaction. *Hypertension 7:* 554–561, 1985.
49. Kelly, R. B. Pathways of protein secretion in eukaryotes. *Science 230:* 25–32, 1985.
50. Kikkawa, R., E. Kitamura, Y. Fujiwara, M. Haneda, and Y. Shigeta. Biphasic alteration of renin–angiotensin–aldosterone system in streptozotocin-diabetic rats. *Renal Physiol. 9:* 187–192, 1986.
51. Kotchen, T. A., W. J. Welch, J. N. Lorenz, and C. E. Ott. Renal tubular chloride and renin release. *J. Lab. Clin. Med. 110:* 533–540, 1987.
52. Kurtz, A. Cellular control of renin secretion. *Rev. Physiol. Biochem. Pharmacol. 113:* 1–40, 1989.
53. Kurtz, A., and R. Penner. Angiotensin II induces oscillations of intracellular calcium and blocks anomalous inward rectifying potassium current in mouse renal juxtaglomerular cells. *Proc. Natl. Acad. Sci. U.S.A. 86:* 3423–3427, 1989.
54. Laragh, J. H. Vasoconstriction-volume analysis for understanding and treating hypertension: the use of renin and aldosterone profiles. *Am. J. Med. 55:* 261–274, 1973.
55. Levy, S. B., L. B. Talner, M. N. Coel, R. Holle, and R. A. Stone. Renal vasculature in essential hypertension: racial differences. *Ann. Intern. Med. 88:* 12–16, 1978.
56. Lilley, J. J., L. Hsu, and R. A. Stone. Racial disparity of plasma volume in hypertensive man. *Ann. Intern. Med. 84:* 707–708, 1976.
57. Lowder, S. C., P. Hamet, and G. W. Liddle. Contrasting effects of hypoglycemia on plasma renin activity and cyclic adenosin 3′,5′-monophosphate (cyclic AMP) in low renin and normal renin essential hypertension. *Circ. Res. 38:* 105–108, 1976.
58. Mitas, J. A., R. Holle, S. B. Levey, and R. A. Stone. Racial analysis of the volume-renin relationship in human hypertension. *Arch. Intern. Med. 139:* 157–160, 1979.
59. Morris, B. J. New possibilities for intracellular renin and inactive renin now that the structure of the human renin gene has been elucidated. *Clin. Sci. 71:* 345–355, 1986.
60. Murakami, K., S. Chino, S. Hirose, and J. Higaki. Specificity and localization of renin-binding protein(s). *Biomed. Res. 1:* 476–481, 1980.
61. Nakamaru, M., T. Ogihara, J. Higaki, K. Masuo, H. Ikegami, K. Shima, and Y. Kumahara. Plasma inactive renin in diabetic patients with neuropathy: a role for the sympathetic nervous system in the conversion in vivo of inactive renin. *Acta Endocrinol. 104:* 216–221, 1983.
62. Nakamura, R., T. Saruta, K. Yamagami, I. Saito, K. Kondo, S. Matsuki. Renin and the juxtaglomerular apparatus in diabetic nephropathy. *J. Am Geriatr. Soc. 26:* 17–21, 1978.
63. Nakane, H., Y. Nakane, P. Corvol, and J. Menard. Sodium balance and renin regulation in rats: role of intrinsic renal mechanisms. *Kidney Int. 17:* 607–614, 1980.
64. New, M. I. The role of steroid hormones in the development of low-renin hypertension in childhood. NHLBI Workshop on Juvenile Hypertension, May, pp. 283–304, 1983.
65. Nishimura, K., F. Alhenc-Gelas, A. White, and E. G. Erdos. Activation of membrane-bound kallikrein and renin in the kidney. *Proc. Natl. Acad. Sci. U.S.A. 77:* 4975–4978, 1980.
66. Nishimura, K., P. Ward, and E. G. Erdos. Kallikrein and renin in the membrane fractions of the rat kidney. *Hypertension 2:* 538–545, 1980.
67. Nugent, C. A. Varieties of low renin hypertension. *Milit. Med. 141:* 519–522, 1977.
68. Ogawa, K., M. Matsunaga, H. Nagai, A. Hara, C. H. Pak, and C. Kawai. Effects of enalapril maleate on plasma level of inactive renin in renovascular hypertension. *Clin. Exp. Hypertens. [A] A7:* 995–1005, 1985.
69. Ogawa, K., C. Nagai, C. H. Pak, C. Kawai, M. Matsunaga, and A. Hara. Studies on the active and inactive renin in reovascular hypertension. *Clin. Exp. Hypertens. [A] A6:* 1641–1651, 1984.
70. Palade, G. Intracellular aspects of the process of protein synthesis. *Science 189:* 347–358, 1975.
71. Park, C. S., P. S. Doh, R. E. Carraway, G. C. Chung, J. C. S. Fray, and T. B. Miller. Stimulation of renin secretion by ethacrymc acid is independent of Na^+-K^+-$2Cl^-$ cotransport. *Am. J. Physiol. 259: (Renal Fluid Electrolyte Physiol. 28):* F539–F544, 1990.
72. Park, C. S., T. W. Honeyman, E. S. Chung, J. S. Lee, D. H. Sigmon, and J. C. S. Fray. Involvement of calmodulin in mediating inhibitory action of intracellular Ca^{2+} on renin secretion. *Am. J. Physiol. 251 (Renal Fluid Electrolyte Physiol. 20):* F1055–F1062, 1986.
73. Pedrinelli, R., A. Clerico, L. Graziadei, S. Teddei, M. D. Chicca, and A. Saluetti. Lack of evidence for NaK-ATPase inhibitor as a cause of low renin human hypertension. *J. Hypertens. 4* (Suppl. 6): 340–342, 1986.
74. Pedrinelli, R., S. Taddei, L. Graziadei, and A. Salvetti. Vascular responses to ouabain and

norepinephrine in low and normal renin hypertension. *Hypertension 8:* 786–792, 1986.

75. Perez, G. O., L. Lespier, J. Jacobi, J. R. Oster, F. H. Katz, C. A. Vaamonde, and L. M. Fishman. Hyporeninemia and hypoadosteronism in diabetes mellitus. *Arch. Intern. Med. 137:* 825–855, 1977.

76. Pinet, F., J. Mizrahi, I. Laboulandine, J. Menard, and P. Corvol. Regulation of prorenin secretion in cultured human transfected juxtaglomerular cells. *J. Clin. Invest. 80:* 724–731, 1987.

77. Pratt, R. E., J. E. Carleton, J. P. Richie, C. Heusser, and V. J. Dzau. Human renin biosynthesis and secretion in normal and ischemic kidneys. *Proc. Natl. Acad. Sci. U.S.A. 84:* 7837–7840, 1987.

78. Pratt, J. H., C. A. Parkinson, M. H. Weinberger, and W. C. Duckworth. Decreases in renin and aldosterone secretion in alloxan diabetes: an effect of insulin deficiency. *Endocrinology 116:* 1712–1716, 1985.

79. Purdon, A. D., A. Y. Loh, and D. H. Osmond. Renin substrate (angiotensinogen) preparations in the determination of prorenin and renin: evidence for extrarenal plasma prorenin and its renal "convertase." *Can. J. Physiol. Pharmacol. 65:* 2319–2328, 1987.

80. Rapp J. P., and S.-M. Wang. Genetic hypertension: classical and molecular genetic concepts as applied to the renin gene. In: *Hypertension,* edited by J. H. Laragh and B. M. Brenner. Raven Press, New York, 1990, pp. 955–964.

81. Resnick, L. M., and J. H. Laragh. Renin, calcium metabolism and the pathophysiologic basis of antihypertensive therapy. *Am. J. Cardiol. 56:* 68H–74H, 1985.

82. Richards, H. K., D. J. Lush, A. R. Noble, and K. A. Munday. Inactive renin in rabbit plasma: effect of furosemide. *Clin. Sci. 60:* 393–398, 1981.

83. Rouiller, C., and L. Orci. The structure of the juxtaglomerular complex. In: *The Kidney, Morphology, Biochemistry, Physiology,* Vol. 4, edited by C. Rouiller and A. F. Muller. Academic Press, New York, 1971, pp. 1–80.

84. Sadoff, L. Neprotoxicity of streptozotocin. *Cancer Chemother. 54:* 457–459, 1970.

85. Sagnella, G. A., P. R. B. Caldwell, and W. S. Peart. Subcellular distribution of low- and high-molecular-weight renin and its relation to a renin inhibitor in pig renal cortex. *Clin. Sci. 59:* 337–345, 1980.

86. Sakamoto, W., K. Yoshikawa, A. Yokoyama, M. Kohri, H. Handa, S. Ueham, A. Hirayama, and H. Izumi. Glandular kallikrein, renin and tonin in tissues of diabetic and hypertensive rats. *J. Clin. Chem. Clin. Biochem. 24:* 437–440, 1986.

87. Saunders, E. Hypertension in blacks. *Med. Clin. North Am. 71:* 1013–1029, 1987.

88. Schalekamp, M. A., M. Lebel, D. G. Beevers, R. Fraser, G. Kolster, and W. H. Birkenhager. Body fluid-volume in low-renin hypertension. *Lancet 1:* 310–311, 1974.

89. Schalekamp, M. A. D. H., M. P. A. Schalekamp-Kuyken, and W. H. Birkenhager. Abnormal renal haemodynamics and renin suppression in hypertensive patients. *Clin. Sci. 38:* 101–110, 1970.

90. Sealey, J. E., S. A. Atlas, and J. H. Laragh. Prorenin and other large molecular weight forms of renin. *Endocr. Rev. 1:* 365–391, 1980.

91. Sealey, J. E., and J. H. Laragh. Searching out low renin patients: limitations of some commonly used methods. *Am. J. Med. 55:* 303–313, 1973.

92. Sigmon, D. H., and J. C. S. Fray. Chemiosmotic control of renin release from isolated renin granules of rat kidneys. *J. Physiol. (Lond.)* 436:237–256, 1991.

93. Simon, C. D., T. W. Honeyman, and J. C. S. Fray. Renin-angiotensin system in hypophysectomized rats. I. Control of blood pressure. *Am. J. Physiol. 246 (Endocrinol. Metab. 10)* E84–E88, 1984.

94. Simon, S. M., and G. Blobel. A protein-conducting channel in the endoplasmic reticulum. *Cell 65:* 371–380, 1991.

95. Skott, O. Do osmotic forces play a role in renin secretion? *Am. J. Physiol. 255 (Renal Fluid Electrolyte Physiol 24)* F1–F10, 1988.

96. Skott, O., and R. Taugner. Effects of extracellular osmolality on renin release and on the ultrastructure of the juxtaglomerular epitheloid cell granules. *Cell Tissue Res. 249:* 325–329, 1987.

97. Sommer, S. C., and J. Melamed. Renal pathology of essential hypertension. *Am. J. Hypertens. 3:* 583–587, 1990.

98. Sullivan, P. A., M. Kelleher, M. Twomey, and M. Dineen. Effects of converting enzyme inhibition on blood pressure, plasma renin activity (PRA) and plasma aldosterone in hypertensive diabetics compared to patients with essential hypertension. *J. Hypertens. 3:* 359–363, 1985.

99. Swales, J. D. Low-renin hypertension: nephrosclerosis? *Lancet 2:* 75–77, 1975.

100. Thurston, H., and J. D. Swales. Low renin hypertension: a distinct entity. *Lancet 2:* 930–932, 1976.
101. Tuek, M. L., M. P. Sambhi, and L. Levin. Hyporeninemic hypoaldosteronism in diabetes mellitus: studies of the autonomic nervous system's control of renin release. *Diabetes 28:* 237–241, 1979.
102. Ueno, N., H. Miyazaki, S. Hirose, and K. Murakami. A 56,000-dalton renin-binding protein in hog kidney is an endogenous renin-inhibitor. *J. Biol. Chem. 256:* 12023–12027, 1981.
103. Veterans Administration Cooperative Study Group on Antihypertensive Agents. Urinary and serum electrolytes in untreated black and white hypertensives. *J. Chronic Dis. 40:* 839–847, 1987.
104. Vlahos, C. J., J. D. Walls, D. T. Berg, and B. W. Grinnell. The purification and characterization of recombinant human renin expressed in the human kidney cell line 293. *Biochem. Biophys. Res. Comm. 171:* 375–383, 1990.
105. Wilson, D. M., and J. A. Luetscher. Plasma prorenin activity and complications in children with insulin-dependent diabetes mellitus. *N. Engl. J. Med. 323:* 1101–1106, 1990.
106. Wright, J. T., and J. G. Douglas. Drug therapy in black hypertensives. In: *Pathophysiology of Hypertension in Blacks,* edited by J. C. S. Fray and J. G. Douglas. Oxford University Press, New York, 1992.
107. Yamamoto, K., and F. Ikemoto. High molecular-weight renin and renin-binding protein. *Trends Pharmacol. Sci. 4:* 381–383, 1983.
108. Zidek, W., C. Karoff, H. Losse, and H. Vetter. Weight reduction and salt restriction in hypertension: effects on blood pressure and intracellular electrolytes. *Klin. Wochenschr. 64:* 1183–1185, 1986.

V

THEORY AND THERAPY . . . THE VOLUME-VASOCONSTRICTION SPECTRUM

11

Pathogenesis of Hypertension in Blacks: Features of an Equilibrium Model

J.C.S. FRAY

At its inception, the mosaic theory was portrayed as an octagon with the then known regulators on each focal point and arrows indicating a closed system in equilibrium.... [genetic, environmental, anatomical, adaptive, neural, endocrine, humoral, hemodynamic]. Clearly, this . . . is not meant to list all of the multiple mechanisms currently adumbrated as constituting the many facets of hypertension considered as a "disease of regulation." Rather, the mosaic concept is intended to provide a logical and orderly way of *thinking* about all forms of hypertension as a subject for research and as a means of analyzing the problem in patients.

I. H. Page

The mosaic theory continues to command the center of hypertension research. Burton (40) was the first to show that any theory for control of blood pressure must rest on some fundamental principles of equilibrium of the arterioles. Page (176) subsequently argued that the problem of hypertension may be "more realistically soluble in terms of *altered equilibria* than by any one of a variety of monistic approaches." He later brought the theory to bear on renal hypertension (175,177), the center being the physical equilibrium of the arteriole, with factors such as *genetic, environmental, anatomical, adaptive, neural, endocrine, humoral,* and *hemodynamic* forming the margin. Thus, most theoretical discourse focuses on renal hypertension, because it has been acknowledged that the pathogenesis is very similar to human essential hypertension (18). The purpose of this chapter is to review the conceptual understanding of the problem of hypertension in general, taking renal hypertension as a marginal model for the pathogenesis of the disease in blacks.

Most theorists have limited their discussion to specific mechanisms but rarely in terms of altered equilibrium. Genetic factors (and animal models) have been identified to play a role (58), and the role of the kidney (18), calcium (140), and salt (56) have all been shown to influence the process, but no comprehensive model as to how genetic factors influence the equilibrium process has been proposed. A recent theory of human hypertension shows this most effectively (215). The growing importance of environmental factors has been well documented and the role of historico-cultural, behavioral, psychological,

239

and social factors reviewed (3,106; see also Chapters 2, 4, and 5). Environmental factors were identified as a contributor to the differences in blood pressure regulation in blacks and whites as early as 1929 (62), and reemphasized recently (see Chapters 4, 5, 6, and 7), but besides the "research paradigms" advanced by Anderson et al. (3) to examine the multidimensional nature of the disease, no unifying view of how environmental factors affect the equilibrium process has been reported. Anatomical factors have also been implicated, and decreased glomerular surface area and porosity along with arteriosclerotic plaques have been proposed as principal sites (172), but data are lacking to evaluate this model, especially in the context of arteriolar equilibrium in blacks. Adaptive changes are now well recognized in theoretical discourse, but the role of structural remodeling (117,129,144,182) and functional characteristics (8,29,73,179,186,210) remain to be centered on physical equilibrium at the arteriole. Several studies have focused on altered characteristics of calcium handling (186,210), but by centering calcium, these theories have marginalized the principle of equilibrium. Perhaps the closest approaches, in terms of theory, to the center of equilibrium are the reviews by Lever (144) showing the etiology of various forms of hypertension, though not hypertension in blacks, and by Aviv (8) showing the interaction of calcium and other factors at the level of the arteriole. The role of a neural component has been discussed and supported, with α-receptor, sodium excretion, natriuretic factor, and cyclic nucleotide metabolism all shown to contribute (2,35,36,44,59,70,151,160), but the theoretical center of neurogenic hypertension remains outside the level of the arteriole. Endocrine control of blood pressure and its involvement in hypertension is well recognized (11,138,184,185,213), but rarely does fundamental mechanism of action recruit physical disequilibrium at the arteriole as a requirement for the pathogenesis of hypertension, except perhaps an interesting theory by Kornel et al. (128). Humoral agents have been suggested to play key roles (21,22,61,116,150,156) and so have hemodynamic influences (27,54, 55,92,141), but except for a few approaches (to be discussed later), the vast majority of these theories are monistic and therefore lack the spirit of the equilibrium approach (176).

Two successful models emerged in the early 1970s: the "vasoconstriction-volume" model of Laragh (138) and the "renal-volume" coupled with "whole-body" autoregulation model of Guyton (92). Both focused on the kidney as a locus of control, a view supported by experimental evidence. Both theories are bipolar in that hypertension results from either vasoconstriction or volume expansion, or both. Both have contributed significantly to the development of the renin–angiotensin–aldosterone system (RAAS), a system now well recognized to play an important role in the pathogenesis of the disease. Both theories, however, view the problem from the systems approach, and thereby circumvent the locus of feedback control—the initiation point—whereby the vasoconstriction and volume forces come to bear on setting, maintaining, and regulating a particular level of blood pressure. And when the locus is actually identified and defined, both models are limited in giving pathogenetic insights of events at the (intra)cellular level. Thus the basic physical (if not philosophical) principle for circulatory control is absent from both models. But despite these deficiencies, both models can be extended to show a unified view of the pathogenesis of hypertension that accounts for most, if not all, of the recent evidence on the role of calcium and other factors on the disease. Because both theories use the concept of *equilibrium* in their formulation, because Page (176) discovered the centrality of the concept, and because stable equilibrium is a physical, as well as physiological concept central to any understanding of circulatory control (40), the extended version has been designated *equilibrium model* (78,149). Because renovascular hypertension has been accorded a privileged position in theoretical studies, it will again be used here as the central example. In fact, Laragh (137) has recently insisted that "renovascular hypertension" should be "a paradigm for *all* hypertension." Understanding the pathogenesis of renovascular hypertension should hasten understanding of the pathogenesis of psychosocial stressor–induced hypertension in blacks, as reviewed in this chapter.

EQUILIBRIUM MODEL IN REVIEW

Table 11.1 summarizes the key equations describing the model (78,149). The approach was first developed by Burton (42) and Azuma and Oka (9), with refinements on the myogenic aspect by Koch (126). Briefly, the model considers a unit length of afferent arteriole subjected to its two main forces: distension and constriction. For stable physical equilibrium the distending force must balance the constricting *(Eq.1)*. The distending force may be calculated from the

TABLE 11.1. Principal Equations Describing the Physical Equilibrium Theory

$T_D = T_p + T_A$	1
$T_D = P_i r_i - P_o r_o$	2
$T_P = T_P^R \exp\left\{\gamma\left(\dfrac{r_i - R}{R}\right)\right\}$	3
$T_A = K_{TA}\left(\dfrac{Ca^2}{K_{Ca} + Ca_i^2}\right)$	4
$Ca_i = Ca_{iH} + Ca_{iS}$	5
$Ca_{iS} = \dfrac{Ca_o}{K_o}\left(\dfrac{S^n}{Q + S^n}\right)$	6
$S = 2\left(\dfrac{1 - 2\gamma}{E}\right)\left\{\dfrac{P_i r_i^2 - P_o r_o^2}{r_o^2 - r^{2i}}\right\}$	7
$Flow = K_F P_i r_i$	8

T_D is the tension responsible for the distending force, whereas, T_P and T_A are the passive and active components of the tension responsible for the constricting force; P_i and P_o are the intravascular and extravascular pressures ($P_o = 5$ mm Hg usually); r_i and r_o are the internal and external radii of the arteriole ($r_i/r_o = 0.75$ usually); T_P^R is the passive tension at radius, R, and is 23.729 dynes/cm, when R is 8.71 μ; τ is a constant, 13.982; K_{TA} is the maximum active tension, 3,000 dynes/cm; K_{Ca} is the square of the intracellular Ca concentration (Ca_i) required for 50% maximum vascular smooth muscle tension, 0.1024 μM^2; Ca_{iS} and C_{iH} are the intracellular Ca pools contributed to by stretch and neurohormones and humoral factors; Ca_o is the extracellular concentration of Ca, 2 mM; K_o is the efflux rate coefficient into which is incorporated all extrusion and sequestration processes, 200; Q and n are constants, 2.9 and 1.5; S is the stretch of the arteriole; v and E are Poisson's ratio and Young's modulus, 0.3 and 10^6 dynes/cm^2. Other terms and constants are previously described (149).

product of the distending stress and the area *(Eq.2)*. The constricting force may be derived from the product of the wall tension and length.

Wall tension is represented by passive (T_p) and active (T_A) components. The passive tension may be exerted by all noncontractile elements in the vessel wall in an effort to resist distension. *Equation 3* shows this tension as a function of radius (101). The active tension component is slightly more complex, but recent theoretical and experimental observations have provided sufficient evidence to justify *Equation 4*. The plasma membrane plays an important role as stretch sensor (78,149) and the fractional activation of calcium channels is governed by stretch (149). Stretch-activated ion channels have been identified and studied in some detail (17,52,65,86,87,110,113,120,136,139,190,197).

The equation chosen to describe stretch-activated channels may be influenced by certain shared characteristics of several well-studied biological control systems (149). The first is that the stretch-sensitive channels are presumably proteins with membrane configurations that dictate the probabilities of whether the channels are opened or closed. Molecular architecture of some of these channel proteins has been described (164) and may be analogous to certain enzymes having a "high" or "low" affinity for substrate (the "substrate" in this case being calcium). Low and high affinity states for the calcium channel were reported (188). The second is that stretch may be postulated, through membrane deformation or rearrangement, to alter the environment of the channel proteins, thus altering their configurations and the fractional probabilities of the channels in the opened state. The third is that since calcium channels are present in the plane of the plasma membrane, it is conceivable that interaction will occur between adjacent channels. This is analogous to cooperativity between the promoters of oligomeric proteins, whose characteristics are typical of allosteric proteins, models of which have been described (163). These are some key reasons that led to *Equation 6,* although other forms of the equation were suggested (52).

Ca_i is divided into a humoral and a stretch-sensitive pool *(Eq.5)*. Calcium inflow into the humoral pool may also be affected by stretch (34,46,104). *Equation 4* estimates active tension development (149), though similar equations have been used in skeletal (201) as well as cardiac (45) muscles. Because *Equation 4* shows T_A as a function of Ca_i it has become useful to describe Ca_i in terms of two components, the component sensitive to stretch (Ca_{is}) and that sensitive to humoral factors (Ca_{iH}) *((Eq.5)*. Multiple calcium entry pathways have been demonstrated (43,108,162,211,217). By combining *Equations 4–7,* an expression may be derived that shows active tension development as a function of several variables $(Ca_o,$ $K_o,$ $K_{iH},$ $S,$ $P_o,$ $P_i,$ $r_i,$ $r_o,$ $v,$ and $E)$. Since active tension is an integral component of the myogenic response, physiological processes such as renin secretion, blood flow, and blood pressure control must be affected by all these factors. Although such considerations point to the complexity of the model in making accurate predictions, they also point to its richness.

At equilibrium:

$$T_D = T_P + T_A \tag{1}$$

In the language of one model (138), the "volume" component (T_D) must counterbalance the vasoconstriction component ($T_P + T_A$).

The logic of the model implies certain consequences of initial disequilibrium that may be approached graphically. Alteration of the left hand side (LHS) of *Equation 1* by increasing P_i (perfusion pressure) leads to changes on the right hand side (RHS) to reestablish a new equilibrium that involves establishing a new internal radius to accommodate the changes initiated by raising P_i (Fig. 11.1). The intermediate steps have been shown to be an increase in perfusion pressure leads to an increase in radius (and thereby an increase in stretch according to *Equation 7*), which leads to an increase in calcium permeability (and thereby an increase in Ca_i, providing calcium is present in the extracellular space), which leads to an increase in active tension development (and consequently decreased radius), decreased blood flow, and increased resistance (78). This sequence of changes in pressure, flow, and resistance was observed experimentally (39,121,158,198). Alterations of the RHS of *Equation 1* also lead to changes on the LHS to reestablish a new equilibrium. Structural remodeling in arterioles influences the equation by altering T_p (75). Factors that raise Ca_i in vascular smooth muscle provoke active tension development, which in turn leads to muscle contraction, radius reduction, and pressure elevation (78). Angiotensin II, vasopressin, endothelin, norepinephrine, and excess potassium are among the most important factors shown to increase active vascular tone by raising Ca_i as a result of increasing calcium inflow through calcium channels or releasing calcium from intracellular stores. Through pharmacological intervention tone can be decreased by blocking inflow of calcium with verapamil, nifedipine, and diltiazem, or by inactivating contractile proteins.

Figure 11.1 is a graphical representation of *Equation 1*. Burton (40) was the first to apply this elastic (or *equilibrium*) diagram to blood vessels. Numerous lines of experimental evidence support the general features of the diagram (39,114,115,198). Points of equilibrium are represented at radii and tensions where the T_D and $T_P + T_A$ curves intersect (149). Figure 11.1 shows that the equilibrium *point* A may be displaced to *point* C by two distinctly different pathways.

The first pathway involves increasing the distending pressure from 100 to 140 mm Hg along *curve* 1 to *point* B. This theoretical view is supported by several experimental observations (39,158,198). The increase in tension from *point* A to *point* B represents mainly an increase in the passive tension of the elastic components of the vessel (149). In hypertension where there is structural remodeling of resistance vessels, the course of *curve* 1 might be different (74). Prevention of active tension makes *point* B the new point of equilibrium (78). Normally, however, an increase in the stretch at *point* B activates stretch-sensitive calcium channels, which provokes the inflow of calcium to raise Ca_i. The increase in Ca_i leads to active tension development and vasoconstriction, which reduces the radius from *point* B to *point* C along *curve* 2. Although *point* C represents the new point of equilibrium, the vasoconstriction induced by a sharp rise in P_i and stretch will "overshoot" to the left along the T_D 140 mm Hg line past *point* C. This overshoot phenomenon has been demonstrated experimentally (10,26,38,39,114,115,121). It is of historical interest that in his

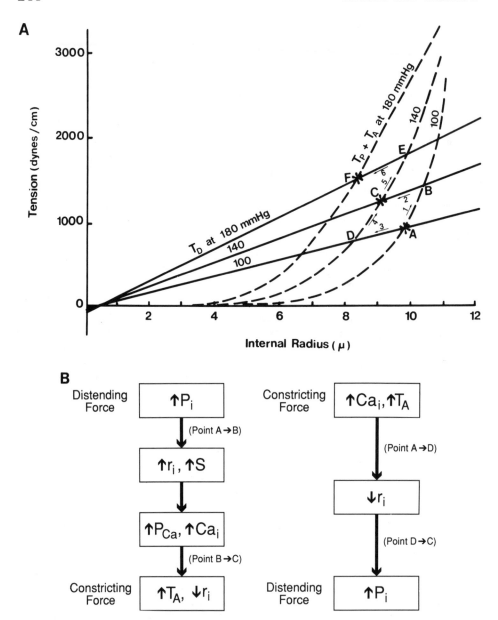

FIGURE 11.1. Elastic (or equilibrium) diagram showing (A) radii at which stable equilibrium of arterioles is achieved and (B) intermediary steps of disequilibrium. A: Tension curves are drawn for designated vales of perfusion pressure. Tissue pressure is taken to be 10 mm Hg for all curves. Radii at which equilibrium occurs are those that show intersection of distending tension (T_D) (solid lines) and constricting tension ($T_P + T_A$) (broken lines) at identical perfusion pressures (*). *Path 1* is increase in pressure from 100 to 140 mm Hg; *path 2* is vasoconstriction in response to the increase in pressure. *Path 3* is neurohormonal-induced vasoconstriction; *path 4* is vasodilation provoked by disequilibrium of forces. *Paths 5* and *6* are similar to *1* and *2*. *Points A, C,* and *F* show vascular equilibrium, whereas *points B, D,* and *E* show disequilibrium. Modified from Fray et al. (87). B: Flow diagram showing reestablishment of equilibrium when the initial disturbance is a rise in *distending force* (left) compared with *constricting force* (right). A computer graphics program of the model is available.

original description of this phenomenon, Bayliss (14) described even the over-shoot: "As the arterial pressure rises the limb is distended passively, but in-stead of merely returning to its original volume [*radius*] when the pressure has come down again, it constricts much below its previous level and only grad-ually returns." *Point* C is the new equilibrium when the initiating imbalance is a rise in P_i (distending force). This may explain why papaverine, an agent believed to prevent tension development, causes vasodilation (194). It may also explain why blockers of calcium influx cause vasodilation and prevent blood flow autoregulation (48,78). In the equilibrium process, changes on the LHS of *Equation 1* are counterbalanced by equal but opposite changes on the RHS.

The second pathway to *point* C (from *point* A) is initiated by directly rais-ing active tension development. Figure 11.1 illustrates the (con)sequence (sequence and the resultant consequence) of initial disequilibrium and subsequent reequilibrium prediction when vascular tone is altered by an in-stantaneous increase in Ca_i. Increasing Ca_i (i.e., preceding any change in pres-sure) shifts *point* A along *curve* 3 to *point* D, which is an "equivalent" vascular wall tension at pressure 140 mm Hg. Although this new point (*point* D in Fig. 11.1) represents a smaller radius (increased total peripheral resistance) at a reduced total wall tension due to vasoconstriction, it is a point (or a radius) whereby the vessel is in disequilibrium with respect to pressure of 100 mm Hg (149). Pressure will increase in response to the increased peripheral vascular resistance. The reduced stretch at *point* D will decrease the calcium influx through the stretch-sensitive calcium channels and thus decrease Ca_i, which thereby tends to relax the muscles (149). The two combined factors of reduced calcium influx and increased pressure shift *point* D along *curve* 4 to *point* C in Figure 11.1, where a new equilibrium is established between constricting and distending tensions. This new equilibrium is established at higher tensions, resistance, and pressure to maintain a constant blood flow, much the same as in the case of reequilibrium initiated by an increase in pressure (149). Note, however, that *point* C was reestablished as the new point of equilibrium due either to the myogenic response (along *curves* 1–2) *or* an increase in active tension (along *curves* 3–4).

An interesting outcome obtains from a disequilibrium initiated by active tension development followed by volume expansion. Figure 11.1 illustrates this sequence as *points* A–D and C–E. *Points* A–D may be characterized as angiotensin II–mediated vasoconstriction, whereas C–E can be seen as aldo-sterone-induced volume expansion. This sequence typifies the core of the va-soconstriction-volume theory (138). Disequilibrium is initiated by angiotensin II–induced increase in active tension (RHS of *Eq.1; point* A–D along *curve* 3 in Fig. 11.1) caused by an increase in the hormone-sensitive component of Ca_i. This powerful effect of angiotensin II on Ca_i and active tension was recently demonstrated (194). *Point* D represents a radius of unstable equilibrium (con-stricting tension of 140 mm Hg vs. distending tension of 100 mm Hg), which rapidly reequilibrates at *point* C (78). Thus *point* C represents a circulation at higher total wall tension maintained by an elevated Ca_i triggered and main-tained exclusively by angiotensin II (78), as demonstrated experimentally (80,200). Volume expansion shifts *points* C–E as it does *points* A–B (see above).

One interesting prediction of the model may be spotlighted. During the second phase (from *point* C–E [Fig. 11.1]) there will be a lower total peripheral resistance at *point* E than at *point* C despite a higher blood pressure (180 mm Hg at *point* E compared with 140 mm Hg at *point* C). The logic of the theory holds that the elevated pressure at *point* E will be maintained by an elevated cardiac output (78). Several reports have confirmed this prediction (19,54,143). Furthermore, some workers showed that in the absence of an increased cardiac output the circulation rapidly moves to *point* F (which is characterized by an elevated total peripheral resistance and normal cardiac output) presumably by a pathway similar to A–D–C (78). In this instance both phases of the sequence are developed and maintained by angiotensin II–induced vasoconstriction and the attendant myogenic response, which may be reversed by angiotensin II blockade (11) or calcium channel antagonism. Thus, stable, long-term physical equilibrium at *point* F is paid for by *physical forces, cellular calcium,* and *structural remodeling.* The physical forces involved are higher pressures and higher wall tensions; the elevated wall tension is maintained by an elevated level of cellular calcium (51,207,219); the structural remodeling involves an elevated wall/lumen ratio (191). Because the long-term maintenance of hypertension is mediated by a heightened resistance, it is expected that the long-term manifestation is characterized by a lower blood flow for a given pressure and by an increased wall thickness. That is to say, the blood pressure–blood flow curve is displaced to the right (78). Sadoshima et al. (191) provided experimental confirmation of these theoretical predictions. At each step the inflow of extracellular calcium is required for the restoration of stable equilibrium (78). This points to the central feature in which calcium plays a key role in the pathogenesis of hypertension (78).

The previous discussion reviews the model in its broad outline. The pathogenesis of renal hypertension has been used to identify data to situate certain general features (78). Essential hypertension in blacks may also be relevant, especially as hypertension is established.

ANALYSIS OF THREE PHASES OF HYPERTENSION

The mechanism responsible for the pathogenesis of renal-induced hypertension in animal models and psychosocial stressor–induced hypertension in blacks may be divided into *three phases* (see Fig. 1.2). This division is useful because different (patho)physiological mechanisms are involved in each phase. Phase I of renovascular hypertension is mediated by angiotensin II–induced peripheral vasoconstriction. Blockade of renin enzymatic activity (196), angiotensin II generation (161), or angiotensin II–induced vasoconstriction (222) prevents initiation. Phase I of essential hypertension in blacks is mediated by one or more physiological stress response molecules (serotonin, ACTH, epinephrine, norepinephrine, dopamine, β-endorphin, angiotensin II, vasopressin, etc.). Phase II of renal hypertension occurs as a consequence of angiotensin II–induced vasoconstriction, by a myogenic component induced by the elevated pressure, or by salt and water retention (78). Phase II in blacks occurs by similar mechanisms, in addition to increased vascular reactivity and genetic predisposition. Phase III represents a continuation of phase II, in addition to structural remodeling (47,82,122,130,144,173), resetting of baroreceptors (6,37, 50,63,131,157), and renal excretory functions (28,29), alteration of responsiveness to vasoactive substances (218), altered ionic transport systems (133), and increased vascular reactivity (see Chapters 3 and 6, this volume). The precise temporal and anatomical details of the transition from outright vasoconstriction to structural changes remain unclear, though it was postulated that the structural changes begin 2 weeks after induction of renal hypertension (182). The general features of these three phases have been well described and experimentally confirmed (19,28,29,57,80,90,92,137,141,144,175,184) and some have stressed the key role of renin (30).

By profiling renin, it is possible to distinguish benign hypertension from malignant hypertension. Barger and coworkers (64) characterized some of the differences. In benign hypertension, there is an immediate rise in renin secretion, blood volume (and consequently, cardiac output), and pressure (Fig. 11.2). Within days, renin returns to normal, resistance rises, and plasma volume remains elevated. The decline in renin secretion and the simultaneous rise in

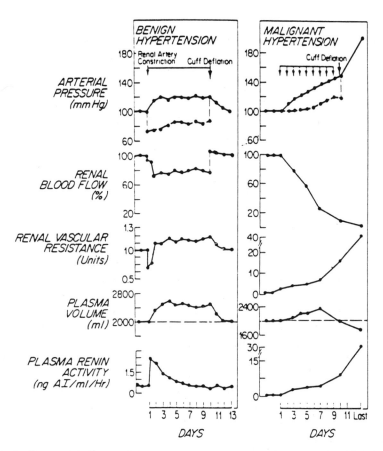

FIGURE 11.2. Sequential changes in systemic and renal hemodynamics, PRA, and plasma volume in experimental benign and malignant hypertension (71).

resistance reflect the rise in Ca_i (78). In malignant hypertension, on the other hand, the blood pressure rises as a consequence of a continually rising PRA without volume excess (Fig. 11.2). Profiling of renin, then, gives indication of different phases of renal hypertension and distinguishes between benign and malignant forms of the disease. A similar picture emerges from studies of renin profile in blacks (see Chapter 10, this volume). The evidence is most complete for phases I and II for renovascular hypertension, so focus will be on this model only.

PHASE I: INITIATION OF HYPERTENSION

Calcium has been shown to play a role in the development of phase I of renal hypertension. Since it is well established and accepted that renin secretion is under the control of calcium (79), focus here will be on one peripheral action of angiotensin II. It was suggested that both the hypertension and general vasoconstriction are mediated by calcium-dependent mechanisms (111). In support of this view, it was demonstrated that reduction of Ca_o lowers the angiotensin II–induced vasoconstriction and hypertension in phase I (222). Regarding the role of Ca_o, a striking correlation between serum calcium and the change in blood pressure during phase I of the hypertension was observed (222). Calcium-channel blockers also reduce the blood pressure in renal hypertension (85). Recent evidence shows that angiotensin II stimulates a dose-dependent increase in Ca_i of vascular smooth muscle cells (169). Thus, phase I appears to be characterized most precisely in terms of angiotensin II–induced mobilization of calcium. Figure 11.1 shows this phase in *curve* 3. Since one prediction of the theory is that *curve* 3 is mediated exclusively by angiotensin II–mediated calcium movement (or mobilization) into cells (specifically vascular smooth muscle), one test of the theory is that *curve* 3 should be absent in renal hypertension (phase I) in the absence of angiotensin II.

PHASE II: DEVELOPMENT OF HYPERTENSION

Phase II is more complex, but calcium plays a role. This phase represents a *rheostasis,* a decisive shift of the set point, of the "resting" level of blood pressure. It is the most subtle, but most significant, therefore it will receive detailed attention. This rheostasis is the core of Guyton's theories (89–92). Brown et al. (29) proposed that angiotensin II is responsible for hypertension in phase II partly because of its direct peripheral vasoconstrictor effect and partly because of its contribution to a resetting of pressure natriuresis with retention of salt and water. The resetting has to do with salt excretion from an increased salt intake and increased filtered load. These issues find support from experimental studies, several of which are important. The first is that increasing the amount of ingested salt has little effect on blood pressure in the short run (100). The second is that the important changes show up in glomerular filtration, renal blood flow, and urinary sodium excretion (100). Angiotensin promotes greater filtration and reabsorption of sodium without altering urinary sodium excretion. Thus in presence of angiotensin II, it takes a higher blood pressure to produce an equivalent amount of salt in the urine compared with control (without angiotensin II) (100). Thus, at least for "normal salt state," the role of salt and water retention and the subsequent increase in cardiac output during phase II of hypertension have been well documented (19,143). For low salt state, however, the increased salt and water retention may be absent (11,80,184).

Angiotensin II–induced stimulation of aldosterone is a primary precursor of salt and water retention, although angiotensin II affects salt and water reabsorption directly (98,99). Weighing both effects prompted the conclusion that "considerable evidence suggests that the intrarenal actions of ANG II are quantitatively more important than changes in aldosterone secretion in the normal day-to-day regulation of Na balance and arterial pressure" (98). In terms of the model, both effects of angiotensin may be calcium-dependent, thereby explaining the indirect calcium-dependency of *curve* 5 (Fig. 11.1). The increase in blood pressure along *curve* 5 is a direct outcome of the increased cardiac output mediated by angiotensin-induced stimulation of aldosterone production and salt and water retention. The model predicts that *curve* 5 represents an elevation of blood pressure due to an elevated cardiac output attended by an initial reduction of resistance. Calcium also plays a role in salt and water retention (112,204,216). Blockage of calcium channels causes a substantial natriuresis (12,67,109,170,220).

Calcium plays an important role in the production of aldosterone by angiotensin II. Two sources of calcium may be involved: 50% comes from intracellular stores, whereas the other 50% comes from the extracellular space (127). Angiotensin II–induced calcium influx from extracellular source may be blocked by verapamil (71,195), methoxyverapamil (76), lanthanum, and lowering Ca_o (71,72,76,195). In at least one study, however, the angiotensin II–induced rise in Ca_i is not blocked by verapamil (41), but angiotensin II requires Ca_o for its full effect (76). More recent studies showed a direct relationship between angiotensin II concentration and Ca_i in adrenal glomerulosa cells (41).

Phase II is therefore characterized by increased cardiac output, which manifests itself at the vascular level as an increase in pressure and thereby distending force. The model predicts that the initial change during this phase is a decreased vascular resistance. This increase proceeds from *point* C–E along *curve* 5 (Fig. 11.1). At *point* E the arteriole is stretched and thereby facilitates the opening of stretch-sensitive calcium channels. The future demonstration of absence of such channels invalidates this aspect of the model. The inflow of calcium through these unique channels initiates the second phase of vasoconstriction. It is interesting that the myogenic construct and the contribution of increased cardiac output were advanced nearly 30 years ago. Ledingham and Cohen (142) were the first to propose the notion that a "myogenic reflex, which maintains constant peripheral blood-flow irrespective of perfusion pressure, constitutes a condition of *unstable equilibrium*. This is because any slight increase in cardiac output would raise pressure and so stimulate vasoconstriction which would thus raise pressure further." This implies that an increase in blood volume, and consequently cardiac output, must precede changes in resistance (1,147). In a recent review of this concept, Hamlyn and Blaustein (102) concluded that "the limited data available indicate that the BV [blood volume] expansion appears to be a prerequisite to alterations in vascular ion metabolism, that both of these changes precede the rise in blood pressure."

In volume depletion the pathogenesis of hypertension is not associated with an increased salt and water retention and cardiac output (80,209). The mechanism whereby angiotensin II–induced vasoconstriction, a manifestation of the entire period of renal artery constriction in sodium-depleted models (80,168), maintains the hypertension, especially during phase II, remains an unsolved problem, though some interesting suggestions have been proposed. Folkow et al. (75) provided one resolution to the dilemma by suggesting that the "intrinsic change of vascular tone is, to some extent at least, due to the mechanical stimulus constituted by the pressure as such, which seems to facilitate the automaticity of the smooth muscles in the small vessels." In other words, hypertension itself is a stimulus for the myogenic reflex observed during hypertension. The model predicts that *curve 6* is myogenetically mediated (Fig. 11.1). Lack of demonstrative active tension development as a result of calcium mobilization during this phase would invalidate this aspect of the model.

Several studies have addressed the issue of myogenically mediated vasoconstriction. Meininger et al. (158,159) provided some evidence concerning its role in renovascular hypertension (Fig. 11.3A). They observed that in several microcirculatory beds of renal hypertensive rats resistance was much greater than that of normal rats. When they placed a constricting cuff around the mesenteric artery, for example, to prevent the vasculature from experiencing hypertension, the resistance was comparable to control. When they released the constricting cuff, however, and thereby exposed these beds to hypertension, there was an immediate and potent myogenic response that increased the resistance to counteract the increased pressure. It is interesting that they observed the initial decrease in resistance *(increased stretch)* and the subsequent increase, as predicted by the equilibrium model (Fig. 11.1). Figure 11.3B shows confirmation at the systemic level (91).

The model predicts that the cascade of the myogenic phase involves an increased radius, increased active tension, and subsequently decreased radius. Baez (10) confirmed these predictions. In addition, Aoki and Sato (7) demonstrated a striking direct relationship between blood pressure and peripheral resistance. Vanhoutte (212) suggested that the myogenic response "depends highly upon the influx of extracellular Ca." He further speculates, "This may be of particular importance in those cases of hypertension in which total body autoregulation the [myogenic reflex mechanism] contributes to the genesis of the disease." In agreement with this view, several workers showed that blockade of calcium influx with calcium channel blockers reverses the hypertension in phase II of hypertension (25,111,125). In isolated arteries, the myogenic response is dependent on Ca_o, especially in the hypertensive range. The response is blunted by lowering Ca_o or by calcium influx blockers (114,115).

Point F represents the final state of hypertension (Fig. 11.1). It is a state in which the circulation, at least at the arteriolar revel, is in a new stable physical equilibrium (78). Compared with "normal," this new state of equilib-

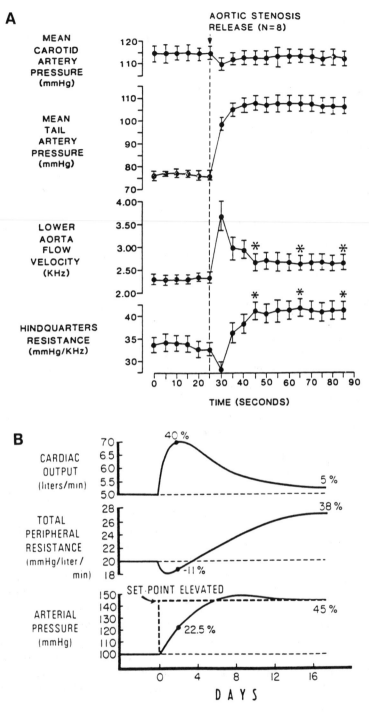

FIGURE 11.3. Acute and chronic reestablishment of equilibrium after an initial disturbance of the distending force. *A:* The effects of sudden deflation (dashed line) of the aortic vascular occluder cuff are shown for two-kidney, one-clip hypertensive rats with normotensive (protected) hindquarters. Data are expressed as the mean ± SEM. Statistical significant changes ($p < 0.05$) are indicated with asterisks (182). *B:* Sequential changes in hemodynamic variables during the onset of volume-loading hypertension. *These are average results from a series of experiments over the past 20 years* (104).

rium is characterized by higher blood pressure, increased resistance, increased active tension, and increased Ca_i. Calcium is central to the reestablishment and maintenance of this new equilibrium, and a higher concentration of Ca_i is required to maintain the higher active contractile tension. The model implies that there are no intrinsic differences in the maximum performance of the contractile machinery in vitro, but that the higher T_A in hypertension is a manifestation of the equilibrium requirement. Arterioles in vitro from normotensive and hypertensive subjects should be exactly alike in terms of their maximum tension development, though factors such as sensitivity and velocity of response may differ. This is an important prediction of the model, which should easily be confirmed or used as a strong line of proof for refutation of this specific aspect. What remains to be addressed is the mechanism(s) responsible for regulating (or maintaining) Ca_i at this elevated level of pressure, which may now be classified as phase III, the established phase of hypertension.

PHASE III: SUSTAINED HYPERTENSION

Recent evidence has pointed to the involvement of calcium in phase III of renal as well as other forms of hypertension, including essential hypertension in blacks. This established phase of hypertension has been "characterized by a rather generalized increase in peripheral vascular resistance and a moderately reduced cardiac output due to a decrease in stroke volume" (25), but a normal cardiac output has also been reported along with the elevated total peripheral resistance. Calcium channel blockers such as felodipine (25), nifedipine (109), and nitrendipine (125) reversed this phase in renovascular hypertension by lowering total peripheral resistance. In addition, Huang (109) showed that nifedipine given during phase III lowered body fluids by promoting salt and water excretion, confirming that the reabsorptive processes during this phase are mediated by a calcium-dependent mechanism. As early as 1966, Tobian and Chesley (207) reported a 13% increase in the calcium content of the arterioles during phase III of renal hypertension. These observations were confirmed qualitatively by others (51,219). The increase in Ca_i reported by Tobian and Chesley (207) is sufficient to sustain a substantial active tension in the myogenic reflex (149). Kwan et al. (133) suggested that the higher calcium content may be explained by an increased calcium permeability or decreased calcium pump activity. Although their studies failed to address the question of increased permeability, they showed a decreased calcium pump activity. It is highly probable that increased permeability to calcium is associated with this phase of hypertension, because the calcium channel blockers reverse the hypertension (25,109,125), presumably by shutting down elevated calcium permeability channels.

Other forms of both clinical and experimental hypertension are also characterized, as is phase III of renal hypertension, by an elevated total peripheral resistance (81). What is very interesting is that the increased resistance is reversed by calcium channel blockers, just as in phase III of renal hypertension (7,13,23,24,123,124,152–154,165,170,171,187,189,192,202,214). Without exception, these calcium channel blockers (nifedipine, nitrendipine, verapamil, diltiazem, tiapamil, nicardipine, niludipine, filodipine, PN200-110, and PY108-068) cause a lowering of blood pressure or a direct vasodilation. What is also very interesting, as in phase III of renal hypertension, Ca_i is elevated in cells (23,28,31–33,38.68,69,148,181,193,199).

Four theoretical possibilities explain the continued increases in Ca_i deserve consideration. The first is an increase in serum (or plasma) ionized calcium, but there is no compelling evidence to support this possibility. The second is an increased release of calcium from intracellular storage (and sequestration) sites. From the limited observations it may be concluded tentatively that increased calcium release from intracellular storage sites may play a role in the elevated Ca_i observed in hypertension, but the relative importance remains unclear. The third is an increased permeability to calcium. The model predicts that the established phase of hypertension is associated with a myogenically induced inflow of extracellular calcium which may be blocked by calcium channel blockers (78). Calcium channel blockers lower Ca_i in platelets of hypertensives, which is associated with a profound hypotension and vasodilation (23,69). Caution should be exercised in interpreting these studies, however, because platelets may not be the cells subjected to the myogenic stress. Calcium inflow into synaptosomes of brain tissue from SHRs is 40% greater than controls (180). Verapamil prevents the calcium inflow. Platelets behave in a manner similar to brain tissue with respect to the effect of calcium uptake and verapamil (180). From these studies it may be concluded that an increased membrane permeability to calcium may be one feature of some membranes in hypertensives. The increased permeability is very likely mediated by, among other factors, membrane depolarization, since Cheung (46) showed a substantial depolarization of arterial smooth muscle as hypertension develops in SHRs. This may explain why voltage-sensitive calcium channel blockers such as verapamil, nefedipine, and nitrendipine prove so effective in hypertensives.

Black hypertensives respond positively to calcium channel blockers, suggesting a role for increased membrane permeability. The most well studied calcium antagonists are verapamil, nifedipine, nitrendipine, and diltiazem (123,155,165,166). Other calcium channel blockers may also be effective, but the fact that these drugs work so effectively on black hypertensives points to the importance of calcium entry in this particular subgroup. It is unclear whether the cellular mechanism in black hypertensives is different from whites, but Cooper et al. (53) showed a striking elevation of Ca_i in black hypertensives, and Kiowski et al. (123) showed a reduction of blood pressure and Ca_i with calcium channel blockers. In fact, these particular observations have prompted Kiowski et al. (123) to suggest that "monotherapy with a calcium antagonist may become a first-line treatment for essential hypertension, particularly in . . . black patients." These observations are consistent with the view that established hypertension is maintained by elevated Ca_i that originates most likely from the extracellular space.

A decreased efflux of calcium is the fourth mechanism whereby cells may maintain an elevated Ca_i during hypertension. The calcium pump and a sodium-calcium exchange (sodium in, calcium out) are two primary mechanisms used by cells to extrude calcium. The calcium-pump of red blood cells has been well studied and a few relevant characteristics may be summarized. It binds calcium with high affinity; it has a calmodulin component on the cytoplasmic face; it is blocked by vanadate, sodium, and several other factors relevant to hypertension (42). In hypertensives, the affinity of the calcium pump is half that in normotensives (180). Calmodulin may correct for the lowered affinity, but even in the presence of excess calmodulin the maximal activity of the calcium-pump is still lower in hypertensives (180). In aortic smooth muscle a calcium-pump with a high affinity for calcium has been described (134). Similarly, in platelets there is also evidence for a calcium pump with high affinity for calcium and which is stimulated by calmodulin (181). Resink et al. (183) showed that the over-all defects in this calcium pump in hypertension are similar to those described for red blood cells (180), and they concluded that "the defective calcium efflux pump activity, as assessed by a decreased degree of calmodulin stimulation, may have contributed to elevated cytoplasmic concentrations in platelets from essential hypertensive subjects." The role of the sodium-calcium exchanger has been widely discussed and supported (20–22,25,27,94,107).

Again, it is unclear whether black hypertensives represent a distinct subgroup, but the calcium pump is sensitive to several maneuvers, including diet (223). It has been shown that the V_{max} and K_m for the calcium-pump of platelets in black hypertensives are 16.5 ± 3.22 nmol P_i·mg protein^{-1}·min^{-1} and 1.87 ± 0.38 µM, respectively (203). These values are only slightly higher than those for whites, but significantly lower than those for normotensives. In another report, the highest level of hypertension was associated with the highest level of Ca_i and calcium pump activity (223). A diet high in calcium and low in sodium reduced Ca_i and calcium pump activity considerably (223). Candidates for the involvement of sodium-calcium exchange in black hypertensives remain to be identified.

The model also provides for the factor(s) responsible for maintaining the generalized increase in Ca_i. Although the myogenic response may adequately explain the maintenance of Ca_i in vascular smooth muscle (78), it is certainly inadequate to explain the increase of Ca_i in red blood cells, adipose tissue, platelets, and other vascular structural cells. This difficulty may be overcome by the proposal that the rise in Ca_i in smooth muscle cells is accompanied by the release of a factor(s) that causes the elevation of Ca_i in other cells. This factor(s) may act by promoting the inflow of calcium through voltage-sensitive channels or by blocking the sodium-potassium pump by a ouabainlike mechanism of action and thereby inhibiting sodium-calcium exchange.

Several laboratories favor the view that a factor is produced during established hypertension and that the factor(s) blocks the sodium-potassium pump by a ouabainlike mechanism. The proposition for such a factor was first advanced by Dahl et al. (56) and subsequently by Haddy and associates (94–97) and DeWardener and MacGregor (60,61), and more recently by Blaustein and coworkers (20–22). The view generally agreed upon is that this natriuretic factor inhibits the sodium-potassium pump in virtually all tissues but especially in vascular smooth muscle, and that this inhibition leads to a rise in intracellular sodium, which in turn raises Ca_i (22,61,94). In support of the final manifestation of this factor, several investigators demonstrated that in established hypertension there is a simultaneous increase in cytosolic sodium and calcium (53,59,148,168,199,224,230). Sodium restriction lowers both Ca_i and sodium (225). The factor is present in animals and humans with established hypertension, and a correlation between the blood pressure elevation and inhibition of sodium-potassium pump activity with the postulated factor(s) was demonstrated (103).

Since hypertension in blacks has been linked to sodium, the role of the pump inhibitor in this postulated subgroup may be of importance. Even when black and white hypertensives have exactly (statistically) the same level of blood pressure, in blacks PRA, serum potassium, and potassium excretion may be statistically significantly lower (84). In addition, sodium to potassium ratio was significantly higher in blacks. These observations are consistent with the presence of a sodium-potassium pump inhibitor. The study of Cooper et al. (53) showing an elevated intracellular sodium in black hypertensives is also consistent with the view of an inhibitor. Grim et al. (84) narrowed the field to focus on sex differences. They showed that although there was no difference between black and white hypertensive men, black women had a lower PRA than white women. Furthermore, black women had the lowest PRA of both sexes and races. They also had the highest systolic blood pressure. It may be of interest that low PRA is usually associated with high Ca_i (79). It was suggested that the presence of the sodium-potassium pump inhibitor may be found in low-renin hypertension (97). Notice, however, that although blacks generally have a lower PRA than whites, there is nothing to suggest that there is something special about low-renin hypertensives, of which blacks have been classified as a subgroup, except the higher Ca_i as predicted from theory.

Thus it appears that in phase III of hypertension a series of reasonable possibilities have been demonstrated. First, Ca_i increases and causes increased resistance. The mechanisms for the increased Ca_i may be increased calcium permeability and decreased calcium pump activity. Both have been documented. Second, some mechanism must be employed to *maintain* the elevated Ca_i. Four mechanisms seem possible: increased serum or plasma calcium, generalized increased membrane permeability to calcium, increased calcium release from intracellular storage sites, and a defect in the calcium efflux mechanism. The generalized increase in calcium permeability and the defective calcium efflux appear to be the most well supported by available evidence. Regarding the increased permeability to calcium, the decrease can be reversed by calcium channel blockers. Regarding the calcium efflux there appears to be a reduced activity of the calcium pump and suppression of the sodium-calcium exchange mechanism. A sodium pump inhibitor is postulated to suppress sodium-calcium exchange by inhibiting the sodium pump.

MECHANISM FOR RENAL RESETTING

The model may be useful in explaining the mechanism for renal "resetting." Brown et al. (28) proposed that "for the resetting processes in essential hypertension, we suggest that increased resistance of preglomerular and postglomerular vessels in the presence of hypertension leads to increased filtration fraction . . . and this raises the oncotic pressure of plasma in the peritubular capillaries, thereby enhancing sodium reabsorption. . . . Changes of renal vascular resistance and filtration fraction have a central role." It was shown that although total renal glomerular filtration rate remains constant in SHRs, renal plasma flow decreases and thereby gives a calculated increase in filtration fraction. It is interesting, however, that at the single nephron level, GFR and blood flow remain the same, thereby preserving constant filtration fraction, and consequently questioning the validity of the theory at the single arteriolar level. Furthermore, whereas Brown et al. (28) suggested that it is purely physical forces that are responsible for the increased sodium reabsorption, Blaustein (20) suggested that a putative humoral factor probably works directly on the sodium reabsorptive process. But is is also possible that both pathways may be of importance. Guyton et al. (90) hold that "the combination of both increased afferent and efferent resistances causes the large reduction in renal blood flow, but because the effects of these resistances on glomerular capillary pressure counterbalance each other, the glomerular filtration rate is still very near normal." This, then, places importance on the afferent and efferent arterioles. Guyton et al. (90) further hold that *"it is the increased afferent arteriolar resistance that causes hypertension,* while the increase in efferent arteriolar resistance increases tubular reabsorption."

Several studies have provided evidence that the afferent arteriole is the key site of resetting (16,47,82,117,118). Some have provided evidence suggesting that "structural" remodeling may be involved (16,47,82), whereas others have shown a shift to the right of the renal blood flow-perfusion pressure curve (118,119). This renal mechanism appears to be important, since the generalized increased cellular sodium and calcium is absent in renal insufficiency (199). Guyton et al. (90) have concluded that

> there are several very clear reasons to believe that essential hypertension, like other types of hypertension, results from *abnormal* renal retention of salt. However, it is still questionable what causes the kidneys to retain salt in essential hypertension. Suggested mechanisms have been . . . [many]. Mathematical model of kidney function is [sic] essential hypertension has shown that only one . . . fits with most of the findings in essential hypertension. . . . This is an intrinsic vascular abnormality of the kidneys in which both afferent arteriolar resistance and efferent arteriolar resistance are increased. The model suggests that it is *increased afferent* arteriolar resistance that causes hypertension.

This view may be extended to suggest that in renal hypertension the process of renal resetting is initiated by a decrease in afferent arteriolar resistance (decreased Ca_i) and is manifested and maintained by an increase in afferent arteriolar resistance (increased Ca_i): disturbed and reestablished equilibrium.

In black hypertensives differences at the afferent arteriolar level have been demonstrated. Renal blood flow is 18% lower in black hypertensives (146). Even during salt deprivation, renal blood flow is lower in black hypertensives (145). Blacks have a higher pressure and a lower afferent arteriolar radius and a thicker arteriolar wall than whites (208).

MECHANISM FOR CAROTID BARORECEPTOR RESETTING

Resetting of aortic and carotid baroreceptors is also involved in the maintenance of hypertension. This resetting phenomenon was first described by
McCubbin and associates (157) and subsequently investigated in greater detail
by several laboratories (6,37,50,63,88,131,167). It is now well established that
the process of resetting occurs within 5 min (131). Physical equilibrium and
calcium have been implicated directly or indirectly in the process (4,5,78,
105,107,131,135,205). As early as 1952, Landgren (135) showed that the carotid sinus demonstrated powerful myogenic responses very similar to those
observed in the renal afferent arterioles (66). Heymans and Delaunois (107)
earlier suggested that "tone and resistance to stretch of the arterial wall where
the pressoreceptors are located are the *fundamental factors* for the reflex au-
tomatic regulation of the systemic arterial pressure." More recently, Munch
and Brown (167) returned to this view and concluded that "since BRs [baro-
receptors] are mechanically coupled to vessel wall structures, resetting may be
due to changes in the wall." The activity of the carotid sinus may be assayed
by increases in neural activity or decreases in peripheral blood pressure. Calcium has been shown to affect both parameters (105,132). The carotid sinus
and aortic arch baroreceptors adapt to changes in calcium and physical forces
(4,15,135). It is not illogical, then, to expect that when arterial pressure is
raised in the areas containing the baroreceptors, the radius and wall thickness
will be altered to reestablish a disturbed equilibrium (131). Because the firing
of the receptors appears to be very sensitive to changes in radius (167), the
resetting phenomenon may be explained by the general view that first and
foremost the vascular structures will aim to achieve a stable physical equilibrium and that all the relevant physiological processes associated with such a
structure will adapt to this law (78). The recent demonstration that chronic
blockade of calcium channels in hypertension reverses the resetting phenomenon provides support for the role of calcium (221).

CONCLUSION AND GENERAL (RE)ORIENTATION

This discussion focused on the pathogenesis of hypertension of renal origin and
offered it as a marginal model for the physiological evolution of the disease in
blacks. In agreement with the mosaic theory, physical equilibrium of the arterioles needs to be the focus of attention in understanding the various phases
of the disease. This discussion, while consistent with the views held by most
practitioners, is aimed primarily at initiates who tomorrow will be the framers
(and solvers) of the problem. It must be stressed that the *concept* of equilibrium
is precisely that, a concept. In itself it cannot be measured, though the physiological (or pathological) manifestations of its presence (or absence) can be
measured. The pathogenesis of hypertension of renal origin is a good example
of these manifestations. Here we will summarize the conclusions reached that
are essential for a (re)orientation (orientation as a consequence of reorienta-
tion) of modern cardiovascular control.

Calcium is involved in the initiation and maintenance of hypertension, and several studies have documented three phases in pathogenesis both for renal hypertension induced by partial renal artery obstruction and for black "essential" hypertension induced by psychosocial stressors. The first phase of renal hypertension is initiated by angiotensin II–mediated vasoconstriction. The angiotensin II results from the renin secreted within seconds of renal artery constriction. Calcium plays a role in both the secretion of renin and the constriction of arterioles. The second phase is represented by a continuation of the first, by a myogenic component, or by salt and water retention, all of which have been shown to involve calcium. The third phase occurs by a continuation of the second phase, in addition to structural remodeling in the blood vessels, resetting of arterial baroreceptors and renal excretory functions, and alteration of responsiveness to vasoactive substances and of ionic transport systems. Calcium has been shown to play a role in third phase processes. The evidence is compelling that calcium channel blockers are effective in reversing or preventing all three phases of renal hypertension. The data provide substantial support for the conclusion that "the systemic haemodynamic and biochemical patterns of chronic renal hypertension are very similar to those of essential hypertension" (18), of which black hypertensives constitute a clearly defined subgroup. In this regard the equilibrium model may be useful in pointing to the similarities and in identifying the factors involved.

Figure 1.1 summarizes intermediary factors involved in the pathogenesis of hypertension, particularly in blacks, where psychosocial stressors have been a key initiating feature (see Chapters 1, 4, 5, and 6, this volume) and where increased total peripheral resistance is the underlying cause of maintaining the disease. Blacks, even children (see Chapter 3, this volume), are at greater risk for the development of hypertension mediated by the physiological stress response molecules triggered by psychosocial stressors (see Chapters 4, 5, and 6, this volume). Psychosocial stressors include low socioeconomic status (SES), poor and overcrowded schools, community violence, unemployment, John Henryism, and negative interpersonal interactions. Interventions to reduce or eliminate any or all of these stressors should attenuate the physiological stress response, which is characterized by increased serotonin, ACTH, cortisol, epinephrine, norepinephrine, renin, angiotensin II, aldosterone, ADH, etc. Brief periods of these interventions may be most valuable during the early phases of the disease and extended periods when the disease is established. Renal impairment in salt and water excretion may be a primary cause of intravascular volume overload. A number of the stress response molecules may induce intravascular volume overload in the early phase of pathogenesis by their physiological role in salt and water homeostasis (ACTH, angiotensin II, aldosterone, and ADH), whereas others may induce vasoconstriction directly by increasing Ca_i (norepinephrine, angiotensin, vasopressin). They all, however, induce hypertension by increasing Ca_i. It is here that volume depletion (sodium-deficient intake or diuretic therapy) and weight reduction and calcium channel blockade become effective because they lower Ca_i (225). Therapeutic agents that selectively inhibit active tension development in vascular smooth muscle are also efficacious, if specificity can be established.

Figure 1.1 also shows specific sites of action for the *mosaic* of genetic, environmental, anatomical, adaptive, neural, endocrine, humoral, and hemodynamic factors in the pathogenesis of black hypertensives. *Genetic* influence may be important in regulating physiological stress response molecules (see Chapter 3, this volume), intravascular volume overload through renal sodium retentional molecules (see Chapter 2, this volume), and increased Ca_i through calcium transporting molecules (see Chapter 9, this volume). *Environmental* influences may influence the psychosocial stressors most profoundly (see Chapters 2, 4, 5, 6, and 7, this volume). It also influences the intravascular volume overload component by dietary alterations (see Chapters 7 and 8, this volume). *Anatomical* influences are important in intravascular volume overload by structural alteration of renal salt retention mechanisms at the afferent and efferent arterioles and proximal tubule, in decreasing stretch of arterioles in general due to decreased vascular compliance, and increased total peripheral resistance due to structural remodeling. *Adaptive* influences may affect psychosocial stressors (see Chapters 4 and 5, this volume), physiological stress response molecules (see Chapters 3, 6, 7, and 8, this volume), intravascular volume overload through renal salt retention molecules (see Chapters 2 and 7, this volume), and increased Ca_i and total peripheral resistance through the equilibrium mechanism (see Fig. 11.1). *Neural* influences may most profoundly influence liberation of physiological stress response molecules to alter vascular reactivity (see Chapter 6, this volume), increase intravascular volume overload through sympathetic control of renal salt retention (see Chapter 7, this volume), increase cardiac output, and increase total peripheral resistance through an "alpha" response (see Chapter 6, this volume). *Endocrine* influences can be seen in the physiological response molecules (see Chapters 3, 7, 8, and 10, this volume), in mediating intravascular volume overload through renal salt and water retention, increasing Ca_i, and total peripheral resistance (see Chapters 3, 6, 7, 8, and 9, this volume). *Humoral* factors such as ions, sugar, and neuropeptides influence liberation of physiological stress response molecules and subsequently all processes along the pathogenetic cascade. *Hemodynamic* influences such as pressure itself influence cardiac output, alter stretch capabilities of the arterioles, and thereby Ca_i, and vascular distensibility and structural remodeling to alter total peripheral resistance. Taken together, the model prompts the conclusion that the term "essential" hypertension in blacks should be replaced by the more accurate *psychosocial stressor–induced hypertension,* giving significance to the evidence that in blacks psychosocial stressors are primary initiating factors and assigning the arterioles as the final pathophysiological manifestation of these stressors.

In its most general form, the model holds that stable physical equilibrium will be achieved providing arterioles display the following main features: *(1)* the force acting to distend (blood pressure) must be equal and opposite to the force acting in the wall to constrict the arteriole (wall tension); *(2)* the wall tension consists of at least passive and active components, the latter of which is defined by the level of Ca_i; *(3)* the stretch of the arterioles (mediated by blood pressure itself) activates the opening of calcium channels in the plasma membrane. This activation leads to increases in Ca_i and thereby to increase in vascular resistance. The implication, therefore, is that calcium functions as the coupling factor that couples stretch to contraction. This endows calcium with a unique role in the pathogenesis of several cardiovascular disorders including psychosocial stressor–induced hypertension in blacks (see Chapter 10, this volume). Maintenance is also a function of calcium. Initially, Ca_i increases and causes increased total peripheral resistance (see Chapter 6, this volume). The mechanisms for the increased Ca_i are increased vascular smooth muscle calcium permeability and decreased calcium pump activity. Subsequently, two mechanisms *maintain* the elevated Ca_i: generalized increased membrane permeability to calcium and a generalized defect in the calcium efflux mechanism. Regarding the increased permeability to calcium the decrease can be reversed by calcium channel blockers. Regarding the calcium efflux there appears to be a reduced activity of the calcium pump and suppression of the sodium-calcium exchange mechanism. A sodium pump inhibitor is postulated to suppress sodium-calcium exchange by inhibiting the sodium pump.

Although the model goes far in explaining the fundamental mechanism of the above processes and the interrelationships among the processes, it goes even further in advancing our understanding of the biophysical mechanisms of hypertension. It provides a theoretical framework for the volume-vasoconstriction approach proposed by Laragh (138), for the autoregulation hypothesis advanced by several workers (27,49,54,83,89,142,178), for the resetting of arterial baroreceptors and renal excretory functions, and for the mosaic approach first proposed by Page (176). The theory has an additional implication, which is primarily philosophic, for it challenges us to view circulatory control in a completely unique way. That is, the physical equilibrium requirement is of importance in any consideration of circulatory control, for it shows that a particular level of blood pressure is not regulated but is *determined* as a consequence of the circulation's search for stable physical equilibria. This further implies that hypertension may be an "ionic disease" whereby the circulation achieves a new state of stable equilibrium. The equilibrium requirement itself may be the "something" that Tobian (206) speculated was manifested in hypertension as a change in the "cell membrane of the arterial muscle cells." The theory provides logical and physiological explanations for the mechanisms whereby calciumchannel blockers, β-adrenergic agonists, diuretics, weight reduction, and sodium deprivation reduce blood pressure in hypertensives: by lowering Ca_i and thereby disturbing physical equilibrium in arterioles.

Other pathogenic mechanisms have been suggested for blacks. The significance of the equilibrium model is that calcium, in association with the physical equilibrium requirement, is central, not marginal. It has become clear that structural remodeling plays an important role, particularly in end organ pathology in blacks. Although in established hypertension, structural remodeling plays a role in establishing stable equilibrium, the decisive factor in initiating the response is calcium. This view receives support from the observation that in the absence of calcium inflow, hypertension (and the subsequent structural remodeling) does not develop. Vessel hypertrophy may feed back on wall tension and consequently influence equilibrium, but details of this mechanism remain speculative. These processes may also influence vascular reactivity, particularly in blacks (see Chapter 6, this volume), but insufficient evidence is available to assess the processes' significance. The equilibrium formulation offers a conceptual framework on which more refined and detailed models can be deconstructed to allow the emergence of new data on essential hypertension in the black population.

Figure 1.2 summarizes the major features of the evidence presented in this book and shows three distinct phases in the pathogenesis of hypertension in blacks when the initial insult is a psychosocial stressor. The initial phase (phase I) is characterized by an increase in physiological stress response molecules. The primary role of total peripheral resistance in psychosocial stressor–induced elevation of blood pressure is well established in blacks (see Chapters 3 and 6, this volume). Intravascular volume may be normal, but cardiovascular reactivity may be high, thereby potentiating the hypertensive effects of the physiological stress response molecules. Genetic predisposition may also begin to play a role in this early phase (see Chapter 3, this volume). The second phase (phase II) represents a continuation of the first, in addition to increased cardiac output as a result of intravascular volume overload, increased vascular reactivity, and renin hyporesponsivity (see Chapter 10, this volume). Phase II is characterized as the stage where genetic predisposition may have significant effect on Ca_i, vascular reactivity, and "salt sensitivity." Impaired renal function and salt excretion may begin to have significant effect in phase II. The final phase (phase III) is established hypertension characterized as a chronic stage of the second phase, in addition to elevated Ca_i, renin hyporesponsivity, and elevated total peripheral resistance. Thus, the pathogenesis of hypertension in blacks, where the initial insult is psychosocial stressors, has much in common with experimental renovascular hypertension where the initial stimulus is partial renal artery obstruction. By centering around Ca_i, the model shows that established hypertension should be associated with a variety of other cardiovascular disorders (see Chapter 10, this volume) in which Ca_i plays a significant role, such as hyperinsulinemia, insulin resistance, obesity, and type II diabetes in blacks.

REFERENCES

1. Ackerman, U. Cardiac output, GFR, and renal excretion rates during maintained volume load in rats. *Am. J. Physiol. 235 (Heart Circ. Physiol. 4)*: H670–H676, 1978.
2. Amer, M. S., I. V. Doba, and D. J. Reis. Changes in cyclic nucleotide metabolism in aorta and heart of neurogenically hypertensive rats: possible trigger mechanism of hypertension. *Proc. Natl. Acad. Sci. U.S.A. 72*: 2135–2139, 1975.
3. Anderson, N. B., H. F. Myers, T. Pickering, and J. S. Jackson. Hypertension in blacks: psychosocial and biological perspectives. *J. Hypertens. 7*: 161–172, 1989.
4. Andresen, M. C., J. M. Krauhs, and A. M. Brown. Relationship of aortic wall and baroreceptor properties during development in normotensive sportaneously hypertensive rats. *Circ. Res. 43*: 728–738, 1978.
5. Andresen, M. C., S. Kuraoka, and A. M. Brown. Individual and combined actions of calcium, sodium, and postassium ions or baroreceptors in the rat. *Circ. Res. 45*: 757–763, 1979.
6. Angell-James, J. E. Characteristics of single aortic and right subclavian baroreceptor fiber activity in rabbits with chronic renal hypertension. *Circ. Res. 32*: 149–161, 1973.
7. Aoki, K., and K. Sato. Pathophysiological background for the use of calcium antagonists. *J. Cardiovasc. Pharmacol. 7*(Supp.4): S28–S32, 1985.
8. Aviv, A. The link between cytosolic Ca^{2+} and the $Na^+ - H^+$ antiport: a unifying factor for essential hypertension. *J. Hypertens. 6*: 685–691, 1988.
9. Azuma, T., and S. Oka. Mechanical equilibrium of blood vessel walls. *Am. J. Physiol. 221*: 1310–1318, 1971.
10. Baez, S. Bayliss response in the microcirculation. *Fed. Proc. 27*: 1410–1415, 1968.
11. Barger, A. C. The Goldblatt memorial lecture, part I: experimental renovascular hypertension. *Hypertension 1*: 447–455, 1979.
12. Bauer, J. H., and G. Reams. Short- and long-term effects of calcium entry blockers on the kidney. *Am. J. Cardiol. 59*: 66A–71A, 1987.
13. Bauer, J. H., S. Sunderrajan, and G. Reams. Effects of calcium entry blockers on renin–angiotensin–aldosterone system, renal function and hemodynamics, salt and water excretion, and body fluid composition. *Am. J. Cardiol. 56*: 62H–67H, 1985.

14. Bayliss, W. M. On the local reactions of the arterial wall to changes of internal pressure. *J. Physiol. (Lond.) 28:* 220–231, 1902.

15. Bell, L. B., J. L. Seagard, E. J. Zuperku, and J. P. Kampine. Mechanical effects of vasoactive drugs on carotid sinus. *Am. J. Physiol. 250 (Regulatory Integrative Comp. Physiol. 20:)* R1074–R1080, 1986.

16. Berecek, K. H., U. Schwertschlag, and F. Gross. Alterations in renal vascular resistance and reactivity in spontaneous hypertension of rats. *Am. J. Physiol. 238 (Heart Circ. Physiol. 8):* H287–H293, 1980.

17. Bevan, J. A. Diltiazem selectively inhibits cerebrovascular extrinsic but not intrinsic myogenic tone. *Circ. Res. 52* (Suppl.I): 104–109, 1983.

18. Bianchi, G., D. Cusi, M. Gatti, G. P. Lupi, P. Ferrari, C. Barlassina, G. B. Picotti, G. Bracchi, G. Colombo, D. Gori, O. Velis, and D. Mazzei. A renal abnormality as a possible cause of "essential" hypertension. *Lancet 1:* 173–177, 1979.

19. Bianchi, G., U. Fox, D. Pagetti, A. M. Caravaggi, P. G. Baer, and E. Baldoli. Mechanism involved in renal hypertension. *Kidney Int. 8:* S165–S173, 1975.

20. Blaustein, M. P. How salt causes hypertension: the natriuretic hormone-Na/Ca exchange-hypertension hypothesis. *Klin. Wochenschr. 63*(Suppl III): 82–85, 1985.

21. Blaustein, M. P. Sodium ions, calcium ions, blood pressure regulation, and hypertension: a reassessment and a hypothesis. *Am. J. Physiol. 232* (Cell Physiol. 2): C165–C173, 1977.

22. Blaustein, M. P., and J. M. Hamlyn. Sodium transport inhibition, cell calcium, and hypertension. The natriuretic hormone/Na^+-Ca^{2+} exchange/hypertension hypothesis. *Am. J. Med. 77*(Supp.4A): 45–59, 1984.

23. Bolli, P., P. Erne, U. L. Hulthen, R. Ritz, W. Kiowski, B. H. Ji, and F. R. Buhler. Parallel reduction of calcium-influx-dependent vasoconstriction and platelet-free calcium concentration with calcium entry and B-adrenoreceptor blockade. *J. Cardiovasc. Pharmacol. 6:* S996–S1001, 1984.

24. Bolli, P., W. Kiowski, P. Erne, L. U. Hulthen, and F. R., Buhler. Hemodynamic and antihypertensive treatment responses with calcium antagonists. *J. Cardiovasc. Pharmacol. 7:* S126–S130, 1985.

25. Bolt, G. R., and P. R. Saxena. Acute systemic and regional hemodynamic effects of felodipine, a new calcium antagonist, in conscious renal hypertensive rabbits. *J. Cardiovasc. Pharmacol. 6:* 707–712, 1984.

26. Borgstrom, P., P-O. Grande, and L. Lindbom. Responses of single arterioles in vivo in cat skeletal muscle to change in arterial pressure applied at different rates. *Acta Physiol. Scand. 113:* 207–212, 1981.

27. Borst, J. G. G., and A. Borst-DeGeus. Hypertension explained by Starling's theory of circulatory homeostasis. *Lancet 1:* 677–682, 1963.

28. Brostrom, C. O. and M. A. Brostrom. Calcium-dependent regulation of protein synthesis in intact mammalian cells. *Ann. Rev. Physiol. 52:* 577–590, 1990.

29. Brown, J. J., A. F. Lever, J. I. S. Robertson, M. A. Schalekamp. Renal abnormality of essential hypertension. *Lancet 1:* 320–323, 1974.

30. Brunner, H. R., J. Nussberger, and B. Waeber. Responsiveness of renin secretion: a key mechanism in the maintenance of blood pressure. *J. Hypertens. 4*(Supp.IV): S89–S94, 1986.

31. Bruschi, G., M. E. Bruschi, A. Cavatorta, and A. Borghetti. The mechanisms of Ca_{i2+} increases in blood cells of spontaneously hypertensive rats. *J. Cardiovasc. Pharmacol. 8*(Supp. 8): S139–S144, 1986.

32. Bruschi, G., M. E. Bruschi, M. Caroppo, G. Orlandini, M. Spaggiari, and A. Cavatorta. Cytoplasmic free [Ca^{2+}] is increased in the platelets of spontaneously hypertensive rats and essential hypertensive patients. *Clin. Sci. 68:* 179–184, 1985.

33. Bruschi, G., M. E. Bruschi, M. Caroppo, G. Orlandini, C. Pavarini, and A. Cavatorta. Intracellular free [Ca2a] in circulating lymphocytes of spontaneously hypertensive rats. *Life Sci. 35:* 535–542, 1984.

34. Bryant, H. J., D. R. Harder, M. B. Pamnani, and F. J. Haddy. In vivo membrane potentials of smooth muscle cells in the caudal artery of the rat. *Am. J. Physiol. 249 (Cell Physiol. 18):* C78–C83, 1985.

35. Buggy, J., S. Huot, M. Pamnani, and F. Haddy. Periventricular forebrain mechanisms for blood pressure regulation. *Fed. Proc. 43:* 25–31, 1984.

36. Buhler, F. R., P. Bolli, Erne, W. Kiowski, F. B. Muller, U. L. Hulthen, and B. H. Ji. Adrenoceptors, calcium, and vasoconstriction in normal and hypertensive humans. *J. Cardiovasc. Pharmacol. 7*(Suppl.6): 130–136, 1985.

37. Burke, S. L., P. K. Dorward, and P. I. Korner. Rapid resetting of rabbit aortic baroreceptors and reflex heart rate responses by directional changes in blood pressure. *J. Physiol. (Lond) 378:* 391–402, 1986.

38. Burrows, M. E., and P. C. Johnson. Arteriolar responses to elevation of venous and arterial pressures in cat mesentery. *Am. J. Physiol. 245 (Heart Circ. Physiol. 14):* H796–H807, 1983.
39. Burrows, M. E., and P. C. Johnson. Diameters, wall tension, and flow in mesenteric arterioles during autoregulation. *Am. J. Physiol. 241 (Heart Circ. Physiol. 10):* H829–H837, 1981.
40. Burton, A. C. On the physical equilibrium of small blood vessels. *Am. J. Physiol. 164:* 319–329, 1951.
41. Capponi, A. M., P. D. Lew, L. Jornot, and M. B. Vallotton. Correlation between cytosolic free Ca^{2+} and aldosterone production in adrenal glomerulosa cells. Evidence for a difference in the mode of action of angiotensin II and potassium. *J. Biol. Chem. 259:* 8863–8869, 1984.
42. Carafoli, E., and M. Zurini. The Ca^{2+}-pumping ATPase of plasma membranes purification, reconstitution and properties. *Biochim. Biophys. Acta 683:* 279–301, 1982.
43. Cauvin, C., S. Lukeman, J. Cameron, O. Hwang, and C. VanBreemen. Differences in norepinephrine activation and diltiazem inhibition of calcium channels in isolated rabbit aorta and mesenteric resistance vessels. *Circ. Res. 56:* 822–828, 1985.
44. Chalmers, J. P., P. M. Pilowsky, J. P. Minson, V. Kapoor, E. Mills, and M. J. West. Central serotonergic mechanisms in hypertension. *Am. J. Hypertens. 1:* 79–83, 1988.
45. Chapman, R. A. Control of cardiac contractility at the cellular level. *Am. J. Physiol. 245 (Heart Circ. Physiol. 14):* H535–H552, 1983.
46. Cheung, D. W. Membrane potential of vascular smooth muscle and hypertension in spontaneously hypertensive rats. *Can. J. Physiol. Pharmacol. 62:* 957–960, 1984.
47. Click, R. L., W. Joyner, and J. P. Gilmore. Reactivity of glomerular afferent and efferent arterioles in renal hypertension. *Kidney Int. 15:* 109–115, 1979.
48. Cohen, A. J., J. C. S. Fray. Calcium dependence of myogenic renal plasma flow autoregulation: evidence from the isolated perfused rat kidney. *J. Physiol. (Lond.) 330:* 449–460, 1982.
49. Coleman, T. G., R. E. Samar, and W. R. Murphy. Autoregulation versus other vasoconstrictors in hypertension. *Hypertension 1:* 324–330, 1979.
50. Coleridge, H. M., J. C. G. Coleridge, M. P. Kaufman, and A. Dangel. Operational sensitivity and acute resetting of aortic baroreceptors in dogs. *Circ. Res. 48:* 676–684, 1981.
51. Constantopoulos, G., M. Kusumoto, J. M. Rojo-Ortega, P. Granger, R. Boucher, and J. Genest. Arterial water, cations, and norepinephrine in early and late renovascular hypertension. *Am. J. Physiol. 228:* 1415–1422, 1975.
52. Cooper, K. E., J. M. Tang, J. L. Rae, and R. S. Eisenberg. A cation channel in frog lens epithelia responsive to pressure and calcium. *J. Membr. Biol. 93:* 259–269, 1986.
53. Cooper, R. S., N. Shamsi, and S. Katz. Intracellular calcium and sodium in hypertensive patients. *Hypertension 9:* 224–229, 1987.
54. Cowley, A. W. The concept of autoregulation of total blood flow and its role in hypertension. *Am. J. Med. 68:* 906–916, 1980.
55. Cowley, A. W., C. Hinojosa-Labourde, B. J. Barber, D. R. Harder, J. H. Lombard, and A. S. Greene. Short-term autoregulation of systemic blood flow and cardiac output. *News in Physiological Sciences 4:* 219–225, 1989.
56. Dahl, L. K., K. D. Knudsen, and J. Iwai. Humoral transmission of hypertension: evidence from parabiosis. *Circ. Res. 24*(Supp.I): 21–33, 1969.
57. Davis, J. O. The pathogenesis of chronic renovascular hypertension. *Circ. Res. 40:* 439–444, 1977.
58. DeJong, W., ed. *Experimental and Genetic Models of Hypertension,* Elsevier, New York, 1984.
59. DeQuattro, V., and Y. Miura. Neurogenic factors inhuman hypertension: mechanism or myth? *Am. J. Med. 55:* 362–378, 1973.
60. DeWardener, H. E., G. A. MacGregor. The relation of a circulating sodium transport inhibitor (the natriuretic hormone?) to hypertension. *Medicine 62:* 310–326, 1983.
61. DeWardener, H. E., and G. A. MacGregor. Dahl's hypothesis that a saluretic substance may be responsible for a sustained rise in arterial pressure: its possible role in essential hypertension. *Kidney Int. 18:* 1–9, 1980.
62. Donnison, C. P. Blood pressure in the African native. *Lancet 1:* 6–7, 1929.
63. Doward, P. K., M. C. Andresen, S. L. Burke, J. R. Oliver, and P. I. Korner. Rapid resetting of the aortic baroreceptors in the rabbit and its implications for short-term and longer term reflex control. *Circ. Res. 50:* 428–439, 1982.
64. Dzau, V. J., L. G. Seiwek, and A. C. Barger. Intrarenal resistance in experimental hypertension. In: *Frontiers in Hypertension Research,* edited by J. H. Laragh, F. R. Buhler, and D. W. Seldin, Springer-Verlag, New York, 1981, pp. 165–168.
65. Edwards, C., D. Ottoson, B. Rydgvist, and C. Swerup. The permeability of the transducer

membrane of the cray fish stretch receptor to calcium and other divalent cations. *Neuroscience 6:* 1455–1460, 1981.

66. Edwards, R. M. Segmental effect of norepinephrine and angiotensin II on isolated renal microvessels. *Am. J. Physiol. 244 (Renal Fluid Electrolyte Physiol.13):* F526–F534, 1983.

67. Ene, M. D., P. J. Williamson, and C. J. C. Roberts. The natriuresis following oral administration of the calcium antagonists-nifedipine and nitrendipine. *Br. J. Clin. Pharmacol. 19:* 423–427, 1985.

68. Erne, P., E. Burgisser, P. Bolli, J. BaoHua, and F. R. Buhler. Free calcium concentration in platelets closely relates to blood pressure in normal and essential hypertensive subjects. *Hypertension 6*(Supp.I): 166–169, 1984.

69. Erne, P., P. Bolli, E. Burgisser, and F. R. Buhler. Correlation of platelet calcium with blood pressure. *N. Engl. J. Med. 310:* 1084–1088, 1984.

70. Esler, M., S. Julius, A. Zweifler, O. Randall, E. Harburg, H. Gardiner, and V. DeQuattro. Mild high-renin essential hypertension: neurogenic human hypertension? *N. Engl. J. Med. 296:* 405–411, 1977.

71. Fakunding, J. T., and K. J. Catt. Dependence of aldosterone stimulation in adrenal glomerulosa cells on calcium uptake: effects of lanthanum and verapamil. *Endocrinology 107:* 1345–1353, 1980.

72. Fakunding, J. L., R. Chow, and K. J. Catt. The role of calcium in the stimulation of aldosterone production by adrenocorticotropin, angiotensin II, and potassium in isolated glomerulosa cells. *Endocrinology 105:* 327–333, 1979.

73. Firth, J. D., A. E. G. Raine, and J. G. G. Ledingham. The mechanism of pressure natriuresis. *J. Hypertens. 8:* 97–103, 1990.

74. Folkow, B. Physiological aspects of primary hypertension. *Physiol. Rev. 62:* 347–504, 1982.

75. Folkow, B., G. Grimby, and O. Thulesius. Adaptive structural changes of the vascular walls in hypertension and their relation to the control of the peripheral resistance. *Acta Physiol. Scand. 44:* 255–272, 1958.

76. Foster, R., M. V. Lobo, H. Rasmussen, and E. T. Marusic. Calcium its role in the mechanism of action of angiotensin II and potassium in aldoesterone production. *Endocrinology 109:* 2196–2201, 1981.

77. Fray, J. C. S. Stretch receptor model for renin release with evidence from perfused rat kidney. *Am. J. Physiol. 231:* 936–944, 1976.

78. Fray, J. C. S., D. J. Lush, and C. S. Park. Interrelationship of blood flow, juxtaglomerular cells, and hypertension: role of physical equilibrium and Ca. *Am. J. Physiol. 251 (Regulatory Integrative Comp. Physiol. 20):* R643–R662, 1986.

79. Fray, J. C. S., C. S. Park, and A. N. D. Valentine. Calcium and the control of renin secretion. *Endocr. Rev. 8:* 1–42, 1987.

80. Freeman, R. H., J. O. Davis, and A. A. Seymour. Volume and vasoconstriction in experimental renovascular hypertension. *Fed. Proc. 41:* 2409–2414, 1982.

81. Frohlich, E. D. Hemodynamic factors in the pathogenesis and maintenance of hypertension. *Fed. Proc. 41:* 2400–2408, 1982.

82. Gothberg, G., and B. Folkow. "Structural autoregulation" of blood flow and GFR two-kidney, one-clip renal hypertensive rats, as compared with kidneys from uni-nephrectomized and intact normotensive rats. *Acta Physiol. Scand. 118:* 141–148, 1983.

83. Granger, H. J., A. C. Guyton. Autoregulation of the total sytemic circulation following destruction of the central nervous system in the dog. *Circ. Res. 25:* 379–388, 1969.

84. Grim, C. E., F. C. Luft, J. Z. Miller, G. R. Meneely, H. D. Battarbee, C. G. Hames, and L. K. Dahl. Racial differences in blood pressure in Evans County, Georgia: relationship to sodium and potassium intake and plasma renin activity. *J. Chronic Dis. 33:* 87–94, 1980.

85. Grossman, E., and T. Rosenthal. The hypotensive effect of nisoldipine in renovascular hypertensive rats. *J. Hypertens. 4* (Suppl. 5): S141–144, 1986.

86. Guharay, F., and F. Sachs. Mechanotransducer ion channels in chick skeletal muscle: the effects of extracellular pH. *J. Physiol. (Lond.) 363:* 119–134, 1985.

87. Guharay, F., and F. Sachs. Stretch-activated single ion channel currents in tissue-cultured embryonic chick skeletal muscle. *J. Physiol. (Lond.) 352:* 685–701, 1984.

88. Guo, G. B., and M. D. Thames. Abnormal baroreflex control in renal hypertension is due to abnormal baroreceptors. *Am. J. Physiol. 245 (Heart Circ. Physiol. 14):* H420–H428, 1983.

89. Guyton, A. C., J. E. Hall, T. E. Lohmeier, R. D. Manning, and T. E. Jackson. Position paper: the concept of whole body autoregulation and the dominant role of the kidneys for long-term blood pressure regulation. In: *Frontiers in Hypertension Research,* ed-

ited by J. H. Laragh, F. R. Buhler, and D. W. Seldin. Springer-Verlag, New York, 1981, pp. 125–134.

90. Guyton, A. C., R. D. Manning, J. E. Hall, R. A. Norman, D. B. Young, and Y.-J. Pan. The pathogenic role of the kidney. *J. Cardiovasc. Pharmacol.* 6(Suppl.1): S151–S161, 1984.

91. Guyton, A. C., R. D. Manning, R. A. Norman, J.-P. Montani, T. E. Lohmeier, and J. E. Hall. Current concepts and perspectives of renal volume regulation in relationship to hypertension. *J. Hypertens.* 4(Supp.4): S49–S56, 1986.

92. Guyton, A. C., T. G. Coleman, and H. J. Granger. Circulation: overall regulation. *Ann. Rev. Physiol. 34:* 13–46, 1972.

93. Haber, E. The role of renin in normal and pathological cardiovascular homeostasis. *Circulation 54:* 849–861, 1976.

94. Haddy, F. J. Abnormalities of membrane transport in hypertension. *Hypertension* 5(Suppl.V): 66–72, 1983.

95. Haddy, F. J., and H. W. Overbeck. The role of humoral agents in volume expanded hypertension. *Life Sci. 19:* 935–948, 1976.

96. Haddy, F., M. Pamnani, and D. Clough. The sodium-potassium pump in volume expanded hypertension. *Clin. Exp. Hypertens. 1:* 295–336, 1978.

97. Haddy, F. J. and M. B. Pamnani. Natriuretic hormones in low renin hypertension. *Klin. Wochenschr.* 65(Suppl. VIII): 154–160, 1987.

98. Hall, J. E. Control of sodium excretion by angiotensin II intrarenal mechanisms and blood pressure regulation. *Am. J. Physiol. 250 (Regulatory Integrative Comp. Physiol. 19):* R960–R972, 1986.

99. Hall, J. E., J. P. Granger, R. L. Hester, and J.-P. Montani. Mechanisms of sodium balance in hypertension: role of pressure natriuresis. *J. Hypertens.* 4(Supp.4): S57–S65, 1986.

100. Hall, J. E., A. C. Guyton, M. J. Smith, and T. G. Coleman. Blood pressure and renal function during chronic changes in sodium intake: role of angiotensin. *Am. J. Physiol. 239 (Renal Fluid Electrolyte Physiol. 8):* F271–F280, 1980.

101. Halpern, W., M. J. Mulvany, and D. M. Warshaw. Mechanical properties of smooth muscle cells in the walls of arterial resistance vessels. *J. Physiol. (Lond.) 275:* 85–101, 1978.

102. Hamlyn, J. M., and M. P. Blaustein. Sodium chloride, extracellular fluid volume, and blood pressure regulation. *Am. J. Physiol. 251 (Renal Fluid Electrolyte Physiol. 20)* F563–F575, 1986.

103. Hamlyn, J. M., R. Ringel, J. Schaeffer, P. D. Levinson, B. P. Hamilton, A. A. Kowarski, and M. P. Blaustein. A circulating inhibitor of (Na^+K^+) ATPase associated with essential hypertension. *Nature 300:* 650–652, 1982.

104. Harder, D. R. Pressure-dependent membrane depolarization in cat middle cerebral artery. *Circ. Res. 55:* 197–202, 1984.

105. Heesch, C. M., B. M. Miller, M. D. Thames, and F. M. Abboud. Effects of calcium channel blockers on isolated carotid baroreceptors and baroreflex. *Am. J. Physiol. 245 (Heart Circ. Physiol. 14):* H653–H661, 1983.

106. Henry, J. P., P. M. Stephens, and D. L. Ely. Psychosocial hypertension and the defence and defeat reactions. *J. Hypertens. 4:* 687–697, 1986.

107. Heymans, C., and A. L. Delaunois. Fundamental role of the tone and resistance to stretch of the carotid sinus arteries in the reflex regulation of blood pressure. *Science 114:* 546–547, 1951.

108. Hogestatt, E. D. Characterization of two different calcium entry pathways in small mesenteric arteries from rat. *Acta Physiol. Scand. 122:* 483–495, 1984.

109. Huang, W. C. Antihypertensive and bilateral renal responses to nifedipine in 2-kidney, 1-clip, Goldblatt hypertensive rats. *Renal Physiol. 9:* 167–176, 1986.

110. Hudspeth, A. J. The hair cells of the inner ear. *Sci. Am. 248:* 54–64, 1983.

111. Huelsemann, J. L., R. B. Sterzel, D. E. McKenzie, and C. S. Wilcox. Effects of a calcium entry blocker on blood pressure and renal function during angiotensin-induced hypertension. *Hypertension 7:* 374–379, 1985.

112. Humes, H. D., C. F. Simmons, and B. M. Brenner. Effect of verapamil on the hydroosmotic response to antidiuretic hormone in toad urinary bladder. *Am. J. Physiol. 239 (Renal Fluid Electrolyte Physiol. 8):* F250–F257, 1980.

113. Hunt, C. C., R. S. Wilkinson, and Y. Fukami. Ionic basis of the receptor potential in primary endings of mammalian muscle spindles. *J. Gen. Physiol. 71:* 683–698, 1978.

114. Hwa, J. J., and J. A. Bevan. A nimodipine-resistant Ca^{2+} pathway is involved in myogenic tone in a resistant artery. *Am. J. Physiol. 251 (Heart Circ. Physiol. 20):* H182–H189, 1986.

115. Hwa, J. J., and J. A. Bevan. Stretch-dependent (myogenic) tone in rabbit ear resistance arteries. *Am. J. Physiol. 250 (Heart Circ. Physiol. 19):* H87–H95, 1986.

116. Insel, P. A., and H. J. Motulsky. A hypothesis linking intracellular sodium, membrane receptors, and hypertension. *Life Sci. 34:* 1009–1013, 1984.
117. Iversen, B. M., L. Morkrid, and J. Ofstad. Afferent arteriolar diameter in DOCA-salt and two-kidney one-clip hypertensive rats. *Am. J. Physiol. 245 (Renal Fluid Electrolyte Physiol. 14):* F755–F762, 1983.
118. Iversen, B. M., and J. Ofstad. Resetting of renal blood flow autoregulation and renin release in spontaneously hypertensive rats. *Contrib. Nephrol. 41:* 415–416, 1984.
119. Iversen, B. M., I. Sekse, and J. Ofstad. Resetting of renal blood flow autoregulation in spontaneously hypertensive rats. *Am. J. Physiol. 252 (Renal Fluid Electrolyte Physiol. 21)* F480–F486, 1987.
120. Johansson, B. Processes involved in vascular smooth muscle contraction and relaxation. *Circ. Res. 43:* I-14–I-20, 1978.
121. Johnson, P. C., and M. Intaglietta. Contributions of pressure and flow sensitivity to autoregulation and mesenteric arterioles. *Am. J. Physiol. 231:* 1686–1698, 1976.
122. Joshua, I. G., F. N. Miller, and D. L. Wiegman. In vivo venular changes with the development of one-kidney, one-clip hypertension in the rat. *Clin. Exper. Hypertens. A8:* 1343–1354, 1986.
123. Kiowski, W., F. R. Buhler, M. O. Fadayomi, P. Erne, F. B. Muller, J. L. Hulthen, and P. Boli. Age, race, blood pressure and renin predictors for antihypertensive treatment with calcium antagonists. *Am. J. Cardiol. 56:* 81H–85H, 1985.
124. Klein, W., D. Brandt, K. Vrecko, and M. Harringer. Role of calcium antagonists in the treatment of essential hypertension. *Circ. Res. 52*(Suppl. I): 174–181, 1983.
125. Knight, D. R., D. A. Kirby, and S. R. Vatner. Effects of a calcium channel blocker on cardiac output distribution in conscious hypertensive dogs. *Hypertension 7:* 380–385, 1985.
126. Koch, A. R. Some mathematical forms of autoregulatory models. *Circ. Res. 14* (Suppl. I): 260–278, 1964.
127. Kojima, I., K. Kojima, and H. Rasmussen. Effects of ANG II and K^+ on Ca efflux and aldosterone production in adrenal flomerulosa cells. *Am. J. Physiol. 248 (Endocrinol. Metabl. 11)* E43, 1985.
128. Kornel, L., N. Kanamarlapudi, and M. M. Von Dreele. The role of arterial mineralocorticoid receptors in the mechanism of hypertension: findings and hypothesis. *Clin. Biochem. 20:* 113–120, 1987.
129. Korner, P. I., G. L. Jennings, M. D. Elser, W. P. Anderson, A. Bobik, M. Adams, J. A. Angus. The cardiovascular amplifiers in human primary hypertension and their role in a strategy for detecting the underlying causes. *Can. J. Physiol. Pharmacol. 65:* 1730–1738, 1987.
130. Kowala, M. C., H. F. Cuenoud, I. Joris, and G. Majno. Cellular changes during hypertension: a quantitative study of the rat aorta. *Exp. Molec. Pathol. 45:* 323–335, 1986.
131. Krieger, E. M. Aortic diastolic caliber changes as a determinant for complete aortic baroreceptor resetting. *Fed. Proc. 46:* 41–45, 1987.
132. Kunze, D. L. Calcium and magnesium sensitivity of carotid baroreceptor reflex in cats. *Circ. Res. 45:* 815–821, 1979.
133. Kwan, C. Y., L. Belbeck, and E. E. Daniel. Characteristics of arterial plasma membrane in renovascular hypertension in rats. *Blood Vessels 17:* 131–140, 1980.
134. Kwan, C. Y., P. Kostka, A. K. Grover, J. S. Law, and E. E. Daniel. Calmodulin stimulation of plasmalemmal Ca^{2+}-pump of canine aortic smooth muscle. *Blood Vessels 23:* 22–33, 1986.
135. Landgren, S. The baroreceptor activity in the carotid sinus nerve and the distensibility of the sinus wall. *Acta Physiol. Scand. 26:* 35–56, 1952.
136. Lansman, J. B., T. J. Hallam, and T. J. Rink. Single stretch-activated ion channels in vascular endothelial cells as mechanotransducers? *Nature 325:* 811–813, 1987.
137. Laragh, J. H. Renovascular hypertension: a paradigm for all hypertension *J. Hypertens.* 4(Suppl. 4):S79–S88, 1986.
138. Laragh, J. H. Vasoconstriction-volume analysis for understanding and treating hypertension: the use of renin and aldosterone profiles. *Am. J. Med. 55:* 261–274, 1973.
139. Larsen, F. L., S. Katz, B. D. Roufogalis, and D. E. Brooks. Physiological shear stresses enhance the Ca^{2+} permeability of human erythrocytes. *Nature 294:* 667–668, 1981.
140. Lau, K., and B. Eby. The role of calcium in genetic hypertension. *Hypertension 7:* 657–667, 1985.
141. Ledingham, J. M. Mechanisms in renal hypertension. *Proc. R. Soc. Med. 64:* 409–418, 1971.
142. Ledingham, J. M., and R. D. Cohen. Hypertension explained by Starling's theory of circulatory homeostasis. *Lancet 1:* 887–888, 1963.

143. Ledingham, J. M., and D. Pelling. Cardiac output and peripheral resistance in experimental renal hypertension. *Circ. Res. 20* (Suppl.2): 187–199, 1967.

144. Lever, A. F. Slow pressor mechanisms in hypertension: a role for hypertrophy of resistance vessels? *J. Hypertens. 4:* 515–524, 1986.

145. Levy, S. B., J. J. Lilley, R. P. Frigon, and R. A. Stone. Urinary kallikrein and plasma renin activity as determinants of renal blood flow. The influence of race and dietary sodium intake. *J. Clin. Invest. 60:* 129–138, 1977.

146. Levy, S. B., L. B. Talner, M. H. Coel, R. Holle, and R. A. Stone. Renal vasculature in essential hypertension: racial differences. *Ann. Intern. Med. 88:* 12, 1978.

147. Liard, J. F. Regional blood flows in salt loading hypertension in the dog. *Am. J. Physiol. 240 (Heart Circ. Physiol. 9):* H361–H367, 1981.

148. Losse, H., W. Zidek, and H. Vetter. Intracellular sodium and calcium in vascular smooth muscle of spontaneously hypertensive rats. *J. Cardiovasc. Pharmacol. 6:* S32–S34, 1984.

149. Lush, D. J., and J. C. S. Fray. Steady-state autoregulation of renal blood flow: a myogenic model. *Am. J. Physiol. 247 (Regulatory Integretative Comp. Physiol. 16):* R89–R99, 1984.

150. MacGregor, G. A. Sodium is more important than calcium in essential hypertension. *Hypertension 7:* 628–637, 1985.

151. Majewski, H., and M. J. Rand. A possible role of epinephrine in the development of hypertension. *Med. Res. Rev. 6:* 467–486, 1986.

152. Marlettini, M. G., T. Salomone, M. Agostini, and M. De Novellis. Long-term treatment of primary hypertension with verapamil. *Curr. Ther. Res. 39:* 59–65, 1986.

153. Massie, B. M. Antihypertensive therapy with calcium-channel blockers: comparison with beta blockers. *Am. J. Cardiol. 56:* 97H–100H, 1985.

154. Massie, B. M., A. J. Hirsch, I. K. Inivye, and J. F. Tubau. Calcium channel blockers as antihypertensive agents. *Am. J. Med.* (Oct. 5): 135–142, 1984.

155. M'Buyamba-Kabangu, J. R., R. Fagard, P. Lijnen, and A. Amery. Nitrendipine and acebutolol in hypertensive African blacks. *J. Cardiovasc. Pharmacol.* 9(Suppl.4): S263–S266, 1987.

156. McCarron, D. A. and Morris, C. D. The calcium deficiency hypothesis of hypertension. *Ann. Intern. Med. 107:* 919–922, 1987.

157. McCubbin, J. W., J. H. Green, and I. H. Page. Baroreceptor function in chronic renal hypertension. *Circ. Res. 4:* 205–210, 1956.

158. Meininger, G. A., V. M. Lubrano, and H. J. Granger. Hemodynamic and microvascular responses in the hindquarters during the development of renal hypertension in rats. Evidence for the involvement of an autoregulatory component. *Circ. Res. 55:* 609–622, 1984.

159. Meininger, G. A., L. K. Routh, and H. J. Granger. Autoregulation and vasoconstriction in the intestine during acute renal hypertension. *Hypertension 7:* 364–373, 1985.

160. Michel, M. C., P. A. Insel, O.-E. Brodde. Renal α-adrenergic receptor alterations: a cause of essential hypertension. *FASEB J. 3:* 139–144, 1989.

161. Miller, E. D., A. I. Samuels, E. Haber, and A. C. Barger. Inhibition of angiotensin conversion in experimental renovascular hypertension. *Science 177:* 1108–1109, 1972.

162. Miller, R. J. Multiple calcium channels and neuronal function. *Science 235:* 46–52, 1987.

163. Monod, J., J. Wyman, J-P. Changeux. On the nature of allosteric transitions: a plausible model. *J. Mol. Biol. 12:* 88–118, 1965.

164. Montal, M. Molecular anatomy and molecular design of channel proteins. *FASEB J. 4:* 2623–2635, 1990.

165. Moser, M., J. Lunn, and B. J. Materson. Comparative effects of diltiazem and hydrochlorothiazide in blacks with systemic hypertension. *Am. J. Cardiol. 56:* 101H–104H, 1985.

166. Moser, M., J. Lunn, D. T. Nash, J. F. Burris, N. Winer, G. Simon, and N. D. Vlachakis. Nitrendipine in the treatment of mild to moderate hypertension. *J. Cardiovasc. Pharmacol. 6:* S1085–S1089, 1984.

167. Munch, P. A., and A. M. Brown. Role of vessel wall in acute resetting of aortic baroreceptors. *Am. J. Physiol. 248 (Heart Circ. Physiol. 17):* H843–H852, 1985.

168. Munoz-Ramirez, H., R. E. Chatelain, F. M. Bumpus, and P. A. Khairallah. Development of two-kidney Goldblatt hypertension in rats under dietary sodium restriction. *Am. J. Physiol. 238 (Heart Circ. Physiol. 7):* H889–H894, 1980.

169. Nabika, T., P. A. Velletri, M. A. Beaven, J. Endo, and W. Lovenberg. Vasopressin-induced calcium increases in smooth muscle cells from spontaneously hypertensive rats. *Life Sci. 37:* 579–584, 1985.

170. Nagao, T., I. Yamaguchi, H. Narita, and H. Nakajima. Calcium entry blockers: antihy-

pertensive and natriuretic effects in experimental animals. *Am. J. Cardiol. 56:* 56H–61H, 1985.

171. O'Rourke, R. A. Rationale for calcium entry-blocking drugs in systemic hypertension complicated by coronary artery disease. *Am. J. Cardiol. 56:* 34H–40H, 1985.

172. Owen, A. The aetiology of essential hypertension: an hypothesis describing two categories. *Med. Hypotheses 19:* 287–290, 1986.

173. Owens, G. K., and S. M. Schwartz. Vascular smooth muscle cell hypertrophy and hyperploidy in the Goldblatt hypertensive rat. *Circ. Res. 53:* 491–501, 1983.

174. Page, I. H. The mosaic theory 32 years later. *Hypertension 7:* 177, 1982.

175. Page, I. H. Initiation and maintenance of renal hypertension. *Am. J. Surg. 107:* 26–34, 1964.

176. Page, I. H. Neural and humoral control of blood vessels. In: *Hypertension,* edited by G. E. W. Wolstenholme and M. P. Cameron. Little, Brown, Boston, 1954, pp. 3–25.

177. Page, I. H., and J. W. McCubbin, eds. *Renal Hypertension,* Year Book, Chicago, 1968.

178. Pickering, T. G., and J. H. Laragh. Autoregulation as a factor in peripheral resistance and flow: clinical implications for analysis of high blood pressure. *Am. J. Med. 68:* 801–802, 1980.

179. Postnov, Y. V. An approach to the explanation of cell membrane alteration in primary hypertension. *Hypertension 15:* 332–337, 1990.

180. Postnov, Y. V., S. N. Orlov, G. M. Kravtsov, and P. V. Gulak. Calcium transport and protein content in cell plasma membranes of spontaneously hypertensive rats. *J. Cardiovasc. Pharmacol. 6:* S21–S27, 1984.

181. Postnov, Y. V., S. N. Orlov, and N. I. Pokudin. Alteration of intracellular calcium distribution in the adipose tissue of human patients with essential hypertension. *Pflugers Arch. 388:* 89–91, 1980.

182. Prewitt, R. L., D. L. Stacy, and Z. Ono. The microcirculation in hypertension: which are the resistance vessels? *News in Physiological Sciences* 2: 139–141, 1987.

183. Resink, T. J., V. A. Tkachuk, P. Erne, and F. R. Buhler. Platelet membrane calmodulin-stimulated calcium-adenosine triophosphate. Altered activity in essential hypertension. *Hypertension 8:* 159–166, 1986.

184. Robertson, J. I. S., J. J. Morton, D. M. Tillman, and A. F. Lever. The pathophysiology of renovascular hypertension. *J. Hypertens.* 4(Suppl. 4): S95–S103, 1986.

185. Robertson, P. W., A. Klidjian, L. K. Harding, G. Walters, M. R. Lee, A. H. T. Robb-Smith. Hypertension due to a renin-secreting renal tumour. *Am. J. Med. 43:* 963–976, 1967.

186. Robinson, B. F. Altered calcium handling as a cause of primary hypertension. *J. Hypertens. 2:* 453–460, 1984.

187. Robinson, B. F., and R. J. W. Phillips. Effects of small increments in plasma calcium concentration on the responsiveness of forearm resistance vessels to verapamil in normal subjects. *Clin. Sci. 67:* 613–618, 1984.

188. Rogart, R. B., A. DeB Kops, and V. J. Dzau. Identification of two calcium channel receptor sites for [³H]nitrendipine in mammalian cardiac and smooth muscle membrane. *Proc. Natl. Acad. Sci. U.S.A. 83:* 7452–7456, 1986.

189. Rubin, L. J., P. Nicod, L. D. Hillis, and B. G. Firth. Treatment of primary pulmonary hypertension with nifedipine. *Ann. Intern. Med. 99:* 433–438, 1983.

190. Sachs, F. Baroreceptor mechanisms at the cellular level. *Fed. Proc. 46:* 12–16, 1987.

191. Sadoshima, S., F. Yoshida, S. Ibayashi, O. Shiokawa, and M. Fujishima. Upper limit of cerebral autoregulation during development of hypertensive rats: effect of sympathetic denervation. *Stroke 16:* 477–481, 1985.

192. Safer, M. E., A. C. Simon, J. A. Leuenson, and J. L. Cazor. Hemodynamic effects of diltiazen in hypertension. *Circ. Res.* 52(Suppl. I): 169–173, 1983.

193. Sang, K. H. L. Q., and M.-A. Devynck. Increased platelet cytosolic free calcium concentration in essential hypertension. *J. Hypertens. 4:* 567–574, 1986.

194. Scheid, C. R., and F. S. Fay. Beta-adrenergic effects of transmembrane 45Ca fluxes in isolated smooth muscle cells. *Am. J. Physiol. 246 (Cell Physiol. 15):* C431–C438, 1984.

195. Schiffrin, E. L., M. Lis, J. Gutkowska, and J. Genest. Role of Ca^{2+} in response of adrenal glomerulosa cells to angiotensin II, ACTH, K+, and ouabain. *Am. J. Physiol. 241 (Endocrinol. Metab. 4):* E42–E46, 1981.

196. Smith, S. G., A. A. Seymour, E. K. Mazack, J. Boger, and E. H. Blaine. Comparison of a new renin inhibitor and enalaprilat in renal hypertensive dogs. *Hypertension 9:* 150–156, 1987.

197. Snowdowne, K. W. The effect of stretch on sarcoplasmic free calcium of frog skeletal muscle at rest. *Biochim. Biophys. Acta 862:* 441–444, 1986.

198. Speden, R. N. Active reactions of the rabbit ear artery to distension. *J. Physiol. (Lond.) 351:* 631–643, 1984.

199. Spieker, C., W. Zidek, H. Lange-Asschenfeldt, H. Losse, and H. Vetter. Essential hypertension versus secondary hypertension discrimination by intracellular electrolytess. *Klin. Worchenschr.* 63(Suppl.): 20–22, 1985.

200. Stephens, G. A., J. O. Davis, R. H. Freeman, J. M. DeForrest, and D. M. Early. Hemodynamic, fluid, and electrolyte changes in sodium-depleted, one-kidney, renal hypertensive dogs. *Circ. Res.* 44: 316–321, 1979.

201. Stienen, G. J. M., T. Blange, and B. W. Treijte. Tension development and calcium sensitivity in skinned muscle fibers of the frog. *Pflugers Arch.* 405: 19–23, 1985.

202. Sunderrajan, S., G. Reams, and J. H. Bauer. Renal effects of diltiazem in primary hypertension. *Hypertension* 8: 238–242, 1986.

203. Takaya, J., N. Lasker, R. Bamforth, M. Gutkin, L. H. Byrd, and A. Aviv. Kinetics of Ca^{2+}-ATPase activation in platelet membranes of essential hypertensives and normotensives. *Am. J. Physiol.* 258 (Cell Physiol. 27): C988–C994, 1990.

204. Taylor, A., and E. E. Windhager. Possible role of cytosolic calcium and Na-Ca exchange in regulation of transepithelial sodium transport. *Am. J. Physiol.* 236 (Renal Fluid Electrolyte Physiol. 5): F505–F512, 1979.

205. Thoren, P., M. C. Andresen, and A. M. Brown. Effects of changes in extracellular ionic concentrations on aortic baroreceptors with nonmyelinated afferent fibers. *Circ. Res.* 50: 413–418, 1982.

206. Tobian, L. Interrelationship of electrolytes, juxtaglomerular cells and hypertension. *Physiol. Rev.* 40: 280–312, 1960.

207. Tobian, L., and G. Chesley. Calcium content of arteriolar walls in normotensive and hypertensive rats. *Proc. Soc. Exp. Biol. Med.* 121: 340–343, 1966.

208. Tracy, R. E. and E. O. Overll. Arterioles of perfusion-fixed hypertension and aged kidneys. *Arch. Pathol.* 82: 529, 1966.

209. Trippodo, N. C., G. M. Walsh, R. A. Ferrone, and R. C. Dugan. Fluid partition and cardiac output in volume-depleted Goldblatt hypertensive rats. *Am. J. Physiol.* 237 (Heart Circ. Physiol. 6): H18–H24, 1979.

210. Van Breemen, C., S. Lukeman, and C. Cauvin. A theoretical consideration on the use of calcium antagonists in the treatment of hypertension. *Am. J. Med.* Oct 5: 26–30, 1984.

211. Van Breemen, C., P. Leijten, H. Yamamoto, P. Aaronson, and C. Cauvin. Calcium activation of vascular smooth muscle. *Hypertension* 8(Suppl. II): II-89–II-95, 1986.

212. Vanhoutte, P. M. Calcium-entry blockers, vascular smooth muscle and systemic hypertension. *Am. J. Cardiol.* 55: 17B–23B, 1985.

213. Vetter, H., W. Vetter, C. Warnholz, J. M. Bayer, H. Kaser, K. Vielhaber, and F. Kruck. Renin and aldosterone secretion in pheochromocytoma. *Am. J. Med.* 60: 866–871, 1976.

214. Weidmann, P., A. Gerber, and K. Laederach. Calcium antagonists in the treatment of hypertension: a critical overview. *Adv. Nephrol.* 14: 197–232, 1984.

215. Williams, R. R., S. C. Hunt, S. J. Hasstedt, P. N. Hopkins, L. W. Wu, T. D. Berry, and H. Kuida. Current knowledge regarding the genetics of human hypertension. *J. Hypertens.* 7(Suppl.6): 8–13, 1989.

216. Windhager, E., G. Frindt, J. M. Yang, and C. O. Lee. Intracellular calcium ions as regulators of renal tubular sodium transport. *Klin. Worchenschr.* 64: 847–852, 1986.

217. Worley, J. F., J. W. Deitmer, and M. T. Nelson. Single nisoldipine-sensitive calcium channel in smooth muscle cells isolated from rabbit mesenteric artery. *Proc. Natl. Acad. Sci. U.S.A.* 83: 5746–5750, 1986.

218. Wright, C. E., J. A. Angus, and P. I. Korner. Vascular amplifier properties in renovascular hypertension in conscious rabbits. Hindquarter responses to constrictor and dilator stimuli. *Hypertension* 9: 122–131, 1987.

219. Wright, G. L., and G. O. Rankin. Concentrations of ionic and total calcium in plasma of four models of hypertension. *Am. J. Physiol.* 243 (Heart Circ. Physiol. 12): H365–H370, 1982.

220. Yokoyama, S., N. Mori, T. Shingu, K. Sakata, T. Iwase, H. Yoshida, S. Takayama, T. Hoshino, and T. Kaburagi. Clinical effects of intravenous diltiazem hydrochloride on renal hemodynamics. *J. Cardiovasc. Pharmacol.* 9: 311–316, 1987.

221. Young, M. A., R. D. S. Watson, and W. A. Littler. Baroreflex setting and sensitivity after acute and chronic nicardipine therapy. *Clin. Sci.* 66: 233–235, 1984.

222. Zawada, E. T., and M. Johnson. Calcium chelation and calcium-channel blockade in anesthetized acute renovascular hypertensive dogs. *Min. Electrolyte Metab.* 10: 366–370, 1984.

223. Zemel, M. B., S. M. Gualdoni, M. F. Walsh, P. Komanicky, P. Standley, D. Johnson, W. Fitter, and J. R. Sowers. Effects of sodium and calcium on calcium metabolism and

blood pressure regulation in hypertensive black adults. *J. Hypertens.* *4*(Suppl. 5): 5364–5366, 1986.

224. Zidek, W., C. Karoff, P. Baumgart, H. Losse, K. J. Fehske, W. Hacker, and H. Vetter. Intracellular sodium and calium during antihypertensive treatment. *Klin. Wochenschr.* *63*(Suppl. III): 147–149, 1985.

225. Zidek, W., C. Karoff, H. Losse, and H. Vetter. Weight reduction and salt restriction in hypertension: effects on blood pressure and intracellular electrolytes. *Klin. Wochenschr.* *64:* 1183–1185, 1986.

12

Drug Therapy in Black Hypertensives

JACKSON T. WRIGHT, JR., AND JANICE G. DOUGLAS

Hypertension is more likely to be resistant to treatment in blacks than in any other segment of the U.S. population (65,73,90). It is also more likely to cause complications. Review of the epidemiology literature reveals hypertension prevalence to be twice as common in blacks, to cause 2–4 times the number of strokes, 4–20 times the rate of progression to end-stage renal disease, and to be associated with at least the same frequency of coronary heart disease deaths as in whites. Black hypertensives are also more apt to have increased renal vascular resistance, renal impairment at presentation, and left ventricular hypertrophy. This further identifies this patient population to be at particular risk of morbidity from the disease. Although there are more similarities of characteristics than differences, black hypertensives are more likely to be characterized by low renin, volume expansion, and abnormal renal sodium handling when compared with whites. Thus hypertension appears to be a more aggressive disease in the black patient and may have some hemodynamic as well as pathophysiological differences that have important implications in the choice of antihypertensive agent.

The goal of antihypertensive therapy is to prevent or reduce as many of the complications of hypertension as safely and with as few side effects as possible. Over the last 25 years, numerous antihypertensive agents have become available, allowing wide flexibility in choice of mechanisms, dose schedules, side effects, and cost. It is assumed that the marker for prevention of hypertensive complications is reduction of blood pressure, although this has not been entirely validated. Furthermore, in spite of observed differences in the characteristics of the disease and its response to treatment in the black hypertensive, until recently data on response of the black hypertensive to therapy have been lacking.

Unlike the treatment of acute diseases, where the effect of therapy is known within a short period of time, in treating hypertension the clinician's prescription to a patient entails a substantial investment in money, time, and risk of medication side effects for a potential benefit that may not become evident until decades later. Because the black hypertensive is at greater risk for the complications of hypertension, including mortality, it is necessary to review the data on the efficacy of various therapies in lowering blood pressure and their success in preventing the complications of the disease in this population.

RACIAL DIFFERENCE IN ANTIHYPERTENSIVE EFFICACY

Diuretics

Although their use has been steadily decreasing, the thiazide diuretics remain a mainstay of therapy in the black hypertensive. Their efficacy in reducing blood pressure, and in reducing hypertension-related morbidity and mortality, is well established (26,39). Their exact antihypertensive mechanism of action remains controversial, even after 30 years of use. Their diuretic action results from their inhibition of sodium reabsorption in the early portion of the distal tubule; however, the precise antihypertensive mechanism of these agents is still uncertain (5,23,64,76,85). They initially reduce plasma and extracellular fluid volume. However, these values return toward, though not completely, to pretreatment levels with chronic treatment while blood pressure control persists. Thus, during chronic use of thiazide diuretics, there is dissociation of their diuretic action from their effect on blood pressure (26). In addition, the loop diuretics, for example, furosemide, which block sodium, potassium, and chloride cotransport in the loop of Henle, are more potent diuretics but are not as effective in lowering blood pressure as the thiazides. Finally, diazoxide, a potent antihypertensive and structurally similar to the thiazides, causes fluid retention rather than diuresis. Its mechanism of action is secondary to arteriolar vasodilation, thereby underscoring the potential diversity in mechanism(s) of action of this class of antihypertensive agents.

Some effect on sodium chloride homeostasis is necessary to the sustained action of thiazide diuretics. Their hypotensive action is antagonized by increased salt intake, and their discontinuation results in increased plasma volume. Diminished sensitivity to vasoactive agonists and reduction of total peripheral resistance by these agents suggest additional mechanisms of lowering blood pressure.

The potassium-sparing diuretics, amiloride and triamterene, are relatively weak antihypertensive agents unless combined with other diuretics (71). They act in the distal nephron to inhibit sodium-potassium exchange. However, spironolactone, a potassium-sparing diuretic that competitively inhibits aldosterone, has demonstrated significant antihypertensive activity even in black hypertensives (33).

Thiazide diuretics have consistently proven their effectiveness in lowering the blood pressure in hypertensive black patients. In comparative trials of diuretics, the thiazides have proven to be more effective than furosemide, amiloride, and triamterene in black hypertensives (34,71). Indapamide is a thiazide type agent that in antihypertensive doses produces less diuresis and metabolic alterations (84). There are few studies evaluating indapamide in black patients. However, Bhigjee et al. (7) in a study of 19 blacks and 18 Indians found similar efficacy between indapamide, chlorthalidone, hydrochlorothiazide, and two preparations using the combination of hydrochlorothiazide and potassium-sparing diuretics.

Some studies have reported an increased efficacy of thiazides in black compared with white hypertensives. However, in most comparative studies, the racial difference in response to the thiazide diuretics is relatively small (7,45,77,79,81). Although there is a dose-response effect in doses up to 200 mg/day of hydrochlorothiazide, the bulk of the antihypertensive effect can be achieved at doses of 50 mg and below (6,45,49,77). Up to 71% of black hyper-tensives can expect to be controlled with thiazide monotherapy and almost 50% on doses of 50 mg/day or less (45,77).

The use of diuretics to treat hypertension has decreased particularly be-cause of reservations resulting from (1) metabolic complications (i.e., hypoka-lemia, hypomagnesemia, and elevations in serum cholesterol and glucose); (2) the failure of these agents in some clinical trials to reduce cardiac events other than congestive heart failure; and (3) other side effects suspected of interfering with long-term compliance (26,89).

Beta Blockers

There are well over a dozen beta blockers now available or in the later stages of clinical development since the introduction of propranolol in this country almost 20 years ago. Like the thiazides, the exact mechanisms of antihyper-tensive action of these agents are controversial. Most of their antihypertensive action can be explained by their ability to decrease cardiac output, inhibit renin release, and decrease sympathetic tone (25). The major clinical differ-ences between drugs of this class relate to differences in their receptor speci-ficity (nonselective, B-1 selective, alpha blockade), presence of agonist activity (intrinsic sympathomimetic activity), duration of action, lipid solubility (asso-ciated with central nervous system effects), and route of elimination. Thus far, no clinical significance can be attached to local anesthetic or membrane sta-bilizing properties, which some compounds of this class may possess.

As a group, beta blockers are reported to be less effective in black than in white hypertensives unless they are combined with a thiazide diuretic (16,28, 36,53,68,70,77,78,87). This conclusion is derived from placebo-controlled stud-ies in black hypertensives and comparison trials with thiazide diuretics and calcium channel blockers in black and white hypertensives (Table 12.1). How-ever, many blacks respond well and most will have some blood pressure reduc-tion with beta blocker antihypertensives. In addition, any racial difference in efficacy has repeatedly been eliminated when beta blockers are combined with a thiazide diuretic (28,70,78,87).

Racial differences in antihypertensive efficacy has been noted with tradi-tional beta blockers, including those that are cardioselective and those with intrinsic sympathomimetic activity (16,36,53,68,70,77). However, labetalol has been reported to be equally effective in black and white hypertensives and more effective in black hypertensives than traditional beta blockers (22,67). Closer review of previous studies with labetalol, however, suggests some resis-tance of black hypertensives to labetalol. Jennings and Parsons (38) reported labetalol to be less effective in black than white hypertensives. Flamenbaum et al. (22) reported labetalol to be significantly more effective than propranolol in decreasing only the standing blood pressure in black hypertensives. Labet-alol and propranolol had similar efficacy in reducing the supine blood pressure in blacks. In a study by Saunders et al. (67) comparing labetalol and propran-olol in an all black study population, labetalol was significantly more effective in reducing sitting and standing diastolic but not systolic blood pressures.

In comparing labetalol with atenolol in black and white hypertensives who were previously renin-profiled, we have recently reported that both labetalol

TABLE 12.1. Response of Black Hypertensives to Beta-Blockers

Drug	Dose	N	Baseline mm Hg	Change mm Hg	Ref.
Monotherapy					
Propranolol	240–360	18	187/119	+1.6/−0.3	(36)
	80–640	196	146/102	−8.2/−9.5	(77)
	120–360	21	152/104	−8.1/−8.6	(16)
	120–640	79	155/102	−6.9/−8.6	(67)
	80–480	35	152/99	+3/−2	(22)
Nadolol	80–240	61	145/101	−5.8/−9.6	(78)
Atenolol	100	19	169/111	−2.2/−6.5	(28)
	100	24	159/103	+2.5/−4.4	(70)
	50–100	14	155/101	−6/−6	(91)
Pindolol	20–60	12	158/105	−15/−5.1	(53)
Labetalol	200–1600	74	153/102	−9.1/−11.2	(67)
	200–1200	30	151/98	−2/−6	(22)
	200–1600	19	155/101	−2/−7	(91)
Combination Therapy					
Atenolol	100	19	169/111	−28.2/−17.8	(28)
Chlorthalidone	25				
Atenolol	100	24	159/103	−14.0/−13.8	(70)
Chlorthalidone	25				
Nadolol	80–240	178	145/101	−27.3/−17.9	(78)
Bendroflumethiazide	5–10				
Labetalol	200–800	36	164/105	−20/−16	(87)
HCTZ	50				

Antihypertensive response of black hypertensives to beta-blockers as monotherapy and in combination with thiazide diuretics.

and atenolol were less effective in black than in white hypertensives (91). However, in contrast to atenolol, the antihypertensive response to labetalol was not related to pretreatment renin activity or renin profile. As with other beta blockers, no racial difference in efficacy was noted in patients when lebetalol was added to diuretic therapy (87).

Potential adverse effects seen with the beta blockers include bronchospasm, decreased cardiac contractility and heart rate, heart block, and vasospastic disease. In addition, the beta blockers without intrinsic sympathomimetic activity produce a consistent significant decrease in HDL-cholesterol.

Non–Beta Blocker Sympatholytics

Non–beta blocker sympatholytics include the centrally active alpha agonists (methyldopa, clonidine, guanfacine, and guanabenz), the peripheral neuronal depleting agents (reserpine, guanethidine, and guanadrel), and the selective alpha-1 blockers (prazosin and terazosin). The adrenergic depleting agents and central alpha agonists were among the earliest antihypertensives utilized. Few comparative trials are available to examine racial efficacy. The few that are available and many years of clinical experience suggest no racial difference in efficacy with these agents (29). However, in one study, there was a tendency for black hypertensives to respond less well and require higher doses of transdermal clonidine than white hypertensives, but the differences failed to reach statistical significance (80). A 10% decrease in seated diastolic blood pressure with the 0.1 mg patch was reported in 26% of white but only 16% of black hypertensives.

The alpha-1 blockers are among the few antihypertensives that have a favorable effect on plasma lipids (increase HDL and the HDL to LDL radio) (40,72). Although racial comparison studies to date have utilized small numbers of patients, they suggest that alpha-1 blockers have a similar effect on blood pressure and lipids in black and white patients (3,41).

Angiotensin Converting Enzyme Inhibitors

The angiotensin converting enzyme inhibitors (ACEI) became available about 12 years ago with the introduction of captopril (83). These agents are becoming increasingly popular because they are very well tolerated with little deterioration in quality of life (14,15).

There are now three ACEIs available in this country, with many more in the final stages of clinical evaluation. They inhibit the conversion of biologically inactive angiotensin I to the potent pressor vasoconstrictor angiotensin II, through inhibition of the converting enzyme. They also prolong the action of the vasodilating kinins by inhibiting their metabolism by angiotensin-converting enzyme (83). There is emerging evidence that inhibition of local tissue angiotensin II production by these agents as well as their effect on plasma angiotensin II concentration are important in the pharmacological action of these drugs (20).

Like the beta blockers, the ACEIs are less effective as monotherapy in black as compared with white hypertensives. Furthermore, as a group they are less effective than thiazide diuretics in black hypertensives (18,79,81). With these agents also, the racial difference in efficacy is eliminated when they are combined with a thiazide diuretic (79,81). The combination of ACEI with a thiazide diuretic also lessens hypokalemia and glucose intolerance, and, in at least one study, alterations in serum cholesterol that occur with thiazide diuretics (81).

Primary prevention data evaluating the efficacy of these agents in preventing hypertension-related morbidity and mortality are as yet unavailable for the ACEI. However, there are secondary prevention data indicating that they slow progression of heart failure in patients with this problem (13). Preliminary data suggest that ACEIs also slow the progression of renal disease in patients with insulin-dependent diabetes mellitus (35,62). Whether the ability of the ACEI to prevent worsening of complications already present (secondary prevention) correlates with any potential of these agents to prevent the complication from developing in the first place (primary prevention) remains an area of controversy. ACEIs have also been reported to induce regression of left ventricular hypertrophy (42,58). However, the effect of this pharmacological property on the natural history of hypertension has not been confirmed.

The major potential adverse effects experienced with these agents are cough (5%–20%), rash (1%–4%), taste disturbance (1%–2%), and angioedema

(0.1%) (83). In addition, they can cause hyperkalemia, especially in patients with diabetes mellitus and renal insufficiency, two frequent concomitant diseases in black hypertensives, as well as a reversible renal failure in patients with bilateral renal artery stenosis or renal artery stenosis to a solitary kidney. The ACEIs do not alter serum lipids (18,79,81).

The ACEIs have been extensively studied for their effect on quality of life (14,15,46). In general, this class of antihypertensive agents is tolerated well and produces little adverse effect on the patient's quality of life (see later).

Calcium Channel Blockers

The calcium channel blockers (CaCB) are heralded as a potentially attractive alternative to diuretic therapy in the black hypertensive. They are effective against concomitant coronary artery disease and are among the agents that will effectively induce regression of left ventricular hypertrophy (LVH), a complication seen more frequently in the black hypertensive (90). They reduce calcium-entry-induced vasoconstriction of vascular smooth muscle cells, and, particularly the phenylalkylamine class of CaCB (verapamil), also decrease cardiac contractility (27).

There are substantial data on the use of CaCB in black hypertensives. These drugs have been compared with thiazides, converting enzyme inhibitors, and beta blockers in both black and white hypertensives [Table 12.2; 16,25,44, 51,52,54,68,86].

In one study, verapamil (up to 160 mg tid) was shown to be significantly more effective than propranolol (up to 120 mg tid) in reducing seated and standing diastolic blood pressure in black hypertensives (16). In a study of

TABLE 12.2. Antihypertensive Response to Calcium Channel Blockers in Black Hypertensives

Drug	N	Baseline mm Hg	Change mm Hg	Ref.
Diltiazem	10	165/104	−34/−18	(54)
HCTZ	10	154/103	−29/−21	
Diltiazem	50	N/A	−11/−11	(44)
Propranolol	45	N/A	−9/−12	
Diltiazem	16	158/101	−15/−12	(86)
Captopril	11	156/100	−9.1/−4.3	
Nitrendipine	30	167/102	−23/−15	(4)
Acebutolol	30	168/104	−10*/−7*	
Verapamil	20	153/100	−17/−13	(16)
Propranolol	21	152/104	−8.1/−8.6*	
Verapamil	100	150/100	−13/−13	(68)
Atenolol	109	152/100	−9.8/−10	
Captopril	98	151/100	−8.2/−9.6	

Comparative clinical trials with CaCB in black hypertensives.
*$p < 0.05$ compared with CaCB

black hypertensives, we compared sustained release verapamil to atenolol and captopril in 393 patients (68). Verapamil monotherapy either normalized supine diastolic blood pressure or reduced it by 10 mm Hg in almost 83% of black patients with mild to moderate hypertension, and it was significantly more effective than monotherapy with either atenolol or captopril.

Similar, though less convincing data are also available for diltiazem. Moser et al. (52) found diltiazem equal to HCTZ in efficacy in a small number (n = 20) of black hypertensives. However, in a comparative trial of 196 hypertensives (101 were black) who were randomized to receive either diltiazem or propranolol, both diltiazem and propranolol produced less systolic and diastolic blood pressure reduction in blacks than in whites, although only the racial difference in response to propranolol reached statistical significance (44). In a study comparing sustained release diltiazem to captopril in black and white hypertensives, diltiazem was more effective than captopril in the black hypertensives, although the number of blacks in the study was small and the difference was not significant (86).

It has been suggested that CaCB are more likely to be efficacious in low-renin hypertension, a characteristic frequently found in blacks and the elderly (10). Several studies have reported alterations in sodium transport and an increase in intracellular sodium in blacks at risk to develop hypertension (90; see Chapter 9, this volume). Such a transport defect is postulated to increase entry of calcium into vascular smooth muscle and facilitate vasoconstriction, which the CaCB theoretically might inhibit (8; see Chapter 9, this volume). However, many of the studies that attempted to discern whether there was increased efficacy in low-renin hypertension used elderly rather than black hypertensives as their source of low-renin patients (4,10). Pharmacokinetic studies of nifedipine and nicardipine have provided data suggesting a correlation of increased efficacy in this population with increased plasma drug levels in elderly patients due to decreased hepatic metabolism (21,66). Additionally, while pharmacokinetic data in blacks are not available, most studies show a lack of resistance rather than increased efficacy when comparing the antihypertensive response of CaCB in black and white hypertensives (Table 12.2).

One area of concern is the extent to which the thiazide diuretics and the CaCB are additive when used together. There are data suggesting that the combination of the CaCB verapamil plus hydrochlorothiazide and nifedipine plus hydrochlorothiazide are less effective than when these agents are used separately (30,59). However, there are other data that demonstrate additivity of these agents when used together and when nitrendipine and diltiazem are used with the thiazides (2,43,52,54,93). In the patient who is apt to require at least two drugs to control blood pressure (more likely to occur in the black hypertensive because of the more frequent greater severity), one would hate to lose the ability to use the thiazide as one of these agents.

Calcium channel blockers are generally well tolerated, and they have not been reported to cause significant adverse metabolic effects. The principal side effects seen with these drugs lie on a continuum based on drug subclass. The dihydropyridines (nifedipine, nicardipine, nitrendipine, and isradipine) are more likely to produce vasodilator symptoms, that is, edema, flushing, headache; while verapamil is more apt to cause conduction abnormalities, decreased cardiac contractility, and constipation. The side effect profile with diltiazem lies in between these two subclasses of CaCB.

Quality of life data are also available for the CaCBs (15,46). The CaCBs generally have no adverse effect on quality of life and compare favorably with ACEIs and the beta blockers in comparison trials where quality of life was measured (46). Clinical trials suggest a lower incidence of sexual dysfunction with CaCBs compared with the thiazide diuretics (46,52).

TREATMENT CONSIDERATIONS

Effect of Therapy on the Natural History of Hypertension

The goal of antihypertensive therapy is to prevent the complications of the disease. The black hypertensive is at greatest risk for hypertensive complications. Therefore, the clinician is challenged more so than in any other population to prescribe for the greatest benefit at the lowest cost.

Antihypertensive therapy has been proven to prevent cardiovascular morbidity and mortality in clinical trials involving tens of thousands of patients (Table 12.3). However, only the HDFP study had sufficient numbers of black

TABLE 12.3. Effect of Antihypertensive Therapy on Cardiovascular Morbidity

Trial[a]	Total cardiovascular		Coronary		Strokes	
	Control	Treat	Control	Treat	Control	Treat
Freis (VA-1) (n = 143)	27	2*	4	1	2	0
Freis (VA-2) (n = 380)	76	22	20	5	13	11
HDFP[b] (n = 10,940)	240	195*	52	29*	69	51*
Oslo (n = 785)	34	25	7	0*	13	20
Australian (n = 3,427)	127	91*	25	12*	88	70
MRFIT[b] (n = 8,012)	—	—	—	—	79	80
MRC (n = 17,245)	351	286*	109	60*	234	222
EWPHE (n = 840)	117	68*	22	16	29	17*

[a]The major clinical trials evaluating the protection against cardiovascular events afforded by antihypertensive therapy. All utilized traditional "Stepped Care" in at least one arm of the study; VA-1, VA-2 = Veterans Administration Cooperative Study Group on Antihypertensive Agents; HDFP = Hypertension Detection and Follow-up Program; OSLO = The Oslo Study; Australian = Management Committee of the Australian National Blood Pressure Study; MRFIT = Multiple Risk Factor Intervention Trial; MRC = Medical Research Council Trial; EWPHE = European Working Party on High Blood Pressure in the Elderly; HAPPHY = Heart Attack Primary Prevention in Hypertensives Trial; MAPHY = Metoprolol Atherosclerosis Prevention in Hypertensives Study; SHEP = Systolic Hypertension in the Elderly Program.
[b]Data reported as mortality only.
From Wright (89).
*$p < 0.05$

subjects to evaluate the effect of antihypertensive therapy on hypertension sequelae in the black hypertensive. In the HDFP, it was the black hypertensives who showed the greatest benefit from treatment. There are no studies evaluating the effect of non-diuretic-based therapy on the complication rate of hypertension in blacks.

Antihypertensive therapy, especially with thiazide diuretics and beta blockers, produces metabolic effects that might adversely affect cardiac risk. The thiazide diuretics (except for indapamide) decrease potassium, increase glucose intolerance, and increase total and LDL cholesterol (85). In fact, this has led some to suggest that the black hypertensive is inappropriately victimized by the extensive use of diuretic antihypertensives in this population. It is necessary, therefore, to review carefully the risk profile data on these agents.

The glucose intolerance with the thiazide diuretics is usually reversible with drug withdrawal and generally appears to be secondary to decreased insulin release produced by the drug's potassium depletion (26,49,89). The glucose intolerance will resolve with correction of serum potassium (89). Elevation of serum glucose has been noted in several of the long-term clinical trials, including the European Working Party on Hypertension in the Elderly (EWP) trial, which used the potassium-sparing hydrochlorothiazide/triamterene combination, and in the Medical Research Council study (1,57). In addition, the thiazides have been reported to produce insulin resistance, which has also been associated with increased cardiovascular morbidity and mortality (63,75). It is noteworthy that in spite of the increase in serum glucose in patients on active treatment during the EWP study, this trial was still one of the few placebo controlled trials that reported decreased coronary heart disease mortality in the treated group (1).

Thiazide diuretics also consistently increase total and LDL cholesterol in the majority of males and postmenopausal females taking the drug, even in doses as low as 12.5 mg/day (49,81). Estrogen appears to protect premenopausal women from the lipid altering effects of the thiazides (9). It is still controversial as to whether the effects of thiazides on plasma lipids are transient or persist after 1 year. Cholesterol values from patients followed in long-term clinical trials return to pretreatment values with prolonged therapy (Table 12.4). In addition, several studies have noted a blunting of the cholesterol increase when the thiazides are combined with alpha blockers, converting enzyme inhibitors, methyldopa, reserpine, metoprolol, and hydralazine (40,41, 45,81). Thus it appears to be only a subset of male and postmenopausal females on thiazide monotherapy who appear to be at risk for the adverse lipid effects of the thiazides.

Diuretic-induced decrease in serum potassium has been proposed to cause cardiac arrhythmias and sudden death, although this too remains controversial (26,85). Increased incidence of sudden death has been reported in several studies in patients treated with diuretics (19,32,56). Post-hoc analysis of the data from these studies suggests that especially in patients with EKG abnormalities, that is, left ventricular hypertrophy, treatment with diuretics increased the likelihood of sudden death. Although in the Oslo study, there were too few events for additional subgroup analyses, in the MRFIT study the increase in sudden death was noted only in patients on diuretics in the special-intervention (SI) group of the trial (56). No increased mortality rate was seen

TABLE 12.4. Long-Term Changes in Serum Cholesterol Induced by Thiazides and Beta Blockers

Study	Drug[a]	Total serum cholesterol in mg/dl					
		Before	3 mo	1 yr	3 yr	5 yr	6 yr
VA	THZ	203.1		213.0			
(n = 610)	PLCB	196.5		196.4			
Oslo	THZ	278			279		
(n = 300)	PLCB	272			270		
EWPHE	THZ/TMP	250.8		247.7			
(n = 335)	PLCB	253.3		243.1			
(n = 90)	THZ/TMP	255.6			238.3		
	PLCB	259.4			238.6		
Berglund	THZ	267		263			255
(n = 106)	PPL	271		263			255
VA	THZ	226.2	231.1	223.3			
(n = 240)	PPL	222.3	217*	217.5*			
HDFP	—	232				223	
HAPPHY		242				242	
MAPHY		244				243	
MRFIT		254				236	
SHEP		238		238			

[a]THZ = thiazide, PPL = propranolol, PLCB = placebo, TMP = triamterene;   VA = Veterans Administration Cooperative Study Group on Antihypertensive Agents; OSLO = The Oslo Study; EWPHE = European Working Party on High Blood Pressure in the Elderly; HDFP = Hypertension Detection and Follow-up Program; HAPPHY = Heart Attack Primary Prevention in Hypertensives Trial; MAPHY = Metoprolol Atherosclerosis Prevention in Hypertensives Study; MRFIT = Multiple Risk Factor Intervention Trial; SHEP = Systolic Hypertension in the Elderly Program.   From Wright (89).   *$p < 0.05$

in patients who received diuretic therapy in the usual-care (UC) group, which received the diuretics from their community physicians. In the study, hydrochlorothiazide and chlorthalidone doses of 50–100 mg were used in the SI group, while 25–50 mg/day was more commonly prescribed by community physicians to the UC patients. However, no dose-response effect was noted and no correlation with degree of hypokalemia was noted (56). Several studies have reported an increase in ventricular irritability on 24-hour electrocardiograms in patients receiving high dose diuretics, but this has been challenged by other data (60,88).

The beta blockers also have adverse metabolic effects that might affect cardiac risk. However, there are four primary prevention studies now available demonstrating the ability of the beta blockers to prevent hypertension-related disease, although significant numbers of black hypertensives were not included in these trials (31,37,50,82). These studies also carefully examined the efficacy of beta blockers in the primary prevention of coronary heart disease. In the Medical Research Council trial, which involved the use of the noncardioselective propranolol, and in the IPPPSH trial, which utilized oxprenolol (a noncardioselective beta blocker with intrinsic sympathomimetic activity), beta blockers failed to protect against coronary heart disease in hypertensives when compared with a thiazide or placebo (37,50). However, total cardiovascular complications were decreased compared with placebo, and post-hoc analysis did reveal a trend toward protection in the subgroup of nonsmokers in these studies. Primary prevention trials involving atenolol, propranolol, and alprenolol (the HAPPHY trial) also found no significant additional protection from coronary heart disease compared with diuretic therapy (31,37,50). However, metoprolol in the MAPHY study (an extension of the HAPPHY trial) was significantly better than thiazide in preventing death from coronary heart disease and stroke and in smokers but not nonsmokers (82).

The ACEIs produce few metabolic abnormalities (except hyperkalemia) and may improve insulin sensitivity. They have been found to decrease cardiovascular mortality in patients with congestive heart failure. Additionally, animal studies and small clinical studies have suggested preservation of renal function by these agents in patients with diabetic nephropathy and insulin-dependent diabetes mellitus (13,35,62). Preservation of renal function has also been noted in the similar patient populations treated with traditional triple therapy consisting of diuretic, metoprolol, and hydralazine (61). However, there are no studies documenting primary prevention of cardiovascular morbid events in patients with asymptomatic hypertension. Therefore, any claim of advantage of converting enzyme inhibitors over standard therapy still remains premature. In any event, combination of an ACEI with a thiazide diuretic is usually indicated in the black hypertensive to increase the drugs' effectiveness in this population.

The CaCBs have only been shown to decrease morbidity in a subset of postmyocardial patients who had suffered a non-Q infarction (55). CaCBs have also been noted to preserve renal blood flow in short-term hemodynamic studies. However, there are no studies documenting preservation of renal function in long-term morbidity–mortality studies (74). While left ventricular hypertrophy has consistently been shown to be an independent risk factor for cardiac events, the therapeutic benefit of medications like the CaCB, which regress LVH, remains theoretical (11). To date, there are no long-term studies to date evaluating the effect of calcium channel blockers in preventing the cardiovascular complications of hypertension.

Adverse Drug Reaction Profile

Adverse drug reaction is often suggested as one of the reasons for the high rate of medication discontinuance. The withdrawal rates for adverse drug reactions in various long-term clinical trials utilizing the Stepped-Care approach are given in Table 12.5. With the exception of the Hypertension Detection and Follow-up Study (HDFP) trial, the rate of withdrawal secondary to medication side effects is relatively low.

The HDFP is also one of the few trials that included significant numbers of black subjects (17). In the HDFP trial, 32.7% of patients had therapy discontinued for possible, probable, or definite adverse drug reactions. However, in only 9.3% of cases was the adverse event felt by the therapist to be "definitely" or "probably" secondary to the drug. Almost 80% of drug withdrawals were felt to be only possibly secondary to the drug. Among blacks in the trial,

TABLE 12.5. Percentages of Patients Withdrawing from Clinical Trials Because of Adverse Drug Reactions

Study[a]		Overall	Active treatment	Control group
VA	(n = 380)	15.0	7.6	7.1
HDFP	(n = 3244)	32.7	32.7	—[b]
USPHS	(n = 389)	5.9	9.8	2.0
OSLO	(n = 785)	1.7	0.4	1.3

[a]VA = Veterans Administration Cooperative Trial; HDFP = Hypertension Detection and Follow-up Study; USPHS = United States Public Health Service Cooperative Study; Oslo = Oslo Study.
[b]Study did not have a control group.
From McCorvey et al. (46).

a total of 22.9% of black women and 26.6% of black men had possible to definite adverse drug reactions severe enough to discontinue therapy.

Although long-term studies are not available for alpha blockers, CaCB, and converting enzyme inhibitors, short-term comparative trials are available comparing them with existing therapies (Table 12.6). Using withdrawal rates as a measure, the newer therapies are at least as well tolerated as the older therapies.

TABLE 12.6. Withdrawal Rates from Antihypertensive Therapy

Drug	Withdrawal rate (%)	Length of follow-up (months)	Ref.
Propranolol	2.3	2.5	(77)
HCTZ	0.6	2.5	
Captopril	3.2	2	(18)
Placebo	2.4	2	
Verapamil	2.7	1	(16)
Propranolol	6.8	1	
Diltiazem	9.2	4	(44)
Propranolol	8.1	4	
Captopril	8.0	6	(14)
Propranolol	12.7	6	
Methyldopa	19.4	6	
Atenolol	7.0	2	(15)
Captopril	4.8	2	
Verapamil	6.8	2	
Diltiazem	2.0	8	(24)
HCTZ	5.3	8	
Diltiazem	7.6	5.5	(86)
Captopril	7.6	5.5	

Utilizing more sensitive measures of drug tolerability—quality of life assessments—the converting enzyme inhibitors and CaCBs have been reported to be better tolerated than sympatholytics such as methyldopa and beta blockers (12,14,15,92). However, these studies were flawed by the lack of a placebo group, poor standardization of instruments, and dosing regimens that biased against the positive control antihypertensive agent(s) used in the studies; in addition, none of the studies made blinded comparisons with the thiazides. Only one controlled trial used significant numbers of black subjects or utilized instruments designed to assess quality of life in black hypertensives.

In a quality of life study in 306 black hypertensives with a culturally adapted instrument, we recently showed that there was no significant difference between atenolol, captopril, and verapamil on quality of life (15). Quality of life actually improved with all three agents, although no placebo group was incorporated. In another double-blind crossover study in elderly hypertensives comparing enalapril, propranolol, and hydrochlorothiazide with placebo, no difference in quality of life compared with placebo was noted (47). However, significantly more complaints occurred with propranolol compared with enalapril. No difference in quality of life or motor or cognitive function was seen between any drug and hydrochlorothiazide.

Cost Considerations

While cost is by necessity a factor when treating any patient population with limited financial resources, a major concern is that cost is overemphasized, minimizing potential hazards. On the other hand, there is extensive marketing of newer, more expensive antihypertensives, which may tend to overemphasize the side effects of popular inexpensive antihypertensives.

The initial choice of antihypertensive will have the greatest financial impact on the patient and will be the most lucrative market for the pharmaceutical industry to attract. While the therapist's overriding concern is to provide for the best therapy regardless of cost, to ignore cost is especially naive in populations where financial resources are limited.

In a survey by Schulman et al. (69), 22.4% of hypertensives reported that medication cost was a problem all or most of the time. Not surprisingly, the lower the economic level, the greater concern cost becomes. Up to 37% of whites and 49% of blacks in this study said medication cost was a barrier to their hypertensive therapy.

While the black hypertensive is more likely to require multiple drug therapy, over half can be controlled on monotherapy (16,45,68,77,91). Control rates from 50% to 70% can be achieved in black hypertensives on monotherapy with the thiazides or a calcium channel blocker (45,68,77), and in spite of the racial resistance 40%–60% of black hypertensives can be controlled even if initial therapy is with a beta blocker or converting enzyme inhibitor (16,67,68,77). Therefore, since most black hypertensives will be controlled by the initial drug prescribed, the initial choice of antihypertensive will play a most important role in determining the results of antihypertensive therapy.

TABLE 12.7. The Cost of Antihypertensive Therapy (selected agents)

Antihypertensive agent	Daily dose range	Cost/month ($)[a]
Hydrochlorothiazide	25 – 50 mg	0.16 – 0.22
Reserpine	0.1 – 0.25 mg	0.07 – 0.15
Hydralazine	50 – 200 mg	0.98 – 3.42
KCl (tabs)	40 – 60 mEq	5.70 – 11.40
Triamterene/HCTZ		
Dyazide	1 – 2 tab	10.21 – 11.40
Maxide		11.12 – 22.24
Generic		6.22 – 12.44
Propranolol		
Inderal LA	80 – 320 mg	18.94 – 30.73
Generic		9.55 – 19.10
Metoprolol (Lopressor)	50 – 200 mg	11.43 – 34.34
Nadolol (Corgard)	40 – 320 mg	18.75 – 76.08
Labetalol (Normodyne/Trandate)	200 – 1200 mg	15.53 – 60.48
Atenolol (Tenormin)	50 – 200 mg	18.95 – 56.97
Prazosin (Minipress)	3 – 20 mg	15.35 – 60.48
Terazosin (Hytrin)	1 – 10 mg	17.91 – 35.82
Alphamethyldopa (generic)	500 – 2,000 mg	12.20 – 45.29
Clonidine		
Catapres tabs	0.2 – 1.2 mg	19.26 – 76.24
Transderm	0.1 – 0.6 mg	20.22 – 94.37
Generic		4.21 – 19.74
Guanfacine (Tenex)	1 – 3 mg	13.53 – 34.90
Captopril (Capoten)	50 – 150 mg	26.56 – 66.40
Enalapril (Vasotec)	5 – 40 mg	21.63 – 63.82
Lisinopril (Prinivil/Zestril)	5 – 40 mg	18.32 – 29.60
Verapamil		
Calan Sr, Isoptin SR	240 – 480 mg	25.40 – 40.80
Generic		1j.88 – 33.76
Nifedipine		
Procardia	30 – 120 mg	38.52 – 135.88
Procardia XL		31.59 – 113.70
Diltiazem (Cardiazem SR)	60 – 360 mg	36.75 – 54.75
Nicardipine (Cardene)	60 – 120	26.30 – 52.60

[a]1990 Red Book (Medical Economics Co., Inc., Oradell NJ) average wholesale price (AWP) for 30 days of therapy in the given dose range. (Does not include pharmacy charges and markup, which may vary.)

The average wholesale costs for one month of therapy with currently available antihypertensive agents are listed in Table 12.7. While regional prices may vary, these costs can be used for comparison. The combination of hydrochlorothiazide 50 mg/day, reserpine 0.25 mg/day, and hydralazine 200 mg/day is effective in normalizing blood pressure in 95% of hypertensives and at an affordable wholesale cost of $3.79/month (Table 12.7). It is also the regimen that was used in many long-term studies that demonstrated that the treatment of hypertension prevents morbidity and mortality. Even using the HDFP data, almost three-quarters of black patients tolerated this regimen and at antihypertensive doses higher than those currently recommended.

RECOMMENDATIONS FOR TREATMENT

The treatment of hypertension in the black hypertensive represents a therapeutic challenge in terms of disease severity, availability of effective agents, and risk to the patient if we fail. The challenge with this population more than any other is to provide the most cost-effective, safest, and best-tolerated therapy.

Tables 12.8–12.11 represent our recommendations for antihypertensive choices in the black hypertensive. Thiazide diuretics remain the drugs of first choice in this population of hypertensives, especially in doses <50 mg/day of hydrochlorothiazide or its equivalent. This is based upon their efficacy in lowering blood pressure, their demonstrated ability to prevent complications in long-term morbidity–mortality trials, their safety record, cost, and convenient dosing schedule.

Therefore, while other agents, that is, calcium channel blockers, may have some theoretical advantages over diuretic-based therapy, this has not yet been established in clinical trials. Diuretic-based therapy decreases cardiovascular morbid and mortal events, including stroke, congestive heart failure, progression of hypertension, and progression of renal deterioration. Therefore, although the concerns about the adverse effects of diuretic-based antihypertensive therapy on cardiac risk factors and their inability to prevent coronary disease in some of the clinical trials are valid, whether therapies without these adverse effects have greater or even equal efficacy in preventing cardiovascular events than diuretic based therapy remains undocumented.

The CaCB are attractive alternatives to the thiazides in patients uncontrolled or intolerant of the thiazides or who have specific indications for these agents (i.e., angina, after non-Q wave myocardial infarction, severe diastolic dysfunction, etc.). They do not affect serum lipids, thus making them excellent choices in patients in whom this is a concern. Finally, they are well tolerated and are effective in black hypertensives. Their cost (although now decreasing, since many are becoming available generically) and especially the lack of primary prevention data at the present time make their use inappropriate as agents of first choice in this high-risk population.

Beta blockers should not be denied to black hypertensives when indications for their use exist. Although they may be less effective as antihypertensives when used as monotherapy, up to 50% of black hypertensives will have significant blood pressure reduction, and resistance to them can be eliminated when they are combined with a diuretic. Excellent primary and secondary prevention data are available for the beta blocker, especially the cardioselective agents without intrinsic sympathomimetic activity. Specific indications for their use in the black hypertensive include angina (along with the CaCB), hypertensives after a Q wave myocardial infarction, and patients requiring migraine prophylaxis.

TABLE 12.8. Specific Indications and Contraindications for Thiazides as Initial Therapy in Black Hypertensives

Indications
Asymptomatic hypertensive without contraindication

Where other antihypertensives are not specifically indicated

Multiple drugs required for blood pressure control

Limited financial resources

Contraindications
Drug intolerance

Creatinine > 2.5

Concomitant diseases, i.e., gout

TABLE 12.9. Specific Indications and Contraindications for Beta Blockers as Initial Therapy in Black Hypertensives

Indications
Post Q wave myocardial infarctions

Concomitant diseases such as angina, migraine headaches

Hypertrophic cardiomyopathies

Contraindications
Drug intolerance

Bronchospasm

Vasospastic disease

Congestive heart failure

The ACEI, like the CaCB, are well tolerated but are lacking long-term primary prevention data. Like the beta blockers, they are less effective but not ineffective in black hypertensives as monotherapy. They have particular value in the black hypertensive with concomitant congestive heart failure. In the future, they may also demonstrate an advantage over existing therapy in the diabetic hypertensive and in the patient with nephropathy; however, these data are still preliminary.

In recommending thiazides as first choice agents in the black hypertensive, this does not mean ignoring the potential of thiazide diuretics to adversely alter cardiac risk factors other than hypertension. The goal of treatment should always be to lower the patient's overall risk profile. In the patient whose risk profile is adversely affected by thiazide therapy (and in patients who are intolerant or uncontrolled), consideration of other therapies is indicated. However, this needs to be put into perspective.

In patients with normal cholesterol values (LDL < 130 mg/dl), there is no evidence that thiazide-induced elevations of LDL cholesterol will substantially affect their risk of coronary heart disease. There is also little reason to be concerned about the use of thiazides in the premenopausal (or postmenopausal on estrogen replacement) black female hypertensive. By the same token, in patients with markedly elevated LDL levels requiring drug therapy, it is even more important that the therapist be aware of the impact of medication cost. In this case, the cautious use of the thiazides in the regimen may lower the

TABLE 12.10. Specific Indications and Contraindications for
ACEI as Initial Therapy in Black Hypertensives

Proven indications
Congestive heart failure

Insufficient evidence but possible indication
Borderline hypercholesterolemia

Left ventricular hypertrophy

??? Diabetic nephropathy

Contraindications
Drug intolerance

TABLE 12.11. Specific Indications and Contraindications for
CaCB as Initial Therapy in Black Hypertensives

Proven indications
Contraindication or intolerance to thiazides

Post non Q wave myocardial infarction

Concomitant angina

Hypertrophic cardiomyopathy/diastolic dysfunction

Insufficient evidence but possible indication
Borderline hypercholesterolemia

Left ventricular hypertrophy

overall cost of care. It is in the patient with borderline cholesterol elevations, especially in the patient where modest alterations in cholesterol may affect lipid-lowering therapy, that consideration for alternatives to thiazide be given if lipid values do not return to expected values with chronic therapy.

In the black hypertensive without MRFIT electrocardiographic criteria for increased risk, concern about sudden death with diuretic therapy (even if the MRFIT data are taken at face value) is also without documentation. Left ventricular hypertrophy is more likely to be encountered in black hypertensives. In these patients, the use of thiazide doses equivalent to less than 50 mg/day of hydrochlorothiazide and the maintenance of normokalemia withstands even the most liberal interpretation of available data.

In the patient with diabetes mellitus, we advise caution about the use of the thiazide only in patients with mild existing glucose intolerance (48). In the patient taking exogenous insulin, it is unlikely that thiazide-induced reduction of insulin release imposes any significant additional risk. Confirmation of the data on the risk of drug-induced insulin resistance is required before its significance on therapy in the black hypertensive can be assessed.

Finally, we recognize a desperate need to get as many black hypertensives as possible into treatment prior to the development of end-organ damage. Access to care needs to be facilitated. Aggressive detection and treatment measures need to be implemented. In addition to markedly reducing morbidity and mortality from hypertension, the cost of treating the disease is substantially less if control can be achieved with thiazide therapy before end-organ damage makes the consideration of more expansive therapies necessary.

REFERENCES

1. Amery, A., P. Berthaux, C. Bulpitt, M. Deruyttere, A. De Schaepdryver, C. Dollery, R. Fagard, F. Forette, J. Hellemans, P. Lund-Johansen, A. Mutsers, and J. Tuomilehto. Glucose intolerance during diuretic therapy. Results of trial by the European Working Party on Hypertension in the Elderly. *Lancet 1:* 681–683, 1978.
2. Anavekar, S. N., N. Christophidis, W. J. Louis, and A. E. Doyle. Verapamil in the treatment of hypertension. *J. Cardiovasc. Pharmacol. 3:* 287–292, 1981.
3. Batey, D. M., M. J. Nicolich, V. I. Lasser, S. S. Jeffrey, and N. L. Lasser. Prazosin versus hydrochlorothiazide as initial antihypertensive therapy in black versus white patients. *Am. J. Med. 86* (Suppl 1B): 74–78, 1989.
4. Ben-Ishay, D., B. Leibel, and J. Stessman. Calcium channel blockers in the management of hypertension in the elderly. *Am. J. Med. 81* (Suppl 6A): 30–34, 1986.
5. Bennett, W. M., W. J. McDonald, E. Kuehnel, M. N. Hartnett, and G. A. Porter. Do diuretics have antihypertensive properties independent of natriuresis. *Clin. Pharmacol. Ther. 22:* 499–504, 1977.
6. Bentsson, C., G. Johnson, R. Sannerstedt, and R. Werko. Effect of different doses of chlorthalidone on blood pressure, serum potassium, and urate. *Br. Med. J. 1:* 197–199, 1975.
7. Bhigjee, A. I., Y. K. Seedat, S. Hoosen, R. M Neerahoo, and K. Naidoo. Biochemical changes in black and Indian hypertensive patients on diuretic therapy. *S. Afr. Med. J. 64:* 969–972, 1983.
8. Blaustein, M. Sodium ions, calcium ions, blood pressure regulation and hypertension: a reassessment and a hypothesis. *Am. J. Physiol. 232 (Cell Physiol. 1):* C165–C173, 1977.
9. Boehringer, K., P. Weidmann, R. Mordasini, H. Schiffl, C. Bachmann, and W. Riesen. Menopause-dependent plasma lipoprotein alterations in diuretic-treated women. *Ann. Intern. Med.* 97: 206–209, 1982.
10. Buhler, F. R., L. Hulthen, W. Kiowski, and P. Bolli. Greater antihypertensive efficacy of calcium channel inhibitor verapamil in older and low renin patients. *Clin. Sci. 63:* 439s–442s, 1982.
11. Casale, P. N., R. B. Devereax, H. Milner, et al. Value of echocardiographic left ventricular mass in predicting cardiovascular morbid events in hypertensives. *Ann. Intern. Med.* 105: 173–178, 1986.
12. Chatellier, G., P. Sassano, A. M. Amiot, P. Corvol, and J. Menard. Efficacy and influence on quality of life of enalapril as a first step treatment of hypertension. *Clin. Exp. Hypertens. A9:* 513–519, 1987.
13. Consensus Trial Study Group. Effects of enalapril in mortality in severe congestive heart failure: results of the Cooperative North Scandinavian Enalapril Survival Study. *N. Engl. J. Med. 316:* 1429–1435, 1987.
14. Croog, S. H., S. Levine, M. A. Testa, et al. The effects of antihypertensive therapy on the quality of life. *N. Engl. J. Med. 314:* 1657–1664, 1986.
15. Croog, S. H., B. W. Kong, S. Levine, et al. Hypertensive black men and women: quality of life and effects of antihypertensive medications. *Arch. Intern. Med. 150:* 1733–1741, 1990.
16. Cubeddu, L. X., J. Aranda, B. Singh, et al. A comparison of verapamil and propranolol for the initial treatment of hypertension: racial differences in response. *J.A.M.A. 256:* 2214–2221, 1986.
17. Curb, J. D., N. O. Borhani, T. P. Blaszkowski, N. Zimbaldi, S. Fotiu, and W. Williams. Long-term surveillance for adverse effects of antihypertensive drugs. *J.A.M.A. 253:* 3263–3268, 1985.
18. Drayer, J. I. M., and M. A. Weber. Monotherapy of essential hypertension with a converting-enzyme inhibitor. *Hypertension* 5(Suppl III): 108–113, 1983.
19. Duke, M. Thiazide-induced hypokalemia: association with acute myocardial infarction and ventricular fibrillation. *J.A.M.A. 239:* 43–45, 1978.
20. Dzau, V. J. Implications of local angiotensin production in cardiovascular physiology and pharmacology. *Am. J. Cardiol. 59:* 59A–65A, 1987.
21. Elliot, H. L. Calcium antagonists in the treatment of hypertension and angina pectoris in the elderly. *J. Cardiovasc. Pharmacol. 13* (Suppl 4): S12–S16, 1989.
22. Flamenbaum, W., M. A. Weber, F. G. McMahon, B. J. Materson, et al. Monotherapy with labetalol compared to propranolol: differential effects of race. *J. Clin. Hypertens. 1:* 59–69, 1985.
23. Fries, E. D., D. J. Reda, and B. J. Materson. Volume (weight) loss and blood pressure response following thiazide diuretics. *Hypertension 12:* 244–250, 1988.
24. Frishman, W. H. Beta-adrenergic blockers. *Med. Clin. North Am. 72:* 37–81, 1988.

25. Frishman, W. H., Z. T. Zawada, L. Kent Smith, et al. Comparison of hydrochlorothiazide and sustained-release diltiazem for mild-to-moderate systemic hypertension. *Am. J. Cardiol. 59:* 615–623, 1987.
26. Frohlich, E. D. Diuretics in hypertension. *J. Hypertens. 5* (Suppl 3): S43–S49, 1987.
27. Godfraind, T., R. Miller, and M. Wibo. Calcium antagonism and calcium entry blockade. *Pharmacol. Rev. 38:* 321–417, 1986.
28. Grell, G. A. C., T. E. Forrester, G. A. O. Alleyne. Comparison of the effectiveness of a beta blocker (atenolol) and diuretic (chlorthalidone) in black hypertensive patients. *South. Med. J. 77:* 1524–1529, 1984.
29. Hall, W. D. Pharmacologic therapy of hypertension in blacks. In: *Hypertension in Blacks: Epidemiology, Pathophysiology, and Treatment,* edited by W.D. Hall, E. Saunders, and N. B. Shulman. Year Book Medical Publishers, Chicago, 1985, pp. 182–208.
30. Hallin, L., L. Anorzin, L. Hansson. Controlled trial of nifedipine and bendroflumethiazide in hypertension. *J. Cardiovasc. Pharmacol. 5:* 1083–1085, 1983.
31. Heart Attack Primary Prevention in Hypertension Trial Research Group. Beta-blockers versus diuretics in hypertensive men: main results from the HAPPHY trial. *J. Hypertens. 5:* 561–572, 1987.
32. Helgeland, A. Treatment of mild hypertension: a five year controlled drug trial: The Oslo Study. *Am. J. Med. 69:* 725–732, 1980.
33. Holland, O. B., C. Gomez-Sanchez, C. Fairchild, and N. M. Kaplan. Role of renin classification for diuretic treatment of black hypertensive patients. *Arch. Intern. Med. 139:* 1365–1370, 1979.
34. Holland, O. B., C. E. Gomez-Sanchez, L. V. Kuhnert, C. Poindexter, and C. Y. C. Pak. Antihypertensive comparison of furosemide with hydrochlorothiazide for black patients. *Arch. Intern. Med. 139:* 1015–1021, 1979.
35. Hommel, E., H. H. Parving, and E. Mathiesin. Effect of captopril on kidney function in insulin-dependent diabetic patients with nephropathy. *Br. Med. J. 293:* 467–470, 1986.
36. Humphreys, G. S., and D. G. Delvin. Ineffectiveness of propranolol in hypertensive Jamaicans. *Br. Med. J. 2:* 601–603, 1968.
37. IPPPSH Collaborative Group. Cardiovascular risk and risk factors in a randomized trial of treatment based on the beta-blocker oxprenolol: the International Prospective Primary Prevention Study in Hypertension (IPPPSH). *J. Hypertens. 3:* 379–392, 1985.
38. Jennings, K., and V. Parsons. A study of labetalol in patients of European, West Indian, and West Indian origin. *Br. J. Clin. Pharmacol. 3* (Suppl. 3): 773–775, 1976.
39. Joint National Committee. The 1988 report of the Joint National Committee on Detection, Evaluation, and Treatment of high blood pressure. *Arch. Intern. Med. 148:* 1023–1038, 1988.
40. Leren, P., O. P. Foss, A. Helgeland, et al. Effect of propranolol and prazosin on blood lipids: the Oslo Study. *Lancet 2:* 4–6, 1980.
41. Luther, R. R., M. J. Klepper, C. J. Maurath, H. N. Glassman, R. Achari, and A. R. Laddu. Efficacy of terazosin in the treatment of essential hypertension in blacks. *J. Hum. Hypertens. 4:* 151–153, 1990.
42. Majais, S. K., G. M. Fouad, and R. C. Tarazi. Reversal of left ventricular hypertrophy with captopril. Hetergeneity of response among hypertensive patients. *Clin. Cardiol. 6:* 595–602, 1983.
43. Massie, B. M., J. F. Tabau, J. Szlachcic, and C. Vollmer. Comparison and additivity of nitrendipine and hydrochlorothiazide in systemic hypertension. *Am. J. Cardiol. 58:* 16D–19D, 1986.
44. Massie, B., E. P. MacCarthy, K. B. Ramanathan, R. J. Weiss, B. A. Eidelson, M. Anderson, D. G. Labreche, J. F. Tubau, D. Ulep. Diltiazem and propranolol in mild to moderate essential hypertension as monotherapy or with hydrochlorothiazide. *Ann. Intern. Med. 107:* 150–157, 1987.
45. Materson, B. J., W. C. Cushman, G. Goldstein, D. J. Reda, E. D. Freis, E. A. Ramirez, F. N. Talmers, T. J. White, D. J. Nunn, R. H. Chapman, et al. Treatment of hypertension in the elderly. I. Blood pressure and clinical changes. Results of a Department of Veterans Affairs Cooperative Study. *Hypertension 15:* 348–360, 1990.
46. McCorvey, E., J. T. Wright, Jr., J. M. McKenney, and J. D. Proctor. Does anti-hypertensive therapy influence quality of life. *Clin. Pharmacol. 8:* 359–364, 1989.
47. McCorvey, E., J. T. Wright, Jr., J. P. Culbert, J. M. McKenney, and J. P. Proctor. The effect of hydrochlorothiazide, propranolol, and enalapril on quality-of-life and cognitive and motor function. (Submitted)
48. McKenney, J. M., R. P. Goodman, and J. T. Wright, Jr. The use of antihypertensive agents in the glucose intolerant hypertensive. *Clin. Pharmacol. 4:* 649–656, 1985.
49. McKenney, J. M., R. P. Goodman, J. T. Wright, N. Rifai, D. Aycock, and M. E. King. The

effect of low-dose hydrochlorothiazide on blood pressure, serum potassium, and lipo-proteins. *Pharmacology 6:* 179–184, 1986.

50. Medical Research Council Working Party. MRC trial of treatment of mild hypertension: principal results. *Br. Med. J. 291:* 91–104, 1985.

51. Mohanty, P. K., L. M. Gonasun, and J. T. Wright, Jr. Isradipine (PN 200-110) vs hydro-chlorothiazide in mild to moderate hypertension: a multicenter study. *Am. J. Hyper-tens. 1:* 241S–244S, 1988.

52. Moser, M. Calcium entry blockers for systemic hypertension. *Am. J. Cardiol. 59:* 115A–121A, 1987.

53. Moser, M., and J. Lunn. Comparative effects of pindolol and hydrochlorothiazide in black hypertensive patients. *Angiology 32:* 561–566, 1981.

54. Moser, M., J. Lunn, and B. J. Materson. Comparative effects of diltiazem and hydrochlo-rothiazide in blacks with systemic hypertension. *Am. J. Cardiol. 56:* 101H–104H, 1985.

55. Multicenter Diltiazem Postinfarction Trial Research Group. The effect of diltiazem on mor-tality and reinfarction after myocardial infarction. *N. Engl. J. Med. 319:* 385–392, 1988.

56. Multiple Risk Factor Intervention Trial Research Group. Baseline rest electrocardio-graphic abnormalities, antihypertensive treatment, and mortality in the Multiple Risk Factor Intervention Trial. *Am. J. Cardiol. 55:* 1–15, 1985.

57. Murphy, M. B., P. J. Lewis, E. Kohner, B. Schumer, and C. T. Dollery. Glucose intolerance in hypertensive patients treated with diuretics: a fourteen year follow-up. *Lancet 2:* 1293–1295, 1982.

58. Nakashima, Y., F. M. Fouad, and R. C. Tarazi. Regression of left ventricular hypertrophy from systemic hypertension by enalapril. *Am. J. Cardiol. 53:* 1044–1049, 1984.

59. Nicholson, J. P., L. M. Resnick, and J. H. Laragh. Hydrochlorothiazide is not additive to verapamil in treating essential hypertension. *Arch. Intern. Med. 149:* 125–128, 1989.

60. Papademetriou, V., J. F. Burris, A. Notargiacomo, R. D. Fletcher, and E. D. Freis. Thiazide therapy is not a cause of arrhythmia in patients with systemic hypertension. *Arch. Intern. Med. 148:* 1272–1276, 1988.

61. Parving, H. H., A. R. Andersen, U. M. Smidt, E. Hommel, E. R. Mathiesen, and Svendsen. Effect of antihypertensive treatment on kidney function in diabetic nephropathy. *Br. Med. J. 294:* 1443–1447, 1987.

62. Passa, P., H. LeBlanc, and M. Marre. Effects of enalapril in insulin-independent diabetic subjects with mild to moderate uncomplicated hypertension. *Diabetes Care 10:* 200–204, 1987.

63. Pollare, T., H. Lithell, and C. Berne. A comparison of the effect of hydrochlorothiazide and captopril on glucose and lipid metabolism in patients with hypertension. *N. Engl. J. Med. 321:* 868–873, 1989.

64. Puschett, J. B. Sites and mechanisms of action of diuretics in the kidney. *J. Clin. Phar-macol. 21:* 564–574, 1981.

65. Report of the Secretary's Task Force on Black and Minority Health. Cardiovascular and cerebrovascular disease. U.S. Department of Health and Human Services, Vol IV, 1986.

66. Robertson, D. R. C., D. G. Waller, A. G. Renwick, and C. F. George. Age-related changes in the pharmacokinetics and pharmacodynamics of nifedipine. *Br. J. Clin. Pharmacol. 25:* 297–305, 1988.

67. Saunders, E., C. Curry, J. Hinds, B. W. Kong, et al. Labetalol compared to propranolol in the treatment of black hypertensive patients. *J. Clin. Hypertens. 3:* 294–302, 1987.

68. Saunders, E., M. Weir, W. Kong, J. T. Wright, Jr., et al. A comparison of the efficacy and safety of a beta blocker, calcium channel blocker and converting enzyme inhibitor in hypertensive blacks. *Arch. Intern. Med. 150:* 1707–1713, 1990.

69. Schulman, N. B., B. Martinez, D. Brogan, et al. Financial cost as an obstacle to hyperten-sion therapy. *Am. J. Public Health 76:* 1105–1108, 1986.

70. Seedat, Y. K. Trial of atenolol and chlorthalidone for hypertension in black hypertensives. *Br. Med. J. 281:* 1241–1243, 1980.

71. Spiekerman, R. E., K. C. Berger, D. L. Thurber, S. W. Gedge, and W. F. McGuckin. Potas-sium-sparing effects of triamterene in treating hypertension. *Circulation 34:* 524–531, 1966.

72. Stamler, R., J. Stamler, F. C. Gosch, D. M. Berkson, A. R. Dyer, and P. Hershinow. Initial antihypertensive drug therapy: final report of a randomized, controlled trial compar-ing alpha-blocker and diuretic. *Hypertension 12:* 574–581, 1988.

73. Subcommittee on Definition and Prevalence of the 1984 Joint National Committee. Hy-pertension prevalence and the status of awareness, treatment, and control in the United States. *Hypertension 7:* 457–468, 1985.

74. Sunderrajan, S., Reams, and J. H. Bauer. Renal effects of diltiazem in primary hypertension. *Hypertension 8:* 238–242, 1986.
75. Swislocki, A. M., B. B. Hoffman, and G. M. Reaven. Insulin resistance, glucose intolerance, and hyperinsulinemia in patients with hypertension. *Am. J. Hypertens. 2:* 419–423, 1989.
76. Tobian, L. Why do thiazide diuretics lower blood pressure in essential hypertension? *Ann. Rev. Pharmacol. 7:* 399–408, 1967.
77. Veterans Administration Cooperative Study Group on Antihypertensive Agents. Comparison of propranolol and hydrochlorothiazide for the initial treatment of hypertension. I. Results of short-term titration with emphasis on racial differences in response. *J.A.M.A. 248:* 1996–2003, 1982.
78. Veterans Administration Cooperative Study Group on Antihypertensive Agents. Efficacy of nadolol alone and combined with bendroflumethiazide and hydralazine for systemic hypertension. *Am. J. Cardiol. 52:* 1230–1237, 1983.
79. Vidt, D. G. A controlled multiclinic study to compare the antihypertensive effects of MK-421, hydrochlorothiazide, and MK-421 combined with hydrochlorothiazide in patients with mild to moderate essential hypertension. *J. Hypertens. 2* (Suppl 2): 81–88, 1984.
80. Weber, M. A., J. I. M. Drayer, F. G. McMahon, R. Hamburger, A. R. Shah, L. N. Kirk. Transdermal administration of clonidine for treatment of high bp. *Arch. Intern. Med. 144:* 1211–1213, 1984.
81. Weinberger, M. Blood pressure and metabolic responses to hydrochlorothiazide, captopril, and the combination in black and white mild to moderate hypertensive patients. *J. Cardiovasc. Pharmacol. 7* (Suppl 1): S52–S55, 1985.
82. Wilkstrand, J., I. Warnold, G. Olsson, J. Tuomilehto, et al. Primary prevention with metoprolol in patients with hypertension: mortality results from the MAPHY study. *J.A.M.A. 259:* 1976–1982, 1988.
83. Williams, G. H. Converting-enzyme inhibitors in the treatment of hypertension. *N. Engl. J. Med. 319:* 1517–1525, 1988.
84. Wilson, P. R., and D. C. Kem. Indapamide. In: *Cardiovascular Drug Therapy,* edited by F. H. Messerli. W. B. Saunders, Philadelphia, 1990, pp. 348–356.
85. Winer, B. M. Antihypertensive mechanisms of salt depletion induced by hydrochlorothiazide. *Circulation 24:* 788–796, 1961.
86. Wolfson, P., D. Abernethy, D. J. DiPette, and R. Zusman. Diltiazem and captopril alone or in combination for treatment of mild to moderate systemic hypertension. *Am. J. Cardiol. 62:* 103G–108G, 1988.
87. Wright, J. T., Jr. Labetalol/Hydrochlorothiazide Multicenter Study Group: Labetalol and hydrochlorothiazide in hypertension. *Clin. Pharmacol. Ther. 38:* 24–27, 1985.
88. Wright, J. T., Jr. Risk factors in the management of the unique hypertensive patient. *J Natl. Med. Assoc. 79*(Suppl): 17–22, 1987.
89. Wright, J. T., Jr. Geriatric hypertension therapy: a guide to cost-effectiveness. *Geriatrics 43:* 55–62, 1988.
90. Wright, J. T., Jr. Profile of systemic hypertension in black patients. *Am. J. Cardiol. 61:* 41H–45H, 1988.
91. Wright, J. T., Jr., D. J. Dipette, R. P. Goodman, R. Townsend, and J. M. McKenney. Renin profile, race, and antihypertensive efficacy with atenolol and labetalol. *J. Hum. Hypertens. 5:* 193–198, 1991.
92. Zachariah, P. K., R. Brobyn, J. Kann, B. Levy, R. Margolis, F. G. McMahon, R. Reeves, D. C. Sperling, D. Sweet, P. Zager, and S. R. Zellner. Comparison of quality of life on nitrendipine and propranolol. *J. Cardiovasc. Pharmacol. 12*(Suppl 4): S29–S35, 1988.
93. Zusman, R., D. Christensen, E. Federman, M. S. Kochar, D. McCarron, J. G. Porush, and S. Spitalewitz. Comparison of nifedipine and propranolol used in combination with diuretics for the treatment of hypertension. *Am. J. Med. 82*(Suppl 3B): 37–41, 1987.

Index